Best of Five MCQs for the Acute Medicine SCE

Best of Five MCQs for the Acute Medicine SCE

Edited by

Nigel Lane
Consultant in Acute Medicine, North Bristol NHS Trust, UK

Louise Powter
Consultant in Acute Medicine, North Bristol NHS Trust, UK

Sam Patel
Consultant in Acute Medicine and Rheumatology,
Clinical Director, Medicine, North Bristol NHS Trust
Training Programme Director, General (Internal) Medicine, Severn Deanery, UK

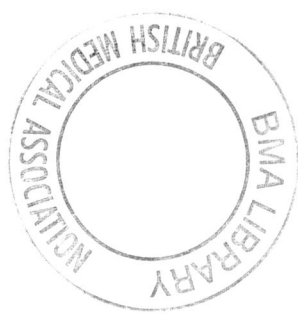

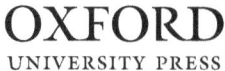

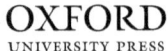
UNIVERSITY PRESS

Great Clarendon Street, Oxford, OX2 6DP,
United Kingdom

Oxford University Press is a department of the University of Oxford.
It furthers the University's objective of excellence in research, scholarship,
and education by publishing worldwide. Oxford is a registered trade mark of
Oxford University Press in the UK and in certain other countries

© Oxford University Press 2016

The moral rights of the authors have been asserted

First Edition published in 2016

Impression: 3

All rights reserved. No part of this publication may be reproduced, stored in
a retrieval system, or transmitted, in any form or by any means, without the
prior permission in writing of Oxford University Press, or as expressly permitted
by law, by licence or under terms agreed with the appropriate reprographics
rights organization. Enquiries concerning reproduction outside the scope of the
above should be sent to the Rights Department, Oxford University Press, at the
address above

You must not circulate this work in any other form
and you must impose this same condition on any acquirer

Published in the United States of America by Oxford University Press
198 Madison Avenue, New York, NY 10016, United States of America

British Library Cataloguing in Publication Data

Data available

Library of Congress Control Number: 2015934703

ISBN 978–0–19–968026–9

Printed in Great Britain by
Ashford Colour Press Ltd, Gosport, Hampshire

Oxford University Press makes no representation, express or implied, that the
drug dosages in this book are correct. Readers must therefore always check
the product information and clinical procedures with the most up-to-date
published product information and data sheets provided by the manufacturers
and the most recent codes of conduct and safety regulations. The authors and
the publishers do not accept responsibility or legal liability for any errors in the
text or for the misuse or misapplication of material in this work. Except where
otherwise stated, drug dosages and recommendations are for the non-pregnant
adult who is not breast-feeding

Links to third party websites are provided by Oxford in good faith and
for information only. Oxford disclaims any responsibility for the materials
contained in any third party website referenced in this work.

CONTENTS

Abbreviations viii
Contributors xv
Introduction xvii

1 Cardiorespiratory arrest and shock
Questions 1
Answers 15

2 Gastroenterology
Questions 27
Answers 42

3 Respiratory
Questions 59
Answers 78

4 Cardiology
Questions 93
Answers 111

5 Diabetes and endocrinology
Questions 127
Answers 143

6 Elderly care and stroke
Questions 157
Answers 170

7	**Renal medicine and urological problems**	
	Questions	183
	Answers	198
8	**Neurology and ophthalmology**	
	Questions	207
	Answers	226
9	**Musculoskeletal medicine**	
	Questions	249
	Answers	269
10	**Oncology and palliative care**	
	Questions	283
	Answers	292
11	**Haematology**	
	Questions	301
	Answers	306
12	**Infectious diseases and HIV**	
	Questions	313
	Answers	330
13	**Poisoning and pharmacology**	
	Questions	351
	Answers	363
14	**Immunology and allergy**	
	Questions	383
	Answers	389
15	**Dermatology**	
	Questions	395
	Answers	400

16 Psychiatry
    Questions   403
    Answers   410

Index   421

ABBREVIATIONS

a-NVH	asymptomatic non-visible haematuria
AAFB	acid and alcohol fast bacilli
ABPA	allergic bronchopulmonary aspergillosis
AchR	acetylcholine receptors
ACR	American College of Rheumatology
ACS	acute coronary syndrome
ACTH	adrenocorticotropic hormone
ADA	adenosine deaminase
AEDs	anti-epileptic drugs
AESs	anti-embolism stockings
AF	atrial fibrillation
ALF	acute liver failure
ALT	alanine transaminase
ANA	antinuclear antibody
ANCA	antineutrophil cytoplasmic antibodies
anti-TNF	anti-tumour necrosis factor
ARDS	acute respiratory distress syndrome
AST	aspartate transaminase
AVN	avascular necrosis
BASDEC	brief assessment schedule depression cards
BASHH	British Society for Sexual Health and HIV
BAUS	British Association of Urological Surgeons
bd	two times daily
BHIVA	British HIV Association
BMI	body mass index
bpm	beats per minute
BPPV	benign paroxysmal positional vertigo
BTS	British Thoracic Society
BSR	British Society for Rheumatology
CAD	coronary artery disease
CBDS	common bile duct stones
CDI	clostridium difficile infection

CF	cystic fibrosis
CHM	Commission on Human Medicines
CI-AKI	contrast-induced acute kidney injury
CINV	chemotherapy-induced nausea and vomiting
CIS	clinically isolated syndrome
CJD	Creutzfeldt-Jakob disease
CMAP	compound muscle action potential
CMT	core medical training (in the UK)
CMV	cytomegalovirus
CNS	central nervous system
COMT	catecol-O-methyl transferase
COPD	chronic obstructive pulmonary disease
CPC	cerebral performance category
CRP	C-reactive protein
CSII	continuous subcutaneous insulin infusions
CTPA	computed tomography pulmonary angiogram
CVID	common variable immunodeficiency
CVP	central venous pressure
CYP450	cytochrome P450
DESMOND	Diabetes Education and Self Management for Ongoing and Newly Diagnosed
DEXA	dual-energy X-ray absorptiometry
DIC	disseminated intravascular coagulation
DIOS	distal intestinal obstruction syndrome
DKA	diabetic ketoacidosis
DSs	dissociative seizures
DTs	delirium tremens
DVLA	Driver and Vehicle Licensing Agency
DVT	deep vein thrombosis
EBV	Epstein–Barr virus
ECG	electrocardiogram
EGDT	early goal-directed therapy
EGPA	eosinophilic granulomatosis with polyangiitis (formerly known as Churg Strauss Syndrome)
EMG	electromyogram
EMR	endomucosal resection
ENT	ear, nose and throat
EPA	Enduring Power of Attorney
ERCP	endoscopic retrograde cholangiopancreatography
ESC	European Society of Cardiology
ESR	erythrocyte sedimentation rate
EULAR	European League Against Rheumatism

EWS	Early Warning Score
F1	foundation year 1 doctor (in the UK)
F2	foundation year 2 doctor (in the UK)
FAST	focused assessment with sonography in trauma
FDIT	faecal donor instillation therapy
FEV	forced expiratory volume
FEV_1	forced expiratory volume in 1 second
FMT	faecal microbiota transplantation
FRAX	Fracture Risk Assessment Tool
FSH	follicle stimulating hormone
FVC	forced vital capacity
GABA	gamma-aminobutyric acid
GBM	glomerular basement membrane
GBS	Guillain–Barré syndrome
GCA	giant cell arteritis
GCS	Glasgow Coma Score
GCSF	granulocyte colony stimulating factors
GDS	geriatric depression scale
GI	gastrointestinal; glycaemic index
GP	general practitioner; glycoprotein
GRACE	Global Registry of Acute Coronary Events
GTN	glyceryl trinitrate
HADS	hospital anxiety and depression scale
Hb	haemoglobin
HHS	hyperosmolar hyperglycaemic state
HIV	human immunodeficiency virus
HONK	hyperosmolar non-ketotic
HPV	human papilloma virus
HRS	hepatorenal syndrome
HSV	herpes simplex virus
IABP	intra-aortic balloon pump
ICD	implantable cardioverter defibrillator
ICH	intracerebral haemorrhage
ICS	inhaled corticosteroid
IDA	iron deficiency anaemia
IGRAs	interferon gamma release assays
IIP	interstitial idiopathic pneumonia
IMCA	independent mental capacity advocate
INR	international normalized ratio
IV	intravenous

IVIG	intravenous immunoglobulin
LABA	long-acting beta agonist
LAMA	long-acting muscarinic antagonist
LEMS	Lambert–Eaton myasthenic syndrome
LH	luteinizing hormone
LMWH	low molecular weight heparin
LPA	Lasting Power of Attorney
LTOT	long-term oxygen therapy
MAOI	monoamine Oxidase Inhibitors
MASCC	Multinational Association for Supportive Care in Cancer
MCM	major congenital malformations
MDAC	multiple-dose activated charcoal
MDR TB	multi-drug resistant tuberculosis
MG	myasthenia gravis
MND	motor neurone disease
MOA-B	monoamine oxidase B
MAOI	monoamine oxidase inhibitor
MRCP	magnetic resonance cholangiopancreatography
MS	multiple sclerosis
MSCC	metastatic spinal cord compression
MSU	mid stream specimen of urine
MUST	Malnutrition Universal Screening Tool
NEAD	non-epileptic attack disorder
NHS	National Health Service
NICE	National Institute for Health and Care Excellence
NIHSS	National Institutes of Health Stroke Scale
NIV	non-invasive ventilation
NNT	number needed to treat
NNTB	number needed to treat to benefit
NOACs	novel oral anticoagulation agents
NOGG	National Osteoporosis Guideline Group
NPH	normal pressure hydrocephalus
NPIS	National Poisons Information Service
NSAIDs	non-steroidal anti-inflammatory drugs
NSIP	non-specific interstitial pneumonia
od	once a day
OGTT	oral glucose tolerance test
OH	orthostatic hypotension
OR	odds ratio
ORS	oral rehydration solution

OSAHS	obstructive sleep apnoea/hypopnoea syndrome
PBC	primary biliary cirrhosis
PCP	pneumocystis pneumonia
PCR	polymerase chain reaction
PD	Parkinson's disease
PE	pulmonary embolism
PEFR	peak expiratory flow rate
PFAPA	periodic fever, aphthous pharyngitis, and cervical adenopathy
PICA	posterior inferior cerebellar artery
PID	pelvic inflammatory disease
PoTS	postural tachycardia syndrome
PPI	proton pump inhibitor
PsA	psoriatic arthritis
PSA	prostate-specific antigen
PSP	primary spontaneous pneumothorax
PCC	prothrombin complex concentrate
PTH	parathyroid hormone
PE	pulmonary embolism
qds	four times daily
RA	rheumatoid arthritis
RCT	randomized controlled trial
RF	rheumatoid factor
RR	relative risk
SABA	short-acting beta agonist
SAH	subarachnoid haemorrhage
SBP	spontaneous bacterial peritonitis
SDAC	single-dose activated charcoal
SIADH	syndrome of inappropriate antidiuretic hormone secretion
SIRS	systemic inflammatory response syndrome
SLE	systemic lupus erythematosus
SNRIs	serotonin–norepinephrine reuptake inhibitors
SpA	spondyloarthritis
SPECT	single-photon emission computed tomography
SSA/Ro	Sjögren's-syndrome-related antigen A, also called Ro
SSB/La	Sjögren's-syndrome-related antigen B, also called La
SSP	secondary spontaneous pneumothorax
SSRIs	selective serotonin re-uptake inhibitors
sTfR	serum transferrin receptor
SUDEP	sudden unexpected death in epilepsy
SVCO	superior vena cava obstructions

TAB	temporal artery biopsy
TB	tuberculosis
TCAs	tricyclic antidepressants
TdP	Torsades de Pointes
tds	three times a day
TIMI	Thrombolysis in Myocardial Infarction
TIPSS	transjugular intrahepatic portsystemic shunt
TRALI	transfusion-associated lung injury
TSH	thyroid stimulating hormone
UC	ulcerative colitis
UK	United Kingdom
UPPP	uvulopalatopharyngoplasty
US	ultrasound
USA	United States of America
UTI	urinary tract infection
VATS	video-assisted thoracic surgery
VKA	vitamin K antagonist
VRII	variable-rate insulin infusion
VT	ventricular tachycardia
VTE	venous thromboembolism
VVIR	ventricular pacing, ventricular sensing, inhibited by a ventricular event, rate-responsive pacemaker
vWF	von-Willebrand factor
WHO	World Health Organization

CONTRIBUTORS

Helen Alexander Consultant in General and Old Age Medicine, Gloucestershire Hospitals NHS Foundation Trust, UK

Louise Beckham Specialty Registrar, Acute Medicine, Severn Deanery, UK

David de Berker Consultant Dermatologist, University Hospitals Bristol NHS Foundation Trust, UK

Begoña Bovill Consultant in Infectious Diseases and HIV, North Bristol NHS Trust, UK

Jeremy Braybrooke Consultant Medical Oncologist, University Hospitals Bristol NHS Foundation Trust, UK

Andrew De Burgh-Thomas Consultant in Genito-urinary medicine and HIV, Gloucestershire Hospitals NHS Foundation Trust, UK

Charlie Comins Consultant Clinical Oncologist, University Hospitals Bristol NHS Foundation Trust, UK

Nerys Conway Speciality Registrar, Acute Medicine, Severn Deanery, UK

Ihab Diab Consultant Cardiologist, University Hospitals Bristol NHS Foundation Trust and Weston Area NHS Trust, UK

Michelle Dharmasiri Consultant Stroke Physician, The Royal Bournemouth and Christchurch Hospitals NHS Foundation Trust, UK

Sara Drinkwater Consultant Immunologist, Central Manchester University Hospitals NHS Foundation Trust, UK

Tomaz Garcez Consultant Immunologist, Central Manchester University Hospitals NHS Foundation Trust, UK

Matthew Hall Consultant Renal Physician, Nottingham University Hospitals NHS Trust, UK

Markus Hauser Consultant in Acute Medicine with an interest in Gastroenterology, Gloucestershire Hospitals NHS Foundation Trust, UK

Roland Jenkins Consultant in Respiratory Medicine, University Hospitals Bristol NHS Foundation Trust, UK

Nigel Lane Consultant in Acute Medicine, North Bristol NHS Trust, UK

Rebecca Maxwell Consultant in Emergency Medicine, University Hospitals Bristol NHS Foundation, Trust UK

Jim Moriarty Consultant Renal Physician, Gloucestershire Hospitals NHS Foundation Trust, UK

Fran Neuberger Specialty Registrar, Acute Medicine, Severn Deanery, UK

Anish Patel Consultant Liaison Psychiatrist, Avon and Wiltshire Mental Health Partnership NHS Trust, UK

Sam Patel Consultant in Acute Medicine and Rheumatology, North Bristol NHS Trust, UK

Justin Pearson Consultant Neurologist, North Bristol NHS Trust, UK

Suzanne Phillips Consultant in Endocrinology and Diabetes, Gloucestershire Hospitals NHS Foundation Trust, UK

Louise Powter Consultant in Acute Medicine, North Bristol NHS Trust, UK

Paul Reavley Consultant in Emergency Medicine, University Hospitals Bristol NHS Foundation Trust, UK

Philip Sedgwick Reader in Medical Statistics and Medical Education, St. George's, University of London, UK

Matthew Sephton Consultant Medical Oncologist, Yeovil District Hospital NHS Foundation Trust, UK

Kanch Sharma Specialty Registrar, Neurology, Severn Deanery, UK

Matt Thomas Consultant in Intensive Care Medicine, North Bristol NHS Trust, Bristol, UK

Rosalind Ward Consultant in Old Age Psychiatry, Avon and Wiltshire Mental Health Partnership NHS Trust, UK

Alastair Whiteway Consultant Haematologist, Southmead Hospital, North Bristol NHS Trust, UK

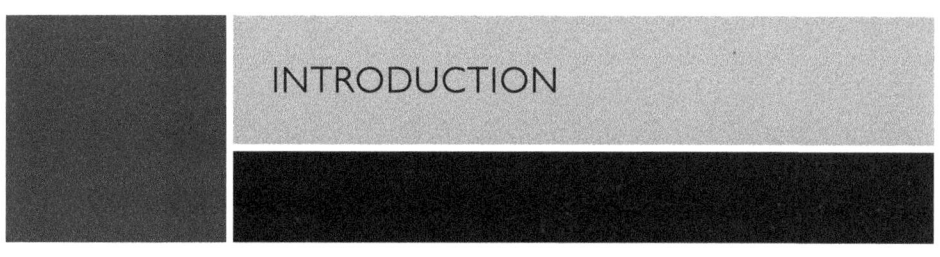

INTRODUCTION

The acute medicine specialty certificate examination (SCE) is the exit exam for acute medicine higher specialty trainees in the UK, which needs to be passed before trainees are awarded a Certificate of Completion of Training. It should be taken towards the end of your registrar training. It consists of two papers, each with 100 questions. The questions are in 'best of five' format. You are given a question stem, which is usually a clinical scenario, and then five possible answers from which you need to choose the most correct one. The exam is computer based, and questions can be flagged for later review. For each paper you have three hours, giving you about 1 minute 45 seconds per question plus 5 minutes for review. Both papers are done on the same day, with a break for lunch.

Nigel and Louise have passed the SCE (in 2012 and 2011 respectively). When it came to revising, it was clear there was a lack of appropriate revision material, hence the need for this book. The book covers the acute internal medicine curriculum (2012) and at the end of each answer you are given relevant additional reading—for instance, national guidelines—so you can easily find additional information. The book is divided into chapters according to subject to make it easier to revise. Of course, in the exam, the questions are random, so you don't know that you are answering a question about cardiology, for example. You can pick questions randomly from the book to more reflect the exam if you choose.

All the questions and answers were correct at the time of writing. However, acute medicine is ever-changing, which is what makes it so exciting, so very new guidance may not be included.

The editors had a lot of help in writing this book from a wide variety of specialists to ensure the questions are accurate and up to date. The editors would like to thank all of the individual chapter editors for their contribution, without which it would not have been possible.

We hope you find this book useful. All that remains is to say good luck!

Nigel Lane, Louise Powter, and Sam Patel

chapter 1

CARDIORESPIRATORY ARREST AND SHOCK

QUESTIONS

1. **A 74-year-old man suffered a cardiorespiratory arrest on a surgical ward four days after an elective sigmoid colectomy (with primary anastomosis) for cancer. His past medical history included hypertension and hypercholesterolaemia for which he took lisinopril, atenolol, and atorvastatin.**

   He had been seen by the surgical foundation year 1 doctor (in the UK) eight hours prior to his cardiorespiratory arrest after an episode of nausea and vomiting. On examination at that time his temperature was 38.0°C, pulse 105 beats per minute, blood pressure 95/40 mmHg, and respiratory rate 28 breaths per minute, with peripheral oxygen saturation of 94% on air. The doctor had noted abdominal tenderness, prescribed intravenous fluids, paracetamol and ondansetron, and performed peripheral blood cultures.

   Which is the most likely cause of the cardiorespiratory arrest?
   A. Anaphylaxis
   B. Hyperkalaemia
   C. Myocardial infarction
   D. Peritonitis
   E. Pulmonary embolus

2. **A 69-year-old man was successfully defibrillated after an episode of ventricular fibrillation secondary to an ST elevation myocardial infarction (STEMI) and transferred to the cardiac catheter laboratory for primary coronary intervention. After the procedure began he had a further episode of ventricular fibrillation.**

   Regarding defibrillation, which is true?
   A. A single direct current shock of 360 joules with a biphasic waveform is the most likely to restore spontaneous circulation
   B. Defibrillation is no more likely to be successful than a properly delivered praecordial thump
   C. It is safe to continue with the coronary angiogram while the shock is delivered to the patient
   D. Three shocks delivered with minimal interruptions should be given before any other intervention
   E. Two minutes of chest compressions before defibrillation is recommended to optimize coronary perfusion

3. A 75-year-old man was admitted via the emergency department with a two-day history of shortness of breath with a productive cough and 12 hours of nausea and vomiting. He had a history of chronic obstructive pulmonary disease and usually took salmeterol and tiotropium inhalers.

   His temperature was 39.3°C, heart rate 112 beats per minute, blood pressure 116/72 mmHg, and respiratory rate 24 breaths per minute. His oxygen saturation was 91% on 2 litres per minute of oxygen via nasal cannulae.

   A venous lactate was measured at 3.3 mmol per litre.

   Which of the following is true?
   A. Elevated lactate always represents tissue ischaemia
   B. Elevated venous lactate identifies a high risk of death
   C. Hyperlactataemia is diagnostic of severe sepsis
   D. Venous and arterial lactate measurements are interchangeable
   E. Venous lactate is not a suitable target for goal directed therapy

4. An 80-year-old woman was admitted to hospital for management of chronic venous leg ulcers. While on the medical ward, she had an asystolic cardiorespiratory arrest. Following resuscitation according to Advanced Life Support guidelines ventricular fibrillation was seen and defibrillation successfully restored spontaneous circulation after 15 minutes.

   What is the patient's chance of having a good neurological outcome?
   A. 5%
   B. 10%
   C. 15%
   D. 20%
   E. 25%

5. A 49-year-old woman was admitted to the intensive care unit after suffering a massive subarachnoid haemorrhage. One week after admission she remained unresponsive and the decision to perform brainstem death tests was made. **What preconditions must be met before the tests are performed?**
   A. Coroner's approval, known irreversible aetiology of coma, exclusion of reversible causes of apnoea
   B. Exclusion of reversible causes of apnoea, known irreversible aetiology of coma, exclusion of reversible causes of coma
   C. Exclusion of reversible causes of coma, 48 hours since onset of coma, structural brain damage on CT scan
   D. Known irreversible aetiology of coma, coroner's approval, evidence of absence of cerebral blood flow (e.g. with angiography)
   E. Twenty-four hours since onset of coma, exclusion of reversible causes of apnoea, absence of contraindications to organ donation

6. A 55-year-old man was admitted to the acute medical unit with a four-day history of increasing shortness of breath and cough productive of green sputum. He was a smoker who took amlodipine for hypertension. On examination his temperature was 35.8°C, pulse rate 85 beats per minute, blood pressure 112/50 mmHg, and respiratory rate 26 breaths per minute. Bronchial breath sounds were heard at the base of his right lung. His capillary refill time was 4 seconds.

```
Investigations:
    haemoglobin             143 g/L             (130-180)
    white cell count        13.9 × 10⁹/L        (4-11)
    neutrophil count        10.1 × 10⁹/L        (1.5-7.0)
    platelets               122 × 10⁹/L         (150-400)
    serum sodium            144 mmol/L          (137-144)
    serum potassium         3.9 mmol/L          (3.5-4.9)
    serum urea              10.5 mmol/L         (2.5-7.0)
    serum creatinine        119 µmol/L          (60-110)
    arterial PO₂ (air)      9.9 kPa             (11.3-12.6)
    arterial PCO₂           4.5 kPa             (4.7-6.0)
    pH                      7.33                (7.35-7.45)
    lactate                 3.3 mmol/L          (0.5-1.6)
```

Which clinical syndrome does he have?

A. Acute kidney injury
B. Acute lung injury
C. Sepsis
D. Septic shock
E. Severe sepsis

7. A 40-year-old man known to have alcoholic liver disease presented with upper gastrointestinal bleeding. While on the medical ward he had a large haematemesis associated with a reduction in conscious level. He had previously had banding of oesophageal varices. On examination his temperature was 36.1°C, pulse rate 135 beats per minute, blood pressure 73/43 mmHg, and respiratory rate 32 breaths per minute. His Glasgow Coma Score was 9 (E3, V2, M5).

```
Investigations:
  haemoglobin                          59 g/L          (130-180)
  white cell count                     14.2 × 10⁹/L    (4-11)
  platelets                            99 × 10⁹/L      (150-400)
  international normalized ratio       1.5 (<1.4)
  activated partial thromboplastin     42 s            (30-40)
    time
  fibrinogen                           2.9 g/L         (1.8-5.4)
  lactate                              5.7 mmol/L      (0.5-1.6)
```

What is your first action in this situation?

A. Activate the massive haemorrhage protocol
B. Call ICU to arrange intubation
C. Give 1 mg of terlipressin intravenously
D. Give 2 litres of 0.9% saline stat
E. Insert a Sengstaken–Blakemore tube

8. **A 60-year-old woman was admitted to the coronary care unit with acute coronary syndrome for which she underwent percutaneous coronary intervention. Her past medical history included type 2 diabetes mellitus, hypertension, osteoarthritis, and a femoro-popliteal bypass six years ago. She was taking metformin, ramipril, amlodipine, paracetamol, codeine phosphate, and aspirin.**

A urinary catheter was inserted during the procedure and over the next 12 hours she passed a total of 140 mL of urine.

On examination her pulse rate was 84 beats per minute, blood pressure 145/85 mmHg, jugular venous pressure 3 cm above the sternal notch, respiratory rate 18 breaths per minute, and oxygen saturation 96% on air. Auscultation of her chest revealed normal breath sounds with occasional fine inspiratory crackles and heart sounds were dual with no murmurs. There was no peripheral oedema and capillary refill time was 2 seconds.

A central venous catheter was inserted and the response to 250 mL of 0.9% saline was assessed:

```
Investigations:
   Central venous pressure (mmHg):
   Pre-treatment                    5
   Post-treatment                   9
```

What is your action based on these results?

A. Insert arterial catheter
B. Repeat fluid challenge
C. Start dobutamine
D. Start furosemide
E. Take the central venous catheter out

9. A 62-year-old man suffered an out-of-hospital cardiac arrest. He was successfully resuscitated in the emergency department and transferred for percutaneous coronary intervention. Following stenting of the left anterior descending artery an intra-aortic balloon pump (IABP) was inserted and he was moved to the coronary care unit.

Two hours after the procedure the patient reported his breathing had become more difficult. The nursing staff had noted that his oxygen saturation had fallen from 96% to 91% on 2 litres per minute of oxygen and that the waveform displayed on the IABP had changed (Figure 1.1). It was switched from a 1:1 to 1:2 ratio for analysis.

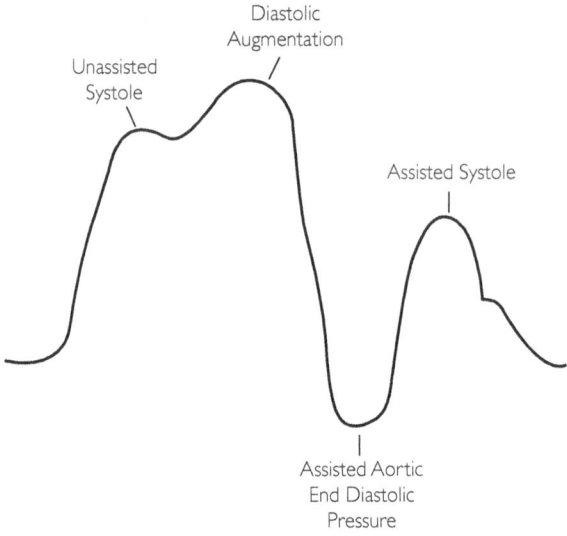

Figure 1.1 Intra-aortic balloon pump (IABP) waveform.

What is the problem with the intra-aortic balloon pump?
A. Early deflation
B. Early inflation
C. IABP kinked
D. Late deflation
E. Slow gas leak

CARDIORESPIRATORY ARREST AND SHOCK | QUESTIONS

10. An 18-year-old woman was admitted to the acute medical unit after having a generalized seizure. While on the ward, she continued to have fits at least hourly despite treatment with lorazepam, phenytoin, and levetiracetam. Between seizures her Glasgow Coma Score ranged from 9 (E2, V2, M5) to 13 (E3, V4, M6). Transfer to the intensive care unit via the CT scanner was arranged.

    Which one of the following would not be considered essential for safe transfer of this patient?
    A. Adrenaline (epinephrine)
    B. Intravenous access
    C. Intubation
    D. Pulse oximetry
    E. Self-inflating bag

11. A 73-year-old man had a cardiac arrest. The rhythm was pulseless electrical activity. Cardiopulmonary resuscitation was started at a rate of 30 chest compressions to 2 ventilations.

    What is the correct rate of chest compressions?
    A. 80–100 per minute
    B. 90–110 per minute
    C. 100–120 per minute
    D. 110–130 per minute
    E. 120–140 per minute

12. A 64-year-old man had a cardiac arrest. The initial rhythm was pulseless electrical activity. During cardiopulmonary resuscitation the rhythm on the monitor was noted to change to VF.

    What is the correct course of action?
    A. Continue cardiopulmonary resuscitation until the two-minute period is completed
    B. Deliver a DC shock then continue chest compressions until the two-minute period is completed
    C. Stop chest compressions and assess the rhythm
    D. Stop chest compressions and check for a pulse
    E. Stop chest compressions and deliver a DC shock

13. A 45-year-old man had a cardiac arrest. Chest compressions were in progress. The anaesthetic trainee intubated the patient, secured the tube at 27 cm at the teeth, and was ventilating the patient using a self-inflating bag with high-flow oxygen. Waveform capnography was attached to the tracheal tube but no end-tidal CO_2 was detected.

    What is the next step in airway management?

    A. Auscultate the chest to check the tube position
    B. Continue ventilation via the endo-tracheal tube
    C. Remove the endo-tracheal tube and establish face-mask ventilation
    D. Replace the waveform capnography with a new monitor
    E. Withdraw the tube by 3 cm then re-secure and continue ventilation

14. A 45-year-old woman collapsed on the neurosurgical ward four days after an elective craniotomy for a meningioma. She had no significant past medical history and was taking paracetamol regularly for post-operative analgesia.

    On the arrival of the medical emergency team her temperature was 37.1°C, pulse rate 119 beats per minute, blood pressure 95/60 mmHg, jugular venous pressure 4 cm above the sternal notch, and respiratory rate 32 breaths per minute. Her Glasgow Coma Score was 13 (E3, V4, M6) and her peripheries were cold. She was complaining of chest pain.

    ```
    Investigations:
      Arterial blood gas analysis (15 litres per minute oxygen via
        face mask):
      pH                   7.19             (7.35-7.45)
      PO2                  8.5 kPa          (11.3-12.6)
      PCO2                 2.9 kPa          (4.7-6.0)
      base excess          -10.4 mmol/L     (±2)
      lactate              5.0 mmol/L       (0.5-1.6)
      oxygen saturation    91%              (94-98)
      ECG showed sinus tachycardia.
    ```

    The appropriate course of action is:

    A. Focused echocardiography and thrombolysis if right ventricular dysfunction
    B. Give low molecular weight heparin and arrange urgent coronary angiography
    C. Measure D-dimer and troponin and start intravenous heparin
    D. Start intravenous heparin and arrange urgent CT pulmonary angiography
    E. Thrombolysis pending CT pulmonary angiography

15. An 18-year-old man was brought to the emergency department on New Year's Eve after an unwitnessed fall into a river on the way home from a nightclub.

    His temperature (rectal) was 28.1°C, pulse rate 31 beats per minute with an irregular rhythm, blood pressure 60/45 mmHg, and respiratory rate 9 breaths per minute. His Glasgow Coma Score was 3. There were no injuries.

    Which of the following is not appropriate for rewarming?
    A. Continuous renal replacement therapy (CRRT)
    B. Extracorporeal membrane oxygenation
    C. Forced air warming blanket
    D. Intravascular cooling device
    E. Warmed humidified oxygen

16. A 75-year-old man was admitted to hospital for an elective revision of a total knee replacement. He had type 2 diabetes and stage 2 chronic kidney disease, and was taking gliclazide. On the orthopaedic ward eight hours after the uneventful procedure he became suddenly unwell with shortness of breath and agitation.

    His temperature was 37.8°C, heart rate 142 beats per minute, blood pressure 70/30 mmHg, and respiratory rate 30 breaths per minute. On auscultation of his chest there were occasional wheezes heard. His peripheries were warm and the capillary refill time was not prolonged. Attached to his intravenous cannula was a 100 mL bag of 0.9% saline containing flucloxacillin. On the bedside table was an empty bag of cell-saver blood.

    ```
    Investigations:
      ECG: sinus tachycardia
      CXR: normal
    ```

    Which diagnosis and therapy is most likely and appropriate?
    A. Anaphylaxis–adrenaline
    B. Myocardial infarction–percutaneous coronary intervention
    C. Pulmonary embolus–heparin
    D. Sepsis–gentamicin
    E. Transfusion reaction–hydrocortisone

17. **A 49-year-old man presented to hospital with a two-day history of sore throat and progressive dyspnoea. He was a heavy smoker but had no other past medical history and took no regular medication.**

    On examination his temperature was 39.0°C, pulse rate 117 beats per minute, blood pressure 155/84 mmHg, and respiratory rate 27 breaths per minute. Oxygen saturations were 88% on room air. He appeared distressed and was drooling. Inspiratory stridor was audible from the end of the bed.

    Which of the following is true:
    A. Antibiotics should be given after tracheostomy
    B. Immediate tracheostomy may be life-saving
    C. Intubation is best attempted before transfer
    D. Oxygen should not be given before intubation
    E. Steroids and antibiotics are first-line therapy

18. **A 45-year-old man with a history of idiopathic dilated cardiomyopathy was admitted after a cardiac arrest at home. The initial rhythm recorded by the ambulance crew was ventricular fibrillation. There was return of spontaneous circulation after 25 minutes of resuscitation following Advanced Life Support guidelines and he was admitted to the intensive care unit for further management including temperature control and haemodynamic support.**

    Which of the following does not apply to the post-cardiac arrest syndrome?
    A. Intra-aortic balloon pumps may be used to support a failing myocardium
    B. Intravascular volume depletion and vasodilatation mimic severe sepsis
    C. Ischaemia-reperfusion injury leads to immunosuppression and coagulopathy
    D. Oxygen saturations of 94% are acceptable to prevent secondary brain injury
    E. Prophylactic phenytoin will reduce the incidence of seizures in the first week

19. An 83-year-old man was admitted to hospital after being unable to cope alone at home with an episode of diarrhoea and vomiting. His past medical history included hypertension, bilateral total hip replacements, and early dementia. He did not smoke but drank 30–40 units of alcohol each week. His medication on admission was amlodipine and donepezil.

He improved with 48 hours of intravenous fluids, at which point the cannula was removed because pus was noticed at the insertion site. His discharge home was delayed because he became increasingly confused.

His temperature was 35.9°C, heart rate 95 beats per minute, blood pressure 105/60 mmHg (having been previously 150/80 mmHg), and respiratory rate 22 breaths per minute. His feet were cold with pitting oedema around his ankles.

```
Investigations:
   Hb                        113 g/L              (130-180)
   WBC                       3.8 × 10⁹/L          (4-11)
   platelets                 98 × 10⁹/L           (150-400)
   INR                       1.6                  (<1.4)
   serum sodium              134 mmol/L           (137-144)
   serum potassium           3.2 mmol/L           (3.5-4.9)
   serum urea                10.1 mmol/L          (2.5-7.0)
   serum creatinine          89 μmol/L            (60-110)
   serum total bilirubin     29 μmol/L            (1-22)
   plasma glucose            8.0 mmol/L
```

Which of the following is the most likely cause of his acute confusional state?

A. Alcohol withdrawal
B. Electrolyte disturbance
C. Hepatic encephalopathy
D. Infection
E. Non-compliance with medication at home

20. A 70-year-old woman had recently been discharged to a medical ward from the intensive care unit after treatment for septic shock secondary to staphylococcal intervertebral disciitis. She was given piperacillin-tazobactam to treat the staphylococcus and a pseudomonas ventilator-associated pneumonia. A call for the medical emergency team was put out after she became apnoeic and unresponsive. Prior to this current acute illness she had been well.

On arrival of the medical emergency team she had a temperature of 38.4°C, a heart rate of 160 beats per minute, a blood pressure of 155/95 mmHg, and a respiratory rate of 39 breaths per minute. Her Glasgow Coma Score was 3 with bilaterally reactive pupils and disconjugate gaze. Shortly after the arrival of the team she had a further apnoeic episode that resolved spontaneously after 20 seconds and was associated with a bradycardia of 35 beats per minute. She remained unresponsive except for facial grimacing during and after painful stimulation and was readmitted to the ICU for further investigation and treatment.

```
Investigations:
  Hb                  104 g/L              (130-180)
  WBC                 11.7 × 10⁹/L         (4-11)
  platelets           433 × 10⁹/L          (150-400)
  serum sodium        150 mmol/L           (137-144)
  serum potassium     2.9 mmol/L           (3.5-4.9)
  serum urea          19.2 mmol/L          (2.5-7.0)
  serum creatinine    90 µmol/L            (60-110)
  serum CRP           30 mg/L              (<10)
  ECG:                normal
  CXR:                bibasal atelectasis
  CT scan of head:    normal
  MR scan of brain:   normal
```

Which of the following is the most likely cause of coma in this case?

A. Brainstem infarction
B. Infective endocarditis
C. Pontine myelinolysis
D. Status epilepticus
E. Venous sinus thrombosis

21. **A 72-year-old man was admitted to the acute medical unit with a diagnosis of sepsis. One week prior to his admission he had undergone a cystoscopy to investigate haematuria. Past medical history included hypertension, obstructive sleep apnoea, and morbid obesity (with an actual body weight of 120 kg). His medication included ramipril and bendroflumethiazide, and had been started on amoxicillin, clarithromycin, and gentamicin intravenously.**

    Twelve hours after admission his urine output was noted to be low at 40 mL over the past six hours. His blood pressure was 85/45 mmHg initially but had increased to 115/60 mmHg after administration of 1500 mL of sodium chloride 0.9%.

    ```
    Investigations:
      Lactate             2.2 mmol/L      (0.5-1.6)
      serum creatinine    211 µmol/L      (60-110)
      serum bilirubin     37 µmol/L       (1-22)
    ```

    Which of the following is recommended by the Surviving Sepsis Campaign Guidelines of 2012?
    A. Give further fluid challenge to exclude occult hypovolaemia
    B. Give regular hydrocortisone to spare vasopressors
    C. Start dobutamine to increase cardiac output
    D. Start low-dose dopamine for renal protection
    E. Start low-dose vasopressin to increase mean arterial pressure

22. **An 80-year-old woman was admitted to the coronary care unit following primary coronary intervention (PCI) for an ST elevation myocardial infarction. On arrival on the coronary care unit she had stopped talking and the attached defibrillator showed a heart rate of 155 beats per minute.**

    Which is not an adverse feature for adult tachyarrhythmia according to the 2015 Advanced Life Support guidelines?
    A. Chest pain
    B. Heart rate >150 bpm
    C. Hypotension
    D. Pulmonary oedema
    E. Unconsciousness

23. A 36-year-old woman was admitted to the emergency department with a two-day history of fever, malaise, and confusion. She had no past medical history, was allergic to penicillin, and worked as a teacher. On examination her temperature was 39.5°C, pulse 122 beats per minute, blood pressure 75/30 mmHg, and respiratory rate 36 breaths per minute. A purpuric rash was evident on her trunk.

Arterial lactate was 6.9 mmol/L (0.6–1.8 mmol/L).

What would you do next?

A. Fluid challenge with crystalloid, insert a central venous catheter, and start vasopressor therapy
B. Give intravenous broad-spectrum antibiotics, fluid challenge with colloid, and insert a central venous catheter
C. Take peripheral blood cultures, give intravenous broad-spectrum antibiotics, and call the intensive care unit
D. Take peripheral blood cultures, give intravenous broad-spectrum antibiotics, and fluid challenge with crystalloid
E. Take peripheral blood cultures, insert a central venous catheter, and start vasopressor therapy

chapter 1

CARDIORESPIRATORY ARREST AND SHOCK

ANSWERS

1. D. Peritonitis

Anastomotic leak occurs in 3–20% of colon resections, reducing with increasing distance of the anastomosis from the anal verge. In this case faecal peritonitis arising from a leak is suggested by the abdominal focus of symptoms, signs elicited and the developing systemic inflammatory response syndrome (SIRS). Although four days is early for a leak to present (median time to presentation is around 12 days), this is the most likely cause in this circumstance.

The incidence of both pulmonary embolus and myocardial infarction is increased post-operatively. 1% of patients undergoing non-cardiac surgery will have an adverse cardiac event (which includes cardiac arrest or myocardial infarction) with the majority occurring in the first week after surgery.

The mnemonic for immediate causes of cardiorespiratory arrest is '4 Hs and 4 Ts':

Table 1.1 '4 Hs and 4 Ts'.

Hypovolaemia	Thrombosis (coronary, pulmonary)
Hypo/hyperkalaemia	Tamponade
Hypoxia	Tension pneumothorax
Hypothermia	Toxic/therapeutic

Reproduced from *Resuscitation*, Monsieurs K, Nolan J, Bossaert L et al., 'European Resuscitation Council Guidelines for Resuscitation 2015. Section 1. Resuscitation 2015'; 95: 1–80.

However, it must be remembered that these may not be diseases in their own right, but reflect underlying pathophysiological processes. Treatment of the underlying process is therefore required as well as resuscitation if patients are to be given the best chance of survival.

Monsieurs K, Nolan J, Bossaert L et al. on behalf of the ERC Guidelines writing group. European Resuscitation Council Guidelines for Resuscitation 2015 Section 1. Resuscitation 2015; 95: 1–80.

2. D. Three shocks delivered with minimal interruptions should be given before any other intervention

The current version of resuscitation guidelines was published in 2015 with an emphasis on maximizing the delivery of good-quality chest compressions. To facilitate this, and to reflect current evidence, single shocks were preferred with compressions continuing while the defibrillator charged.

However, in a few special circumstances the option to deliver 'stacked shocks' (i.e. three shocks in sequence with minimal delays) should be considered, namely:

1. VF/VT occurring during cardiac catheterization
2. VF/VT occurring early after cardiac surgery (where early is defined as still in hospital)
3. VF/VT arrest where the patient is already connected to a manual defibrillator.

Although there is no evidence to support the use of stacked shocks, it is the opinion of the Resuscitation Council that chest compressions are unlikely to improve the already high chance of restoring spontaneous circulation when shocks are delivered very early in these special circumstances.

The 2015 guidelines emphasise minimising interruptions in chest compressions to less than 5 seconds to attempt defibrillation. The 2015 guidelines on compression depth and rate have not changed. While charging the defibrillator during compressions is safe, conclusive evidence for safety during shock delivery (even with gloves on) does not yet exist. There should be no contact with the patient while shocks are delivered.

Monsieurs K, Nolan J, Bossaert L et al. on behalf of the ERC Guidelines writing group. European Resuscitation Council Guidelines for Resuscitation 2015 Section 1. Resuscitation 2015; 95: 1–80.

3. B. An elevated venous lactate identifies a high risk of death

Multivariate regression analysis has shown that elevated venous lactate on presentation to hospital is an independent predictor of increased 28-day mortality. Multiple mechanisms result in an increased lactate in sepsis, including catecholamine-stimulated glycolysis and pyruvate production, pyruvate dehydrogenase inhibition, and reduced lactate clearance, all of which can occur in the presence of adequate oxygen. Under ischaemic conditions lactate may rise secondary to continued glycolysis and mitochondrial dysfunction, but in sepsis there is often increased oxygen delivery to tissues with elevated cardiac output. The block to oxygen transport and utilization is at the capillary and cellular level (cytopathic hypoxia).

Hyperlactatemia is not diagnostic of the syndrome of severe sepsis, but does identify patients with cardiovascular organ dysfunction and add prognostic information, especially if the level does not fall with therapy. Targeting lactate clearance instead of central venous oxygen saturation in a haemodynamic goal-directed resuscitation protocol is associated with similar outcomes.

Venous lactate is more easily obtained than arterial in the absence of an arterial catheter. Although a high venous lactate may indicate a high arterial lactate, there is a bias towards higher readings with peripheral samples. If venous lactate is high this is worth confirming with arterial samples to avoid unnecessary interventions. A low venous lactate is more reassuring.

Bakker J, Jansen T. Don't take vitals, take a lactate. Intensive Care Medicine 2007; 33: 1863–1865.

4. A. 5%

The American National Registry of Cardiopulmonary Resuscitation (see Table 1.2) demonstrates that while 11.9% of those suffering asystolic cardiorespiratory arrests will survive to discharge only 8.8% have a good neurological outcome (defined as a cerebral performance category (CPC) of 1 or 2, or no change from baseline CPC). They also observed that asystole followed by a period of ventricular fibrillation or tachycardia was associated with 7.5% survival to discharge and 5% had a good neurological outcome.

In the United Kingdom the National Cardiac Arrest Audit (NCAA) analysed data from 144 hospitals between 2011 and 2013. 8.7% of patients presenting in asystole after in-hospital cardiac arrest survived to discharge. Of the survivors to discharge in whom CPC could be assessed 96.7% had a good neurological outcome. There was significant variation in outcome between hospitals and with age and time and day of cardiac arrest. The American data is preferred as a more conservative estimate of prognosis in an elderly patient with comorbidity.

Table 1.2 Event survival after first-documented rhythm.

n = 51,919	Survive >24 hours (%)	Survive to discharge (%)	Good neurological outcome (%)
VT	53.3	36.9	31.2
VF	50.6	37.3	31.6
PEA	30.9	13.8	9.9
PEA + VF/VT	19.0	6.5	4.5
Asystole	26.2	11.9	8.8
Asystole + VF/VT	22.5	7.5	5.0

Reproduced from *Critical Care Medicine*, Meaney P et al., 'Rhythms and outcomes of adult in-hospital cardiac arrest', 38, pp. 101–108, Copyright (2010) with permission from Wolters Kluwer Health, Inc.

The CPC categories are:
1. Normal or mild cerebral disability (able to work)
2. Moderate cerebral disability (able to live independently)
3. Severe cerebral disability (dependent on others for daily support)
4. Coma or vegetative state
5. Brain death

http://www.fda.gov/ohrms/dockets/ac/05/briefing/2005-4100b1_03_CPC%20Scale.pdf

Meaney P, Nadkarni V, Kern K, Indik J, Halperin H, Berg R. Rhythms and outcomes of adult in-hospital cardiac arrest. Critical Care Medicine 2010; 38: 101–108.

Nolan J, Soar J, Smith G, Gwinnutt C, Parrott, Power S, Harrison D, Nixon E, Rowan K on behalf of the National Cardiac Arrest Audit. Incidence and outcome of in-hospital cardiac arrest in the United Kingdom National Cardiac Arrest Audit. Resuscitation 2014; 85: 987–992.

5. B. Exclusion of reversible causes of apnoea, known irreversible aetiology of coma, exclusion of reversible causes of coma

The Academy of Royal Medical Colleges document on the diagnosis of death states that three preconditions must be met before proceeding to test for death by irreversible cessation of brainstem function:

1. Irreversible brain damage of known aetiology
2. Exclusion of reversible causes of coma
3. Exclusion of reversible causes of apnoea.

There is no time restriction on when the tests may be performed. In practice the irreversibility of damage may be apparent earlier after some injuries (e.g. subarachnoid haemorrhage) than others (hypoxic brain injury post-cardiac arrest). While in the UK there is no requirement to demonstrate the absence of cerebral blood flow this may be a useful corroborative test where clinical doubt remains about the irreversible nature of the coma; Doppler or CT or MRI angiography could substitute for a formal cerebral angiogram. There is also no requirement for a structural brain lesion, but in these cases it is more difficult to be sure that the coma is truly irreversible.

The coroner's approval does not have to be given before brainstem tests are performed, but will be required in many circumstances if organ donation is to follow (for example, in cases of trauma or neglect).

Reversible causes that must be considered include:

1. Hypothermia (i.e. core temperature <34°C)
2. Drugs: sedation, analgesia (opioids), neuromuscular blockade

3. Metabolic and endocrine function (especially sodium, glucose, potassium, magnesium, phosphate, thyroid, and adrenal)
4. Neuromuscular disease (including spinal cord injury in trauma cases).

The tests themselves are standardized to examine cranial nerves for signs of brainstem function and include disconnection of the ventilator to confirm apnoea in the face of an adequate carbon dioxide stimulus. Two sets of tests are performed with the time of death recorded as the time of the first set of tests. One of the two doctors involved must be a consultant and both must have been registered for more than five years, be competent in the procedure, and have no conflict of interest (e.g. as a member of a transplant team).

A Code of Practice for the Diagnosis and Confirmation of Death. Academy of Medical Royal Colleges. PPG Design and Print, London, 2008.

6. E. Severe sepsis

The diagnosis of acute kidney injury is discussed in chapter 7. Acute lung injury is defined most simply as a P:F ratio (PaO_2/FiO_2) <40 kPa, or <300 mmHg (in this case the PaO_2 is 9.9 kPa and FiO_2 is 21% or 0.21 therefore 9.9/0.21 = 47.1). The definition of the acute respiratory distress syndrome has recently been revised, although the fundamental reliance on P:F ratio is unchanged.

Sepsis is the systemic inflammatory response syndrome resulting from proven or suspected infection. To have SIRS, two of the six criteria must be met:

1. Temperature <36 or >38.3°C
2. Heart rate >90 beats per minute
3. Respiratory rate >20 breaths per minute or PCO_2 <4.3 kPa
4. White blood cells <4 or >12 × 10^9/L or >10% immature band forms
5. Glucose >7.7mmol/L (in the absence of known diabetes)
6. New onset confusion or altered mental state

If there is evidence of end-organ dysfunction (e.g. poor peripheral perfusion demonstrated by prolonged capillary refill or raised lactate, acute lung injury, confusion, acute kidney injury) then the sepsis is said to be severe. Septic shock is the most severe end of the spectrum and is said to exist when hypotension persists despite adequate fluid resuscitation. Hypotension is usually defined as systolic blood pressure <90 mmHg or a >20% drop from baseline; adequate fluid resuscitation is much less clear but a rough rule of thumb would be at least 20 mL/kg given in under an hour.

Ferguson N, Fan E, Camporota L et al. The Berlin definition of ARDS: an expanded rationale, justification and supplementary material. Intensive Care Medicine 2012; 38: 1573–1582.

Levy M, Fink M, Marshall J et al. 2001 SCCM/ESICM/ACCP/ATS/SIS international sepsis definitions conference. Critical Care Medicine 2003; 31: 1250–1256.

Mehta R, Kellum J, Shah S et al. Acute Kidney Injury Network: report of an initiative to improve outcomes in acute kidney injury. Critical Care 2007; 11: R31.

7. A. Activate the massive haemorrhage protocol

The working diagnosis is hypovolaemic shock secondary to variceal bleeding. Where bleeding is the cause of shock then there are two priorities in management: resuscitate to prevent multi-organ failure or death, and stop ongoing bleeding.

In recent years the concept of damage control resuscitation has become popular. This originated in military trauma protocols and is now widely used in civilian trauma and surgical cases of massive haemorrhage. Essentially, damage control resuscitation aims to minimize complications of resuscitation and limit ongoing blood loss until control of bleeding is achieved. Behind this is the recognition that high-volume crystalloid and colloid resuscitation carries risks of coagulopathy and renal injury, and that attempts to restore normal haemodynamic parameters before definitive control of bleeding may prevent clot formation and increase blood loss. To avoid these problems early use of blood and blood products (fresh frozen plasma and platelets) is advised, with a much lower blood: fresh frozen plasma ratio than previously given to prevent development of coagulopathy associated with clotting factor loss. Monitoring of clotting using laboratory analysis is also less important. The immediate goal of resuscitation is to restore a palpable radial pulse, rather than normal blood pressure, until the bleeding is controlled.

All hospitals will have a major haemorrhage policy and the haematology laboratory will maintain a massive transfusion pack. This contains packed red cells, fresh frozen plasma, and platelets (e.g. in a 4:4:1 ratio), and can be requested urgently. Group O negative blood will also be immediately available, but the use of type-specific blood (ready in 10–15 minutes) is preferred if possible.

In this situation the patient will need endoscopy with banding for control of the bleeding point; given the reduction in conscious level and large blood load this will be best done with airway control (i.e. intubation). Terlipressin will reduce the risk of re-bleeding after banding and is recommended by NICE. In the clinical context as previously discussed, resuscitation with blood products has priority, especially since the products would take longer to obtain than the terlipressin. If control cannot be achieved with banding then tamponade with a Sengstaken tube is a second-line option for temporary control, but is not definitive. Interventional radiology for embolization or transjugular intrahepatic portosystemic shunting should be considered if banding fails.

Jansen J, Thomas R, Loudon M, Brooks A. Damage control resuscitation for patients with major trauma. British Medical Journal 2009; 338: b1778.

NICE Clinical Guideline 141: Acute upper gastrointestinal bleeding management. http://www.nice.org.uk/nicemedia/live/13762/59549/59549.pdf

Young P, Cotton B, Goodnough L. Massive transfusion protocols for patients with substantial haemorrhage. Transfusion Medicine Reviews 2011; 25: 293–303.

8. E. Take the CVC out

In this situation the central venous pressure response to a fluid bolus is commonly used to assess intravascular volume. Hypovolaemia may be contributing to oliguria, and hypervolaemia risks pulmonary oedema; it is also a marker for worse outcome in acute kidney injury. However, this strategy is flawed for two reasons. First, the necessary information is available in the history and examination. Given the history, hypovolaemia is unlikely; there has been no ongoing and unreplaced fluid loss. A patient who is not tachycardic with a normal blood pressure, and warm peripheries has an adequate cardiac output. In the absence of peripheral or pulmonary oedema (the latter very unlikely with normal saturations and respiratory rate) there is no evidence of fluid overload either. Finally, the likely renal injury is contrast medium-related and therefore unlikely to respond to fluid loading after the event. Second, the central venous pressure (CVP) is not a measure of intravascular volume. It is a pressure measurement that is determined by the relationship between cardiac performance and venous return. Poor function and low return cannot be distinguished from good function and normal return or hyperdynamic function and increased return on the basis of a static reading.

Similarly, the change in CVP reading in response to a fluid challenge may be related to changes in cardiac contractility or changes in venous return. Without simultaneous measurement of cardiac output (or echocardiography) it is difficult if not impossible to tease out the contributions of each to the observed change in CVP. Even then, the question that has actually been answered is 'Is this patient fluid-responsive (or not)?' and not 'Does this patient need fluid?'

Kumar A, Anel R, Bunnell E et al. Pulmonary artery occlusion pressure and central venous pressure fail to predict ventricular filling volume, cardiac performance, or the response to volume infusion in normal subjects. Critical Care Medicine 2004; 32: 691–699.

Magder S. Central venous pressure: a useful but not-so-simple measurement. Critical Care Medicine 2006; 34: 2224–2227.

9. B. Early inflation

The waveform shows overall reduction in diastolic augmentation that encroaches on systole with no visible dicrotic notch. Assisted diastole and systole are unaffected. The balloon is inflating before the aortic valve is closed causing aortic regurgitation, reduction in cardiac output, increased left ventricular volumes and pressures, and increased myocardial oxygen demand.

Intra-aortic balloon pumps (IABPs) are designed to inflate in diastole (increasing coronary perfusion) and deflate in systole (improving ejection fraction and cardiac output). Timing is usually taken from the patient's ECG, although this can be changed manually. In the medical setting, intra-aortic balloon pumps are primarily indicated for myocardial support in cardiogenic shock post-myocardial infarction where they have the advantage of improving haemodynamics without increasing myocardial oxygen demand. Recent evidence suggests that routine use of IABPs in cardiogenic shock after percutaneous coronary intervention does not improve outcome in patients managed with best medical therapy and early revascularization.

There are several significant complications associated with IABP use, including:
1. Limb ischaemia +/− compartment syndrome
2. Bleeding
3. Thrombocytopenia and anaemia
4. Infection
5. Aortic dissection

In addition, poor positioning or timing may worsen coronary perfusion and overall cardiac performance. This makes their use a specialist area and advice from cardiologists, cardiac surgeons, or perfusionists experienced in their management is essential.

Maquet Cardiac Assist Educational Programme http://ca.maquet.com/clinician-information/educational-materials/ (accessed 1 November 2012).

Thiele H, Zeymer U, Neumann F et al. for the IABP-SHOCK II Trial Investigators. Intra-aortic balloon support for myocardial infarction with cardiogenic shock. New England Journal of Medicine 2012; 367: 1287–1296.

10. C. Intubation

In this case it is arguable that intubation is not required as the patient recovers to an acceptable level of consciousness between seizures. The frequency is such that it would be a reasonable assumption that a short transfer (such as to ICU via radiology) could be accomplished in the interval between fits.

There are a number of things that are required for all patient transfers, no matter how short. Oxygen must always be available (in sufficient quantity for the whole transfer), airway adjuncts, a means of ventilation, working intravenous access, monitoring (pulse oximetry, non-invasive blood pressure, and ECG as a minimum for the non-intubated patient), and at least two healthcare providers. Also to hand should be appropriate emergency drugs (including adrenaline if there is a risk of cardiorespiratory arrest) and intravenous fluids for hypotensive patients. If any intravenous pumps are in use then battery life should be checked before leaving; the same applies to the monitor. And don't forget the notes! A simple mnemonic when preparing to transfer a patient (whether inter- or intra-hospital) is ACCEPT: assess, control, communicate, evaluate, prepare, transfer. The essence of this is that transfer only occurs when the patient is stable and everything is ready; it should not be rushed.

AAGBI Safety Guideline: Interhospital transfer. The Association of Anaesthetists of Great Britain and Ireland, London, 2009.

Macartney I, Nightingale P. Transfer of the critically ill adult patient. Continuing Education in Anaesthesia, Critical Care and Pain 2001; 1: 12–15.

11. C. 100–120 per minute

ALS guidelines 2015 state CPR should be started immediately on confirmation of cardiac arrest, at a ratio of 30 chest compressions to two ventilations and a rate of 100–120 compressions per minute. The correct hand position for chest compression is the middle of the lower half of the sternum, at a depth of 5–6 cm and a rate of 100–120 compressions per minute. Allow the chest to completely recoil after each compression and minimize interruptions to chest compressions. The quality of chest compressions is an important determinant of outcome.

Monsieurs K, Nolan J, Bossaert L et al. on behalf of the ERC Guidelines writing group. European Resuscitation Council Guidelines for Resuscitation 2015 Section 1. Resuscitation 2015; 95: 1–80.

12. A. Continue CPR until the two-minute period is completed

On the non-shockable side of the ALS algorithm (PEA or asystole), CPR should be performed at a rate of 30:2 for two minutes and the rhythm rechecked after every two-minute cycle. Adrenaline 1 mg should be given as soon as intravascular or intraosseous access can be obtained then every 3–5 minutes (every other cycle). If a shockable rhythm is seen on the monitor during the two-minute cycle, continue CPR until the two minutes is complete then be fully prepared to deliver a shock if the rhythm is still shockable.

Monsieurs K, Nolan J, Bossaert L et al. on behalf of the ERC Guidelines writing group. European Resuscitation Council Guidelines for Resuscitation 2015 Section 1. Resuscitation 2015; 95: 1–80.

13. C. Remove the endo-tracheal tube and establish face-mask ventilation

Waveform capnography is the most reliable way to verify positioning of an endo-tracheal tube. End-tidal CO_2 is detected and displayed as a graph which varies with respiration. Even though the patient is in cardiac arrest, chest compressions will be creating some circulation; therefore, some CO_2 will be detected. A sudden rise in end-tidal CO_2 may indicate return of spontaneous circulation. Other CO_2 monitors include infrared spectrometers displaying a number, or disposable colorimetric detectors which use litmus paper which changes colour according to the amount of CO_2 detected. End-tidal CO_2 detectors cannot detect whether the tube is in the trachea or the left main bronchus. If no CO_2 is detected the tube is not in the respiratory tree and is most likely in the oesophagus. Unrecognized oesophageal intubation is common in patients in cardiac arrest and it is important to recognize it. If in doubt, take it out.

Monsieurs K, Nolan J, Bossaert L et al. on behalf of the ERC Guidelines writing group. European Resuscitation Council Guidelines for Resuscitation 2015 Section 1. Resuscitation 2015; 95: 1–80.

14. D. Start intravenous heparin and arrange urgent CT pulmonary angiography

CT pulmonary angiography will make a definitive diagnosis and importantly the brain can also be scanned at the same time to exclude bleeding before formal anticoagulation. Unfractionated heparin is preferred as it has the greatest reversibility if bleeding does occur. An inferior vena cava filter is another option to reduce the risk of subsequent pulmonary emobli, but will not help with any clot already in the lung.

Transthoracic echocardiography is useful to assess right ventricular size and function. Evidence of right ventricular (RV) strain or failure, even in the absence of gross haemodynamic compromise, is associated with a greater risk of adverse events. However, evidence for thrombolysis on the basis of RV dysfunction is equivocal and this is a high-risk setting (i.e. recent intracranial neurosurgery).

D-dimers are less useful as a diagnostic test post-operatively, and do not make an immediate diagnosis in any case. Similarly, troponin may be elevated, and is a marker of risk if so, but it is not diagnostic and is associated with a delay in obtaining a result.

In the absence of risk factors and ECG changes coronary ischaemia is unlikely, but again focused echocardiography is useful to assess regional wall motion abnormalities and look for tamponade.

National Institute for Health and Care Excellence. Clinical Guideline 144. Venous thromboembolic diseases: diagnosis, management and thrombophilia testing. June 2012.

15. C. Forced air warming blanket

The cornerstone of management of severe hypothermia (core temperature <30°C) is core rewarming. Invasive methods offer the most effective means of increasing temperature, so cardiopulmonary bypass, continuous renal replacement therapy (CRRT), and use of an intravascular cooling device (which, of course, can also rewarm patients) are all options depending on local availability and expertise. A lower-tech invasive option is cavity lavage with warmed fluids (pleural, peritoneal, and bladder), but it is not the method of choice when the others are available.

Warming and humidifying inspired gases is essential to prevent further heat loss from the respiratory tract, although it will not produce core rewarming if used as the sole technique.

A forced air warming blanket depends on peripheral circulation to carry heat to the core and is a suitable technique for less severe hypothermia. In this situation it will not be effective and may produce thermal injury to the skin.

Rewarming may be associated with problems including haemodynamic instability, electrolyte imbalance (especially potassium, magnesium, and phosphate), and diuresis. As the core temperature nears normal levels shivering may begin and require treatment with sedation and analgesia. Hypothermia per se is associated with complications such as pancreatitis, immune suppression and infection, and coagulopathy.

Do not forget to look for an underlying cause which could be a medical or surgical illness, or trauma- or drug-related.

Brown D, Brugger H, Boyd J, Paal P. Accidental hypothermia. New England Journal of Medicine 2012; 367: 1930–1938.

16. A. Anaphylaxis–adrenaline

Anaphylaxis may not present on the first administration of the offending drug. It is the most likely diagnosis in this situation given the temporal association with administration of a common trigger agent and the clinical findings of cardiovascular collapse and bronchospasm. Warm peripheries argues against cardiogenic, obstructive, or hypovolaemic shock. Sepsis is unlikely though not impossible given that prophylactic antibiotics are routine. A transfusion reaction too is possible, but most transfusions after knee surgery is autologous and therefore not associated with major incompatibility reactions.

It is not always an easy diagnosis to make especially as confirmation depends on mast cell tryptase collected after the event and ultimately immunological challenge when fully recovered. A high index of suspicion should be maintained as immediate treatment with oxygen, fluids, and adrenaline is essential. The dose of adrenaline is 0.5 mg intramuscularly, which may be repeated if there is no response.

Monsieurs K, Nolan J, Bossaert L et al. on behalf of the ERC Guidelines writing group. European Resuscitation Council Guidelines for Resuscitation 2015 Section 1. Resuscitation 2015; 95: 1–80.

17. E. Steroids and antibiotics are first-line therapy

Epiglottitis carries a significant risk of mortality (approximately 7%), which may be secondary to airway obstruction or severe sepsis. Inspiratory stridor is associated with extra-thoracic airway obstruction and may be rapidly progressive. In this case respiratory distress, drooling (representing inability to swallow), and hypoxia suggest that obstruction is well advanced and measures to secure the airway are urgently needed.

Usually, this means intubation under inhalational anaesthesia by a consultant anaesthetist, with another consultant capable of performing emergency tracheostomy (ENT or occasionally intensive care medicine) scrubbed in theatre. Tracheostomy is the second-line airway plan and while it might be life-saving it is not the primary airway intervention.

Intubation is merely supportive and does not treat the condition itself: this requires antibiotics to treat infection and steroids to reduce airway swelling.

Inspiratory stridor is the hallmark of upper-airway obstruction whatever the cause: trauma, infection, oedema (angio-oedema or anaphylaxis), or foreign body. Treatment options will vary according to cause; for example, antibiotics, or adrenaline nebulizers. A definitive airway will be needed for imminent total obstruction and early referral to intensive care is essential.

Charles R, Fadden M, Brook J. Acute epiglottitis. British Medical Journal 2013; 347: f5235.

18. E. Prophylactic phenytoin will reduce the incidence of seizures in the first week

The post-cardiac arrest syndrome describes the multi-organ failure resulting from a period of whole body ischaemia-reperfusion. Any and all organs may be affected and organ support for post-cardiac arrest dysfunction is not significantly different to that for organ failure from any other cause.

There is no evidence either for or against the use of prophylactic anticonvulsants.

Nolan J, on behalf of the Council of the Intensive Care Society. Cardiac Arrest—management post return of spontaneous circulation. The Intensive Care Society, 2008.

19. D. Infection

Sepsis may present insidiously, especially in the elderly and immunocompromised. A wide range of symptoms and signs may be associated with infection (including those traditionally thought of as markers of sepsis, such as a high white cell count or C reactive protein); for example, altered mental state, fluid retention, ileus, tachypnoea, and poor peripheral perfusion.

In this case a probable source of infection (the intravenous cannula) can be identified. In association with this, SIRS is present (tachycardia and low white cell count) as well as thrombocytopenia, altered mental status, hyperglycaemia in the absence of diabetes, and coagulopathy; hence, sepsis is the most likely diagnosis. Blood cultures should be drawn and broad-spectrum antibiotics started to cover likely pathogens (staphylococcus and streptococcus in this situation).

None of the other options can explain the full clinical picture although they may have a contribution to his confusion (especially alcohol withdrawal).

Dellinger R, Levy M, Rhodes A et al. for the Surviving Sepsis Campaign Guidelines Committee. Surviving Sepsis Campaign: International Guidelines for the management of severe sepsis and septic shock: 2012. Critical Care Medicine 2013; 41: 580–637.

20. D. Status epilepticus

The causes of coma are extensive, as are the sequelae of severe sepsis. In this situation the normal CT and MRI suggest a non-structural cause of coma, and infective endocarditis, while always possible with staphylococcal septicaemias, is less likely given the low inflammatory markers, normal ECG and absence of embolic lesions on brain imaging. Status epilepticus may occur with partial or non-convulsive seizures as well as generalized ones.

National Institute for Health and Care Excellence. Clinical Guideline 137. Epilepsies: diagnosis and management. January 2012.

21. A. Give further fluid challenge to exclude occult hypovolaemia

Severe sepsis is the combination of known or suspected infection and organ dysfunction. In this case urosepsis is likely and it is associated with multi-organ dysfunction. The correct response is to give further fluid to a total of 30 mL/kg as initial resuscitation. Crystalloid is preferred although albumin may also be used as a resuscitation fluid if requirements are significantly greater than this. Starch solutions should not be used.

Low-dose dopamine is associated with harm and should not be used. If, after adequate fluid resuscitation, hypotension or organ failure persists then noradrenaline (norepinephrine) is the first-line vasoactive agent. Second-line or additional options include adrenaline, dobutamine, or vasopressin depending on the haemodynamic situation. Hydrocortisone is considered if the combination of fluid and vasopressor is insufficient to maintain blood pressure.

Dellinger R, Levy M, Rhodes A et al. for the Surviving Sepsis Campaign Guidelines Committee. Surviving Sepsis Campaign: International Guidelines for the management of severe sepsis and septic shock: 2012. Critical Care Medicine 2013; 41: 580–637.

22. B. Heart rate >150 bpm

Assessment of the patient using an ABCDE approach should be the immediate response to this situation ('treat the patient, not the ECG'). Full non-invasive monitoring should be applied, oxygen administered, and reversible causes sought.

Then management of tachyarrhythmias in the adult patient depends on an assessment of haemodynamic stability. Signs that the cardiac output is inadequate (myocardial ischaemia, syncope, shock, or heart failure) should prompt treatment of the tachyarrhythmia with synchronized DC cardioversion after appropriate sedation and analgesia. The heart rate is no longer used in this situation to determine therapy.

Monsieurs K, Nolan J, Bossaert L et al. on behalf of the ERC Guidelines writing group. European Resuscitation Council Guidelines for Resuscitation 2015 Section 1. Resuscitation 2015; 95: 1–80.

23. D. Take peripheral blood cultures, give intravenous broad-spectrum antibiotics, and fluid challenge with crystalloid

The clinical picture is most likely to be due to sepsis, which can be considered severe with evidence of end-organ failure (confusion, hypotension, and hyperlactataemia). The Surviving Sepsis Campaign publish guidelines (revised in 2012) and resuscitation bundles (revised in 2015) for management of severe sepsis. Step one is measurement of serum lactate. Arterial lactate is considered the gold standard, but many emergency departments use peripheral venous lactate for convenience. This must be viewed with caution in the overall clinical context as they are not completely interchangeable. There are three further steps in the three hour bundle: obtain blood cultures, give broad-spectrum antibiotics, and deliver 30 mL/kg crystalloid for hypotension or lactate >4 mmol/L (updated from 20 mL/kg in 2012). Further actions in the six hour bundle are: administer vasopressors if no response to fluid to maintain mean arterial pressure (MAP) ≥65 mmHg (first-choice vasopressor is noradrenaline (norepinephrine)), to reassess volume status and tissue perfusion if hypotension remains after initial fluid administration and to remeasure lactate if initial lactate elevated.

In this situation the three most appropriate are peripheral blood cultures, fluid resuscitation with crystalloid, and broad-spectrum intravenous antibiotics. Colloid should not be used for resuscitation in severe sepsis as there is no evidence of benefit (and there is evidence of harm). The updated 2012 guidelines advise avoidance of hetastarch formulations, and to consider albumin if large quantities of crystalloid are needed.

Antibiotics and source control if appropriate are the only therapeutic interventions for infections and delayed or inappropriate administration is associated with a worse outcome. A central venous catheter would be required if there is no response to the initial fluid bolus for the safe administration of vasopressors.

In the UK the Sepsis Trust promotes the use of the 'Sepsis Six' bundle. For high risk patients (called 'red flag sepsis') the following interventions should be completed within the first hour:

1. High flow oxygen
2. Blood cultures, consider source control
3. Intravenous antibiotics
4. Intravenous fluid resuscitation
5. Check haemoglobin and serial lactates
6. Hourly urine output measurement

Monitoring of the central venous pressure and measurement of central venous oxygen saturation or mixed venous oxygen saturation was recommended by the Surviving Sepsis Guidelines based on a single centre trial; however, the validity of these as resuscitation goals has been questioned and the whole package of early goal directed haemodynamic therapy has undergone further trials in the UK, Australia and New Zealand, and the USA. In none of the three trials did early goal directed therapy with specific central venous pressure (CVP) and central venous oxygen saturation resuscitation goals produce clinical benefit when compared to usual care, and evidence from the UK shows it to be associated with increased use of intensive care resources.

Changes in other aspects of critical care over the last decade may have contributed to an overall lower mortality, and 'usual care' may have changed due to heightened awareness of sepsis, reducing any marginal benefit of EGDT.

ARISE Investigators and the ANZICS Clinical Trials Group. Goal-directed resuscitation for patients with early septic shock. New England Journal of Medicine 2014; 371: 1496–1506.

Dellinger R, Levy M, Rhodes A et al. Surviving Sepsis Campaign: International Guidelines for Management of Severe Sepsis and Septic Shock: 2012. Critical Care Medicine 2013; 41/2: 580–637.

Mouncey P, Osborn T, Power G et al for the ProMISe Trial Investigators. Trial of early goal-directed resuscitation for septic shock. New England Journal of Medicine. 2015; 372: 1301–1311.

Sepsis Trust http://sepsistrust.org/

Surviving Sepsis Campaign http://www.survivingsepsis.org/Pages/default.aspx

Yearly D, Kellum J, Huang, D et al. A randomized trial of protocol-based care for early septic shock. The ProCESS investigators. The New England Journal of Medicine, 2014; 370: 1683–1693.

chapter 2

GASTROENTEROLOGY

QUESTIONS

1. A 76-year-old woman was admitted to the acute medical unit with a one-week history of diarrhoea. She was opening her bowels four times per day. She had recently started a new medication.

   On examination, her temperature was 36.4°C, pulse was 74 beats per minute, and blood pressure was 134/78 mmHg. She had a resting tremor in the right upper limb. Her abdomen was soft, with mild generalized tenderness.

   Which of the following drugs is most likely to have caused her diarrhoea?
   A. Bisoprolol
   B. Co-careldopa
   C. Omeprazole
   D. Paracetamol
   E. Simvastatin

2. A 55-year-old man was admitted to the acute medical unit with abdominal distension. He drank 12 units of alcohol per day. An ultrasound scan of his abdomen showed liver cirrhosis and ascites. He underwent therapeutic paracentesis and a total of 3.5 L of ascites was drained.

   Which is the most important step to be undertaken during paracentesis?
   A. Administer 100 mL 20% human albumin solution
   B. Administer piperacillin/tazobactam intravenously 4.5 g eight-hourly for seven days
   C. Give alcohol reduction advice to the patient
   D. Refer to the local liver unit for a transjugular intrahepatic portsystemic shunt (TIPSS) procedure
   E. Send ascitic fluid for neutrophil count and culture

GASTROENTEROLOGY | QUESTIONS

3. A 20-year-old woman was admitted to the acute medical unit following an overdose of an unknown quantity of paracetamol. She did not take any other substances or alcohol and took all the tablets together.

   Four hours after ingestion, her plasma paracetamol concentration was 120 mg/L. She had taken a paracetamol overdose six months previously and was treated with intravenous acetylcysteine, and had an adverse reaction to this with a rash and wheezing.

   What is the best course of action?
   A. Administer oral-activated charcoal via a nasogastric tube
   B. Prescribe intravenous acetylcysteine
   C. Prescribe oral methionine
   D. Recheck her paracetamol levels in two hours
   E. Refer for urgent haemodialysis

4. A 62-year-old man was admitted to the acute medical unit following a large haematemesis. He had a history of liver cirrhosis.

   He had a pulse rate of 100 beats per minute and a blood pressure of 90/60 mmHg. He had spider naevi on his chest and gynaecomastia.

   ```
   Investigations:
     haemoglobin         76 g/L          (130-180)
     serum sodium        135 mmol/L      (137-144)
     serum potassium     4.3 mmol/L      (3.5-4.9)
     serum creatinine    120 µmol/L      (60-110)
   ```

   Which of the following treatments is not appropriate?
   A. Intravenous ceftriaxone
   B. Intravenous sodium chloride 0.9%
   C. Intravenous terlipressin
   D. Oral chlordiazepoxide
   E. Two-unit red cell transfusion

5. An 80-year-old woman was admitted to the acute medical unit with constipation.

   Which of the following does not commonly cause constipation?
   A. Hypophosphataemia
   B. Hypothyroidism
   C. Panhypopituitarism
   D. Primary hyperparathyroidism
   E. Uraemia

6. A 55-year-old man presented to the acute medical unit via his GP with epigastric pain, coffee-ground vomiting and recurrent iron deficiency anaemia. He had previously had upper and lower gastrointestinal endoscopy which was normal. Duodenal biopsies were normal and helicobacter pylori urease test was negative. He was taking ferrous sulphate 200 mg twice daily and tolerating it well; however, he still needed recurrent blood transfusions and received a transfusion of two units of packed red cells four weeks ago.

```
Investigations:
   haemoglobin      82 g/L       (130-180)
   MCV              76 fL        (80-96)
   MCH              24 pg        (28-32)
   serum ferritin   10 µg/L      (15-300)
```

He had a repeat oesophagogastroduodenoscopy (OGD), which again showed no relevant pathology that could account for his anaemia.

What is the most appropriate investigation?

A. Bone marrow biopsy
B. Capsule endoscopy
C. CT scan of abdomen
D. Laparoscopy
E. Tissue transglutaminase antibody serology

7. A 65-year-old man presented to the acute medical unit with weakness and lethargy and was found to have iron deficiency anaemia. He had no history of blood loss and had no symptoms of gastrointestinal disturbance or weight loss. He had an oesophagogastroduodenoscopy (OGD) which showed oesophagitis. Coeliac serology was negative.

What is the next step?

A. Colonoscopy
B. CT colonography
C. CT scan of abdomen
D. Helicobacter pylori eradication
E. Proton pump inhibitor

8. A 38-year-old man with alcoholic liver disease presented to the acute medical unit with haemetemesis. He had mild epigastric pain.

    On examination he had spider naevi over his chest wall and was clinically jaundiced. There was no hepatomegaly and no ascites on examination. His heart rate was 110 beats per minute, blood pressure 90/50 mmHg, respiratory rate 20 and oxygen saturation 96% on room air.

    ```
    Investigations:
      haemoglobin                      110 g/L          (130-180)
      white cell count                 10.5 × 10⁹/L     (4.0-11.0)
      platelet count                   35 × 10⁹/L       (150-400)
      international normalized         1.4              (<1.4)
        ratio
      activated partial                44 s             (30-40)
        thromboplastin time
      fibrinogen                       1.9 g/L          (1.8-5.4)
    ```

    What is the most appropriate way to manage his coagulopathy?
    A. Cryoprecipitate
    B. Fresh frozen plasma
    C. Platelet transfusion
    D. Prothrombin complex concentrate
    E. Vitamin K

9. An 82-year-old woman presented to the acute medical unit with two episodes of dark vomit. The staff at her nursing home said this looked like coffee grounds. She had a past medical history of COPD and ischaemic heart disease for which she was taking aspirin, ramipril, furosemide, and inhalers. She had mild epigastric tenderness.

    On examination she had a heart rate of 90 beats per minute, blood pressure 120/82 mmHg, respiratory rate 20, and oxygen saturation 93% on air. Intravenous access was established, she was kept nil by mouth, and upper gastrointestinal endoscopy requested.

    Before endoscopy is performed what is the most appropriate treatment?
    A. Intravenous H_2-receptor antagonist
    B. Intravenous proton pump inhibitor
    C. No acid suppressant therapy
    D. Oral H_2-receptor antagonist
    E. Oral proton pump inhibitor

10. **A 75-year-old woman presented to the acute medical unit with two episodes of coffee-ground vomiting and epigastric pain. She had a past medical history of ischaemic heart disease and had previously had two myocardial infarctions. She had symptomatic angina about once a month. She was taking regular aspirin 75 mg, ramipril 5 mg, bisoprolol 5 mg, simvastatin 40 mg, and nicorandil 20 mg bd.**

    On examination she had mild epigastric tenderness to palpation. Her heart rate was 68 beats per minute, blood pressure 120/82 mmHg, respiratory rate 20, and oxygen saturation 96% on air.

    Upper gastrointestinal endoscopy was performed, which showed a duodenal ulcer. Haemostasis was achieved at endoscopy. She was started on a proton pump inhibitor.

    What is the best management of her anti-platelet therapy?
    A. Continue aspirin
    B. Discontinue aspirin
    C. Discontinue aspirin for one week then restart
    D. Discontinue aspirin until repeat endoscopy in six weeks
    E. Switch to clopidogrel

11. **A middle-aged man presented to the emergency department with mild epigastric pain and a single episode of coffee-ground vomit. He had no past medical history and was not on any medication.**

    On examination his heart rate was 70 beats per minute and regular. His blood pressure was 132/80 mmHg, respiratory rate 12, and oxygen saturation 99% on air. Physical examination was normal.

    ```
    Investigations:
      haemoglobin         145 g/L              (130-180)
      platelet count      120 × 10⁹/L          (150-400)
    ```

    What further information is required to calculate his Blatchford score?
    A. Age
    B. Creatinine
    C. Platelets
    D. Prothrombin time
    E. Urea

12. It is recommended to calculate the Blatchford score in all patients admitted to hospital with a current or recent history of upper gastrointestinal blood loss.

    Which statement is <u>incorrect</u> regarding the Blatchford score?
    A. The Blatchford score assists in the clinical management of patients presenting with gastrointestinal haemorrhage
    B. The Blatchford score helps identify which patient is likely to benefit from endoscopic intervention
    C. The Blatchford score helps identify which patients are likely to require endoscopic intervention for their GI bleed
    D. The Blatchford score is helpful to identify which patients should be sent home
    E. The Blatchford score predicts 30 day mortality

13. A 26-year old woman was referred to the acute medical unit with colicky abdominal pain and bloating. She had had these symptoms on and off for six months, and had occasional loose stool and occasional constipation. She found the pain was often relieved by defecation, and when she got pain she found her stool frequency increased. She had no blood or mucous on per rectum (PR) examination, no weight loss, and no change in appetite.

    Her observations were normal and examination was unremarkable. Blood tests including full blood count, urea and electrolytes, serum calcium, liver function tests, thyroid function tests, and tissue transglutaminase antibodies were all normal.

    What is the next step in investigation?
    A. Abdominal X-ray
    B. Colonoscopy
    C. CT scan of abdomen
    D. Flexible sigmoidoscopy
    E. No further investigations

14. A 75-year-old man presented to the acute medical unit with a collapse. On arrival of the ambulance he was hypotensive with a blood pressure of 80/40 mmHg, but this spontaneously resolved. He had a history of hypertension and was taking amlodipine.

    On examination his Glasgow Coma Score was 15/15, heart rate was 80 beats per minute, and blood pressure was 110/50 mmHg.

    A FAST (focused assessment with sonography in trauma) ultrasound scan was performed in the emergency department, which showed no free fluid in the abdomen. The aortic diameter was 6.4 cm.

    Which statement is true?
    A. A FAST scan can rule out an abdominal aortic aneurysm if the diameter is less than 4 cm
    B. A trace of free fluid in the pouch of Douglas can be seen in normal women
    C. Blood can be differentiated from ascites in the abdomen on FAST scanning
    D. The abdominal aortic aneurysm hasn't ruptured as there is no free fluid in the abdomen
    E. The presence of an abdominal aortic aneurysm on a FAST scan should be confirmed by CT before proceeding to surgery

15. A 45-year-old man presented to the ambulatory care clinic with mild epigastric pain and an episode of coffee-ground vomit. He had no past medical history and was not on any medication. On examination his heart rate was 70 beats per minute and regular, blood pressure was 132/80 mmHg, respiratory rate 12 breaths per minute, and oxygen saturation 99% on air. Physical examination was normal. His haemoglobin was 145 g/L (130–180) and serum urea was 4.5 mmol/L (2.5–7.0). His Blatchford score was 0.

    What is the next step in management?
    A. Calculate the Rockall score
    B. Discharge home for outpatient endoscopy
    C. Discharge home with oral proton pump inhibitor
    D. Routine inpatient endoscopy
    E. Urgent inpatient endoscopy

16. A 57-year-old woman was referred to the acute medical unit with right upper quadrant pain. On examination she was afebrile, her heart rate was 64 beats per minute and blood pressure was 124/75 mmHg. She had right upper quadrant tenderness on palpation.

```
Investigations:
    white cell count                  4.5 × 10⁹/L      (4.0-11.0)
    serum C-reactive protein          6 mg/L           (<10)
    serum total bilirubin             83 µmol/L        (1-22)
    serum alkaline phosphatase        243 U/L          (45-105)
    serum alanine aminotransferase    64 U/L           (5-35)
    serum albumin                     42 g/L           (37-49)

    Ultrasound scan of abdomen: common bile duct measures 8 mm
    in diameter.
```

What is the next stage in management?

A. Abdominal X-ray
B. CT scan of abdomen
C. Endoscopic Retrograde Cholangiopancreatography
D. Intravenous antibiotics
E. Magnetic Resonance Cholangiopancreatography

17. An 86-year-old woman was admitted to the acute medical unit with a four-day history of diarrhoea. On further questioning it became apparent that she didn't have a fridge and kept meat in her larder, which she said stayed cool.

A stool culture grew campylobacter.

Which statement is true?

A. Antibiotics should be started
B. Campylobacter is not contagious
C. Campylobacter is gram negative
D. The Health Protection Team should be notified
E. The incubation period is 7–14 days

18. A 36-year-old man presented to the acute medical unit with a seven-day history of abdominal pain and bloody diarrhoea, passing 10–12 stools per day. He had no past medical history and was not on any medication. Examination revealed lower abdominal tenderness and digital rectal examination showed some soft stool with blood. Stool samples for microscopy and culture, clostridium difficile and norovirus were negative after ten days.

What is the next step in management?

A. CT scan of abdomen
B. Colonoscopy
C. Flexible sigmoidoscopy
D. Stool for ova, cysts, and parasites
E. Tissue transglutaminase antibodies

GASTROENTEROLOGY | QUESTIONS

19. A 24-year-old woman was admitted to the acute medical unit following a paracetamol overdose. She had been treated with intravenous acetylcysteine. On day three after the overdose her blood tests were as follows.

```
Investigations:
   serum bilirubin          320 µmol/L      (1-22)
   serum alanine            2340 U/L        (5-35)
   aminotransferase
   serum creatinine         183 µmol/L      (60-110)
   prothrombin time         88 s            (11.5-15.5)
   pH                       7.29
```

Which variable fulfils criteria for liver transplantation?

A. pH
B. Prothrombin time
C. Serum alanine aminotransferase
D. Serum bilirubin
E. Serum creatinine

20. A 60-year-old man with alcoholic liver disease was admitted to the acute medical unit with ascites. He asks you about liver transplantation, what should you tell him?

A. Abstinence from alcohol for six months is mandatory
B. Alcoholic cardiomyopathy is a major determinant of outcome
C. Most patients start drinking again after transplantation
D. One-year survival is around 65%
E. Patients more than 60 years old are not eligible

21. A 42-year-old woman presented to the ambulatory care clinic with skin discolouration. She had a one-month history of fatigue and pruritis, and noticed yellowing of her skin for the last week. On examination she was jaundiced, her observations were normal, and her abdominal examination was unremarkable.

```
Investigations:
   serum bilirubin                   94 µmol/L       (1-22)
   serum alanine aminotransferase    86 U/L (5-35)
   serum alkaline phosphatase        286 U/L         (45-105)
   antinuclear antibodies            positive
   antimitochondrial antibodies      positive
   ultrasound scan of biliary tree   common bile duct 3 mm
```

What test would you do to enable you to stage her disease?

A. CT scan of abdomen
B. ERCP
C. Liver biopsy
D. MRCP
E. Ultrasound scan with portal flow studies

22.
A 34-year-old man presented to the acute medical unit with abdominal pain and jaundice. He had been on an alcohol binge and over the last three days had drunk approximately 120 units of alcohol. He had a history of drinking this amount regularly for the last 20 years. On examination his heart rate was 110 beats per minute and blood pressure was 120/74 mmHg. He was tender in the right upper quadrant.

```
Investigations:
    serum bilirubin                     310 µmol/L      (1-22)
    serum alanine aminotransferase       37 U/L         (5-35)
    serum aspartate aminotransferase    103 U/L         (1-31)
    serum alkaline phosphatase          110 U/L         (4-105)
    prothrombin time                     22 s           (11.5-15.5)
    serum creatinine                     80 µmol/L      (60-110)
    haemoglobin                         140 g/L         (130-180)
    platelets                           160 × 10⁹/L     (150-400)

    Maddrey's discriminant function      48
```

What treatment is most likely to decrease his chance of death?

A. Acetylcysteine
B. Antibiotics
C. Cholestyramine
D. Parenteral vitamins B and C (Pabrinex®)
E. Steroids

23.
A 54-year-old man with alcoholic liver disease presented to the acute medical unit with general malaise and worsening ascites. On examination his temperature was 36.8°C, heart rate was 100 beats per minute, blood pressure was 100/70 mmHg, and respiratory rate was 18 breaths per minute. He had tense ascites.

```
Investigations:
    haemoglobin          130 g/L            (130-180)
    white cell count     11.5 × 10⁹/L       (4.0-11.0)
    platelets            100 × 10⁹/L        (150-400)
    prothrombin time     18.5 s             (11.5-15.5)
    serum bilirubin      32 µmol/L          (1-22)
    serum albumin        22 g/L             (37-49)
    serum urea           13.3 mmol/L        (2.5-7.0)
    serum creatinine     230 µmol/L         (60-110)
```

Management should not include:

A. Drainage of ascites
B. Human albumin solution
C. Sodium chloride 0.9%
D. Steroids
E. Terlipressin

24. A 72-year-old man presented to the acute medical unit with abdominal pain and vomiting. He had a past medical history of hypertension and ischaemic heart disease and had had an appendicectomy many years before. His abdominal X-ray showed dilated loops of small bowel.

    A CT scan of his abdomen was reported as showing a small bowel transition point with free fluid in the abdomen.

    What is the most appropriate management?
    A. Intravenous fluids and flatus tube
    B. Intravenous fluids and light diet
    C. Intravenous fluids and narrow bore nasogastric tube
    D. Intravenous fluids and surgical exploration
    E. Intravenous fluids and wide bore nasogastric tube

25. A 26-year-old woman presented to the ambulatory care clinic with intermittent abdominal pain, bloating, and diarrhoea for six months. There was no blood or mucous per rectum and no weight loss. She had had recent negative stool cultures, a normal full blood count, and negative anti-transglutaminase antibodies. Her C-reactive protein was 40 mg/L (<10).

    What is the next best test to help distinguish between inflammatory or non-inflammatory bowel diseases?
    A. Colonoscopy
    B. CT abdomen
    C. Erythrocyte sedimentation rate
    D. Faecal calprotectin
    E. Flexible sigmoidoscopy

26. A 42-year-old man attended the emergency department with dyspepsia for two weeks. There was no weight loss, no difficulty swallowing, and no evidence of any gastro-intestinal blood loss. His symptoms had not resolved with as-required over-the-counter alginate therapy. He was not taking any regular medications.

    What should you advise?
    A. As-required proton pump inhibitor
    B. Offer full course of proton pump inhibitor treatment for 4 weeks
    C. Outpatient upper gastro-intestinal endoscopy
    D. Regular histamine type-2 receptor antagonist
    E. Regular sodium alginate (antacids)

GASTROENTEROLOGY | QUESTIONS

27. A 33-year-old woman with known ulcerative colitis presented to the acute medical unit with diarrhoea and abdominal pain. She was opening her bowels up to ten times per day, for the last six days. There was mucous and occasional blood in her stool. On examination her heart rate was 110 beats per minute, blood pressure was 120/70 mmHg, and respiratory rate was 18 breaths per minute. She had generalized abdominal tenderness but there was no guarding or rebound.

What is the most appropriate next step?

A. Flexible sigmoidoscopy
B. Intravenous hydrocortisone
C. Intravenous metronidazole
D. Oral prednisolone
E. Stool samples for microscopy

28. A 64-year-old woman presented to the acute medical unit with epigastric pain. She had no significant past medical history and was not taking any regular medication. She drank about 30 units of alcohol per week. On examination her heart rate was 120 beats per minute, blood pressure was 134/84 mmHg, respiratory rate was 32 breaths per minute, and oxygen saturation was 88% on air. On examination she had bilateral crackles on her chest and epigastric pain to palpation.

```
Investigations:
    haemoglobin              110 g/L            (115 -165)
    white cell count         23 × 10⁹/L         (4.0-11.0)
    platelets                265 × 10⁹/L        (150-400)
    serum corrected calcium  2.20 mmol/L        (2.20-2.60)
    serum albumin            18 g/L             (37-49)

    Arterial blood gas on air:
    pH           7.36
    pO2          7.6 kPa    (11.3-12.6)
    pCO2         4.5 kPa    (4.7-6.0)
    bicarbonate  22 mmol/L  (35-45)
    lactate      2.4 mmol/L (0.5-1.6)
```

What in the next step in management?

A. Continuous positive airways pressure
B. CT scan of abdomen
C. Intravenous albumin
D. Intravenous broad-spectrum antibiotics
E. Intravenous vitamin B + C compound (Pabrinex®)

29. An 83-year-old woman presented to the acute medical unit with difficulty swallowing. She was known to have a benign oesophageal stricture. She had an upper gastrointestinal endoscopy, which was her 12th procedure since the stricture was diagnosed 18 months ago. She was reviewed prior to discharge and was complaining of chest pain. She had a temperature of 38.0°C, heart rate of 110 beats per minute, blood pressure of 110/70 mmHg, respiratory rate of 24 breaths per minute, and oxygen saturation 94% on air.

    Which test is likely to give you the diagnosis?

    A. Arterial blood gas
    B. Chest X-ray
    C. D-dimer
    D. ECG
    E. Troponin T

30. A 32-year-old man was diagnosed with coeliac disease on duodenal biopsies.

    Which is true?

    A. Anti-tissue transglutaminase antibodies will stay positive on a gluten-free diet
    B. Any oats are safe to eat
    C. Food containing less than 20 parts per million of gluten can be labelled as gluten-free
    D. He should be prescribed calcium supplements and a bisphosphonate
    E. HLA-DQ8 Gene expression is present in 95% of patients who suffer from coeliac disease

31. A 46-year-old man was admitted to the acute medical unit with diarrhoea six times per day. He described streaks of blood in the stool. He had a history of Crohn's disease. He was mobile. His haemoglobin was 120 g/L (130–180).

    Which is true regarding thromboprophylaxis?

    A. He should be prescribed aspirin for thromboprophylaxis
    B. He should be prescribed prophylactic dose low molecular weight heparin
    C. He should be prescribed treatment dose low molecular weight heparin as he is at high risk
    D. He should not be prescribed low molecular weight heparin as he has bloody stool
    E. He should not be prescribed low molecular weight heparin because he is mobilizing

32. A 75-year-old man was referred to the acute medical unit with abdominal pain and intermittent rectal bleeding. He had had these symptoms on and off for three months. Over that time he had lost 3 kg in weight. He had no significant past medical history. His GP had arranged a flexible sigmoidoscopy, which was normal.

    What is the best management strategy?

    A. Barium enema
    B. Colonoscopy
    C. CT colonography
    D. CT scan of abdomen
    E. Repeat flexible sigmoidoscopy

33. An 82-year-old woman presented to the acute medical unit via her GP with a small amount of coffee-ground vomit. She was diagnosed with oesophageal cancer which was being treated palliatively and she had an oesophageal stent in situ. On her chest X-ray the stent looked well placed. She was cardiovascularly stable. Her haemoglobin was 90 g/L (115–165) and had been at this level for several weeks. She had had multiple previous endoscopies and was not keen on a further procedure.

    What should you advise her?

    A. She should be allowed home with symptomatic management
    B. She should be transfused to a haemoglobin of 100 g/L
    C. She should have a barium swallow to assess the stent
    D. She should have a further endoscopy to investigate the bleeding
    E. She should have palliative radiotherapy

34. A 43-year-old woman had extensive but quiescent ulcerative colitis shown on her last colonoscopy. Her father had colorectal cancer diagnosed at the age of 55 years.

    What would you advise her regarding colorectal cancer surveillance?

    A. Colonoscopy every year
    B. Colonoscopy every 2 years
    C. Colonoscopy every 3 years
    D. Colonoscopy every 4 years
    E. Colonoscopy every 5 years

35. A 55-year-old woman with known alcohol dependence presented to the acute medical unit with confusion and ataxia.

    What dose of thiamine should she receive?

    A. Oral thiamine 100 mg twice daily
    B. Parenteral vitamins B + C (Pabrinex®) one pair once daily
    C. Parenteral vitamins B + C (Pabrinex®) one pair three times daily
    D. Parenteral vitamins B + C (Pabrinex®) two pairs once daily
    E. Parenteral vitamins B + C (Pabrinex®) two pairs three times daily

36. A 46-year-old man was brought to the emergency department via ambulance having a tonic-clonic seizure. He was known to be a heavy drinker usually consuming 40 units of alcohol per day. He had not been seen in his usual pub for the last two days.

    What is the best management for his seizures?

    A. Chlordiaxepoxide
    B. Haloperidol
    C. Lorazepam
    D. Phenytoin
    E. Vitamin B + C complex (Pabrinex®)

37. A 26-year-old woman with anorexia nervosa was transferred from the psychiatric unit to the acute medical unit for initiation of nasogastric feeding. She weighed 38 kg and her body mass index was 13 kg/m². A feeding regime was started with feed of 1 kcal/mL running at 50 mL/hr for 20 hours in every 24 hours.

    What are the risks of this feeding regime?

    A. Hyperglycaemia
    B. Hyperkalaemia
    C. Hypernatraemia
    D. Hyponatraemia
    E. Hypophosphataemia

38. An 82-year-old woman was admitted to the acute medical unit with diarrhoea. She had recently had a course of coamoxiclav for a urine infection. She had no other past medical history. She was opening her bowels six times per day. On examination her temperature was 38.0°C, heart rate 90 beats per minute, and blood pressure 124/75 mmHg. Her abdomen was soft but mildly tender. Her white cell count was 19 × 10⁹/L (4.0–11.0). Her stool was positive for clostridium difficile toxin.

    What is the first-line treatment?

    A. Intravenous metronidazole 500 mg three times daily
    B. Intravenous vancomycin 500 mg twice daily
    C. Oral fidoximicin 200 mg twice a day
    D. Oral metronidazole 500 mg three times daily
    E. Oral vancomycin 125 mg four times daily

39. A 75-year-old woman presented to the acute medical unit with constipation. She was taking regular codeine for osteoarthritis.

    Which laxative has an osmotic effect?

    A. Docusate sodium
    B. Ispaghula husk
    C. Macrogol
    D. Senna
    E. Sodium picosulphate

40. A 65-year-old man presented to the acute medical unit with progressive dysphagia. Subsequent investigations confirmed adenocarcinoma of the oesophagus, stage 2a. He did not have any other past medical history.

    What is the best management option?

    A. Chemotherapy
    B. Endoscopic mucosal resection
    C. Oesophageal stenting
    D. Oesphagectomy
    E. Radiotherapy

chapter 2

GASTROENTEROLOGY

ANSWERS

1. B. Co-careldopa

This case highlights important aspects of side effects of medication. There are a number of drugs that may be associated with diarrhoea and tenderness in the abdomen. The patient is 76 years old and has a unilateral, asymmetrical tremor of the right upper limb and is likely suffering from Parkinson's disease. Co-caredopa or Sinemet® is a combination of levodopa and carbidopa. Levodopa is broken down into dopamine by dopa-decarboxylase in the substantia nigra, and as a result boosts dopaminergic transmission in the brain to reduce symptoms. Only 5–10% of levodopa crosses the blood–brain barrier; the rest is usually metabolized to dopamine peripherally resulting in side effects. The carbidopa inhibits the peripheral dopa-decarboxylase reducing the peripheral breakdown of levodopa. Side effects of the drug are multiple including hypostatic dysregulation, blood pressure drop, rash, angioedema, balance or coordination problems, and neuroleptic malignant syndrome. There are a multitude of other side effects including neurological and psychiatric symptoms such as sleep disturbance, depression, and psychosis with suicidal ideation.

Gastrointestinal symptoms include dry mouth, bitter taste, nausea, abdominal discomfort, indigestion, pain, flatulence, diarrhoea, and ulcers. When treating a patient with Parkinson's disease one should start at the lowest possible level to reduce side effects related to the drug.

A number of other drugs listed are also associated with diarrhoea. Omeprazole has side effects that include bloating and predominantly watery diarrhoea. It is also associated with an increased risk of clostridium difficile associated diarrhoea, especially in the combination with antibiotics.

Bisoprolol is generally well tolerated, and side effects are mild and transient. These include dizziness, fatigue, depression, headache, nausea, abdominal cramps, diarrhoea, cold extremities, sore throat, and shortness of breath or wheezing.

Simvastatin has a multitude of side effects and may cause persistent elevation in liver function tests. Liver function test should be closely monitored and the drug should be discontinued in patients with persistent elevations (three times normal). Other side effects include fatty changes in the liver, cirrhosis, hepatic failure, and fulminant hepatic necrosis.

Gastrointestinal side effects are common, tend to be mild and transient in nature, and often resolve under continued therapy. Side effects include constipation, nausea, flatulence, diarrhoea, dyspepsia, and abdominal pain.

Paracetamol has been associated with diarrhoea but it is less common than with other non-steroidal anti-inflammatories.

Chassany O, Michaux A, Bergmann J. Drug-induced diarrhoea. Drug Safety January 2000; 22(1): 53–72.

2. E. Send acitic fluid for neutrophil count and culture

The patient's medical history and presenting complaint is that of abdominal distension. Ultrasound confirms liver cirrhosis with ascites. The question is, what is the most important step to be undertaken *during* paracentesis?

Antibiotics such as piperacillin/tazobactam 4.5 g intravenously eight-hourly for seven days should always be administered if spontaneous bacterial peritonitis (SBP) is diagnosed. This is confirmed by sending ascitic fluid for neutrophil count and culture. SBP is usually due to escherichia coli or streptococcus pneumoniae in cirrhotic patients with ascites. It does not always present with the clinical features of pain, rebound tenderness, and absent bowel sounds but often presents with decompensated liver disease and encephalopathy. Antibiotics should be started if the neutrophil count in the ascitic fluid is greater than 250 mm^3.

Giving alcohol advice is vital and important, but not necessary during therapeutic paracentesis.

Referral for a transjugular intrahepatic portsystemic shunt (TIPSS) procedure should be considered in diuretic resistant ascites requiring repeated paracentesis and in uncontrolled bleeding from gastric or oesophageal varices. Control of bleeding is effective (approaching 100%) but one-month mortality is high (30–40%) owing to the underlying liver cirrhosis. Late complications, which are common, include encephalopathy and blocked stents.

The clinical history does not support the use of a TIPSS procedure as it does not highlight a resistant ascites requiring repeated paracentesis.

Administration of human albumin solution is only recommended in larger ascitic taps over 5 L.

Moore K and Aithal G. Guidelines on the Management of Ascites in Cirrhosis Gut. 2006; 55, 1–12. doi:10.1136/gut.2006.099580.

3. B. Prescribe intravenous acetylcysteine

The Commission on Human Medicines (CHM) has changed the guidelines for treatment of paracetamol overdose (2012) (Figure 2.1). Hypersensitivity is no longer a contraindication to treatment with acetylcysteine. The other change is that the duration of administration of the first dose of acetlycysteine has increased from 15 minutes to one hour.

Paracetamol cannot be removed by dialysis but is naturally secreted out of the body through the kidneys. 75% is secreted through the kidneys; 25% through the liver. The half-life of paracetamol is five hours and it can be significantly prolonged in overdose. Rechecking her paracetamol levels is not beneficial in making a decision regarding treatment.

The newest guidelines by the CHM does not differentiate between high-risk and low-risk paracetamol overdose; there is now only one treatment line. The licensed indication for acetylcysteine is now:

- Paracetamol overdose irrespective of the plasma paracetamol level in circumstances where the overdose is staggered or there is doubt over the time of paracetamol ingestion.
- Paracetamol overdose with a timed plasma paracetamol concentration on or above a single treatment line joining points of 100 mg/L at four hours and 15 mg/L at 15 hours, regardless of risk factors of hepatotoxicity.

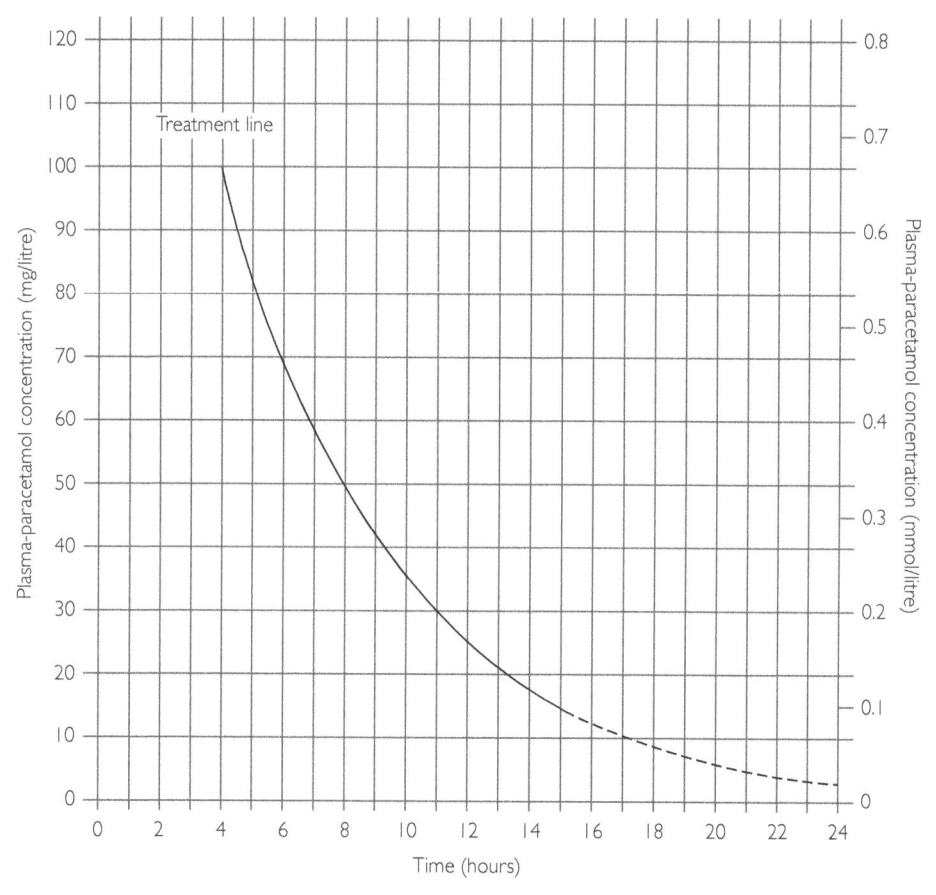

Figure 2.1 Paracetamol treatment graph.

Reproduced from Drug Safety Update, 6, 2:A1, Medicines and Healthcare products Regulatory Agency (MHRA), 'Treating paracetamol overdose with intravenous acetylcysteine: new guidance', Copyright (2012) with permission from MRHA.

Commission on Human Medicines. Paracetamol overdose: new guidance on use of intravenous acetylcysteine. September 2012. http://www.mhra.gov.uk/Safetyinformation/Safetywarningsalertsandrecalls/Safetywarningsandmessagesformedicines/CON178225.

4. D. Oral chlordiazepoxide

The patient is suffering from upper gastrointestinal bleeding and is in hypovolaemic shock. In view of his medical history the most likely cause of bleeding is a variceal haemorrhage. Latest NICE (National Institute for Health and Care Excellence) guidance published in 2012 highlight the following recommendations:

- Offer terlipressin to patients with suspected variceal bleeding when they first present.
- Offer prophylactic antibiotic therapy at presentation to patients with suspected or confirmed variceal bleeding.
- Patients with massive haemorrhage should be transfused with blood and blood products in accordance with local protocols for the management of massive bleeding.
- A haemoglobin level of 80 g/L should be used as the threshold for triggering consideration of transfusion.

No information is given about this man's alcohol intake and there are no signs of alcohol withdrawal described. All the other treatments are indicated in acute variceal haemorrhage.

It is important to consider the risk of alcohol withdrawal treatment in this patient, but this is the least important issue in the context of this acute upper gastrointestinal haemorrhage.

National Institute for Health and Care Excellence, Clinical Guideline 141. Acute upper gastrointestinal bleeding in over 16s: management. June 2012.

5. A. Hypophosphataemia

Hypothyroidism, uraemia, and primary hyperparathyroidism can all lead to the development of constipation.

Uraemia is the condition in which there are abnormally high concentrations of urea and nitrogenous substances in the blood as a result of kidney failure. Gastric and gastrointestinal motility is deranged in some patients with uraemia. Serum levels of several polypeptide hormones such as gastrin, cholecystokinin, and neurotensin are raised as a consequence of renal insufficiency subsequently having an effect on modulation of gastrointestinal motility. Several other abnormalities are also common in uraemia including hypercalcaemia, hypokalaemia, and acidosis. These have a direct effect on the smooth muscle of the gut contributing to dysmotility and constipation.

Panhypopituitarism is a condition of inadequate or absent production of all anterior pituitary gland hormones. These include Growth Hormone, the Gonadotropins including LH (luteinizing hormone) and FSH (follicle stimulating hormone), ACTH (adrenocorticotropic hormone) and TSH (thyroid stimulating hormone). Constipation is a common feature of panhypopituitarism.

Hypophosphataemia may be caused by diarrhoea, but the converse is not true. B to E can all cause constipation.

Peppas G, Alexiou V, Mourtzoukou E et al. Epidemiology of constipation in Europe and Oceania: a systematic review. BMC Gastroenterology 2008; 8: 5 (ISSN: 1471–230X).

6. B. Capsule endoscopy

Iron deficiency anaemia (IDA) is common in 2–5% of men and post-menopausal women in the developed world. Both upper and lower gastrointestinal (GI) cancer as well as malabsorption in coeliac disease are important causes that need to be excluded. Causes of IDA can be multifactorial and management is often suboptimal due to incomplete investigations. Concurrent pathology in both the upper and lower GI tract occur in 1–10% of all patients. Both upper and lower GI investigations should be considered in all post-menopausal female and all male patients. Patients should be tested for coeliac disease with serology screening which includes testing for total IgA and IgA tTG (tissue transgultaminase). If the IgA tTG is weakly positive, also test for IgA EMA (endomysial antibodies). Duodenal biopsies should be taken if IgA EMA or IgA tTG antibodies are positive and/ or if patients present with symptoms consistent with coeliac disease such as diarrhoea, fatigue, unexpected weight loss, abdominal pain and discomfort.

British Society of Gastroenterology guidance highlights that small bowel investigations should be considered if a cause of bleeding cannot be established on upper and lower investigation and there are symptoms suggestive of small bowel pathology. This includes if the haemoglobin cannot be maintained despite iron substitution and transfusion.

In summary, this patient presented with an IDA and history of recurrent GI blood loss. He has undergone both upper and lower GI investigations. IgA EMA and IgA tTG antibodies should be performed for completeness as duodenal pathology can be segmental and biopsies should be taken from both D1 (Duodenal bulb) and pars II duodeni.

Helicobacter pylori serology is negative. Helicobacter pylori colonization can contribute to impaired iron absorption and increased iron loss but this would not explain his history of haematemesis.

CT scan has the benefit of identifying extra luminal and extra intestinal pathology such as renal cell carcinoma and lymphomas but has very little sensitivity in identifying luminal/mucosal pathology which is often flat and small in the small bowel.

Capsule endoscopy of the small bowel is sensitive in identifying these lesions, which may account for this patient's symptoms of haematemesis and continuous anaemia despite transfusions and iron supplementation.

National Institute for Health and Care Excellence. NICE Guideline 20. Coeliac disease: recognition, assessment and management. September 2015.

7. A. Colonoscopy

Iron deficiency anaemia (IDA) is the most common cause for anaemia in the world. The most common cause of IDA in the UK is heavy menstrual bleeding. Haemoglobin (Hb) levels below the normal lower range for the laboratory performing the test should be used to define anaemia. The World Health Organization (WHO) defines anaemia as Hb concentration below 130 g/L in men, below 120 g/L in non-pregnant women, and below 110 g/L in pregnant women.

The NICE referral guidelines for suspected lower GI cancer suggest that only patients with Hb concentrations below 110 g/L in men and 100 g/L in women be referred. This is likely to miss patients with colorectal cancer and it is recommended that any level of anaemia should be investigated in the context of IDA.

The full blood count identifies a hypochromic (MCH <27 pg) and microcytic (MCV <80 fL) picture which is likely due to an IDA but can also be due to chronic disease, thalassaemia, or sideroblastic anaemia.

Serum ferritin (<30 µg/L) should always be used to confirm IDA. However, ferritin is an acute-phase protein, which may be elevated in the context of chronic inflammation. Levels >50 µg/L can still be consistent with IDA. Serum iron levels and total iron-binding capacity should be measured to confirm IDA. Increased serum transferrin receptor (sTfR) is believed to be a good marker for iron deficiency in healthy people. Several studies have shown that the Log sTfR to serum ferritin index provides a good discrimination to either test alone in the context of chronic disease. This has not been established in the clinical context due to limited availability of sTfR levels.

Bone marrow investigations can be used to assess iron deposits and give estimations of iron concentration by histochemical method. This may be useful to discriminate between iron deficiency and impaired iron release from the monocyte-macrophage system. Due to its invasive form of investigation it remains seldom performed in this context.

Concurrent pathology in both the upper and lower gastrointestinal (GI) tract occur in 1–10% of all patients. A result of this knowledge highlights the need that both upper and lower GI investigations are preformed.

Colonoscopy is usually the investigation of choice. It has advantages over radiological investigations as it allows visualization of mucosa and improved identification of lesions that are not seen on CT scans. These include flat lesions and superficial pathology such as angiodysplasia. A colonoscopy also enables biopsies to be taken to confirm diagnosis or offer definite treatment for adenomas that can be removed by endomucosal resection (EMR).

CT colonography is useful in the elderly patient who may struggle with the bowel preparation needed for colonoscopy and physiological stress related to the investigation. It is also used where colonoscopy is contraindicated. The sensitivity of CT colonography for lesions >10 mm in size is >90%. Smaller lesions and smaller flat mucosal pathology is readily overseen. CT colonography is not useful in post-operative situations where the ileocaecal valve has been removed due to the limitations to create double contrast of the bowel with barium and carbon dioxide. Barium enema is less reliable but useful when colonoscopy and CT colography are not available.

Goddard AF, James MW, McIntyre AS, Scott BB. Guidelines for the management of iron deficiency anaemia. On behalf of the British Society of Gastroenterology, 2011. Gut 2011;60:1309e1316. doi:10.1136/gut.2010.228874.

8. C. Platelet transfusion

When patients are admitted to hospital with upper gastrointestinal (GI) bleeding it is important to establish if they are suffering from a severe life-threatening bleed that requires activation of the hospital's massive transfusion policy. For bleeding of lesser severity the role of blood transfusion is less clear.

His coagulopathy identifies a borderline raised INR, a moderately raised aPTT, and fibrinogen levels within normal limits. His Hb and WBC are within acceptable levels in the context of an upper GI bleed but his platelet count is very low at 35×10^9/L.

Current evidence is limited but the consensus gained in the 2012 NICE Guideline on the management of upper GI bleeding developed pragmatic and sensible guidance to manage coagulopathy.

Fresh frozen plasma should be given when the fibrinogen levels are less than 1 g/L or if the aPTT is greater than 1.5 times the normal level. Both these criteria are not met in our case. Over correction of coagulopathy is not necessary and cost-intensive with no improvement in outcome.

Prothrombin complex concentrate (PCC) is not indicated in this patient, as he is not taking warfarin. The NICE guidance highlights PCC's use in the active bleeding patient who is taking warfarin.

Vitamin K can be given to reverse the effects of vitamin K deficiency brought about by the anticoagulant warfarin or in cases of biliary obstruction when vitamin K has not been effectively absorbed. Vitamin K-dependent clotting factors include prothrombin (factor II) factor VII, IX, and X as well as the protein C, S, and Z. Its effect on re-instituting coagulation is delayed and has no immediate effect in the actively bleeding patient.

Cryoprecipitate, also called 'Cryoprecipitated Antihaemophilic Factor' typically contains 100 IU of factor VIII, and 250 mg of fibrinogen. It also contains von-Willebrand factor (vWF) and factor XIII. It has its place in the management of haemophilia, von Willebrand's disease, and hypofibrinogenaemia in the context of life-threatening bleeds which have massive transfusion requirements.

NICE guidance does advise offering platelet transfusions to patients who are actively bleeding and have a platelet count of less than 50×10^9/L.

National Institute for Health and Care Excellence. Clinical Guideline 141. Acute upper gastrointestinal bleeding in over 16s: management. June 2012.

9. C. No acid suppressant therapy

Latest NICE guidance advises that all patients admitted with upper gastrointestinal (GI) bleeding have a pre-endoscopy Blatchford score and a post-endoscopy Rockall score calculated. Our 82-year-old patient is clinically stable with a stable blood pressure, heart rate of 90, and a respiratory rate of 20. Her abbreviated Early Warning Score (EWS) is not relevantly raised accepting her low oxygen saturation in the context of COPD. Her pre-endoscopy Rockall score is 4/7 and calculates her predicted mortality at 24.6% based on her age and co-morbidities.

Acid-suppressing drugs have been studied in multiple clinical trials of peptic ulcer bleeding. The rationale behind the use of acid-suppressing agents is that a pH >6.5 stabilizes the blood clot that plugs the bleeding defect and could lead to a reduced risk of continuing bleeding, re-bleeding, need for blood transfusions, and overall mortality. Although proton pump inhibitors (PPIs) and H_2-receptor antagonists can achieve a sustained rise of pH in the gastric cavity when used, the results of these trials have not confirmed the benefits of their use in a heterogeneous population of 'upper GI bleeders'.

Offering all patients pre-endoscopy acid-suppressive treatment is unnecessary and wasteful since approximately 80% of ulcers stop bleeding without any form of intervention. Offering acid-suppressive treatment pre-endoscopy may well contribute to a reduced incidence of major stigmata but this did not translate into a clinical benefit such as a reduced mortality rate.

Clinical benefit of PPI treatment was shown to be effective in those patients who underwent endoscopy that showed evidence of current or recent non-variceal bleeding.

On the basis of the available evidence, the NICE guidance does not advise the use of acid-suppressive agents pre-endoscopy but did endorse its use in those patients identified on endoscopy who had evidence of current or recent bleeding. There is evidence that their use results in improved outcome, and reduction in length of stay.

National Institute for Health and Care Excellence. Clinical Guideline 141. Acute upper gastrointestinal bleeding in over 16s: management. June 2012.

10. A. Continue aspirin

Sung et al. (2010) in a randomized controlled trial (RCT) compared the outcomes of patients with known cardiovascular disease and endoscopic-confirmed peptic ulcers showing signs of active bleeding, adherent clot, or visible vessel on the base of an ulcer. They were either randomized to continue or discontinue their aspirin for established cardiovascular or cerebrovascular disease once haemostasis with endoscopic therapy was achieved. Mortality rates were significantly lower in those patients who continued their aspirin therapy. Although bleeding rates were higher in those who continued aspirin, this did not reach statistical significance.

There is currently no evidence available regarding the continued use of clopidogrel (or any other thienopyridine antiplatelet agents) in the context of an acute upper gastrointestinal bleed. NICE guidance advises that the risks and benefits are discussed with the appropriate specialist and patient regarding its continued use. No general consensus is available and each patient needs to be considered individually depending on co-morbidities and risks.

Sung JJ, Lau JY, Ching JY et al. Recommencing continuation of low-dose aspirin therapy in peptic ulcer bleeding: a randomized trial. Annals of Internal Medicine 2010; 152: 1–9.

11. E. Urea

Latest NICE guidance advises that all patients admitted with upper gastrointestinal (GI) bleeding have a pre-endoscopy Blatchford score (Table 2.1) and a post-endoscopy Rockall score calculated.

Table 2.1 The Blatchford bleeding score.

Blood Urea (mmol/L)	6.5–7.9 mmol/L	2
	8.0–9.9 mmol/L	3
	10.0–25.0 mmol/L	4
	>25 mmol/L	5
Haemoglobin	120–129 g/L	1
- men (g/L)	100–119 g/L	3
	<100 g/L	6
Haemoglobin	100–109 g/L	1
- women (g/L)	<100 g/L	6
Systolic BP (mmHg)	100–109 mmHg	1
	90–99 mmHg	2
	<90 mmHg	3
Other markers	Pulse >100/min	1
	Presentation with melaena	1
	Presentation with syncope	2
	Hepatic disease	2
	Cardiac disease	2

Reprinted from *The Lancet*, 356, Blatchford W et al., 'A risk score to predict need for treatment for uppergastrointestinal haemorrhage', pp.1318–1321, Copyright (2000), with permission from Elsevier

GASTROENTEROLOGY | ANSWERS

The Blatchford score is based on simple clinical and laboratory variables. Its advantage over the Rockall score, which assesses the risk of mortality in patients with upper gastrointestinal bleeding, is that it does not require a subjective evaluation of variables such as the severity of systemic disease nor an endoscopy to have been preformed to complete it.

Blood urea, haemoglobin, systolic blood pressure, and pulse rate are calculated and allocated points depending on results. History or clinical evidence of chronic or acute liver or heart failure contributes to the overall score. This does not require a subjective assessment of the severity of disease such as the Rockall score requires.

Blatchford O, Murray WR, Blatchford M. A risk score to predict need for treatment for upper-gastrointestinal haemorrhage. Lancet 2000 14 Oct; 356(9238): 1318–1321.

12. A. The Blatchford score assists in the clinical management of patients presenting with gastrointestinal haemorrhage

The Blatchford score predicts the need for endoscopic intervention or likely mortality. Low scores are associated with low mortality rates and help identify those patients *who may* be suitable for outpatient management.

It does not replace good clinical judgement and is only used to assist clinicians to decide who is safe to be considered for discharge. There are multiple other criteria that need to be considered if a patient is safe to be discharged.

Blatchford O, Murray WR, Blatchford M. A risk score to predict need for treatment for upper-gastrointestinal haemorrhage. Lancet 2000 14 Oct; 356(9238): 1318–1321.

13. E. No further investigations

Irritable bowel syndrome is very common, the hallmark features being chronic abdominal pain and altered bowel habit, without structural bowel disease. It is not associated with the development of any bowel pathology or increased mortality. Different diagnostic criteria exist, centring around the presence of relapsing abdominal pain or discomfort which is relieved by defecation or its onset is associated with a change in stool consistency or frequency. Patients have often had symptoms for more than six months, and report that stress makes symptoms worse. Symptoms are often aggravated by food. Further investigation beyond a thorough history and examination, and basic blood tests including full blood count, ESR, CRP, and a coeliac screen, is not needed unless there are any alarm features. These include rectal bleeding, unintentional weight loss, a family history of bowel or ovarian cancer, a change to more frequent or looser stools for more than six weeks in patients aged more than 60 years, anaemia, an abdominal or rectal mass, or raised inflammatory markers.

Spiller R, Aziz Q, Creed F et al. British Society of Gastroenterology. Guidelines on the irritable bowel syndrome: mechanisms and practical management. Gut 2007; 56: 1770–1798. doi: 10.1136/gut.2007.119446.

National Institute for Health and Care Excellence. Clinical Guideline 61. Irritable bowel syndrome in adults: diagnosis and management. February 2008. (updated February 2015).

14. B. A trace of free fluid in the pouch of Douglas can be seen in normal women

Focused assessment with sonography in trauma (FAST scanning) can also be very useful in non-trauma situations. It is not the same as full diagnostic ultrasonography, and seeks to answer a single question—i.e. is there free fluid in the abdomen (or is the aorta dilated)?—rather than looking for a diagnosis. Any free fluid in the abdomen in a trauma situation is assumed to be blood; you cannot tell the difference between blood and ascites. The abdominal aorta is abnormally dilated if the diameter is more than 3 cm (the whole of the abdominal aorta must be imaged). The aorta is retroperitoneal so you don't see free intraperitoneal fluid when it ruptures; ultrasound is not accurate in determining the presence of leak from an abdominal aortic aneurysm (AAA). If the aorta is dilated in an unstable patient, the patient is assumed to have a ruptured aneurysm and should go straight to theatre. If the patient is stable and a ruptured AAA is suspected, the patient can go to CT for assessment. A trace of free fluid in the pouch of Douglas in women can be normal, especially around ovulation. Practitioners should be appropriately trained and assessed and continue to practise appropriately to maintain competence in bedside ultrasonography.

Royal College of Emergency Medicine. Core (level 1) Ultrasound Training curriculum, 2013. http://www.rcem.ac.uk

15. B. Discharge home for outpatient endoscopy

This patient is stable so does not need hospital admission. He does, however, need an endoscopy to investigate the cause for his upper GI bleeding. A Glasgow Blatchford score of 0 is highly sensitive in predicting no death or re-bleeding, making it appropriate to use to enable outpatient management, as long as no other features warrant admission.

National Institute for Health and Care Excellence. Clinical Guideline 141. Acute upper gastrointestinal bleeding in over 16s: management. June 2012.

16. C. Endoscopic Retrograde Cholangiopancreatography (ERCP)

The likely diagnosis is common bile duct stones (CBDS). In patients with suspected CBDS, initial investigations should be liver function tests and transabdominal ultrasound. However, ultrasound is not very sensitive for ductal stones. Endoscopic ultrasound and MRCP are more sensitive in confirming the presence of CBDS, and further investigation should be based on likelihood of CBDS. In over 55-year-olds, with a bilirubin more than 30 μmol/L, and a dilated common bile duct on ultrasound, as in this case, the likelihood of CBDS is 72%; therefore, ERCP is recommended and further investigation with MRCP is not required. When patients have symptoms and investigations suspect ductal stones, extraction should be performed if possible. Unnecessary biliary instrumentation should be avoided as there are risks involved (pancreatitis, haemorrhage, cholangitis, perforation).

Williams E, Green J, Beckingham I et al. British Society of Gastroenterology. Guidelines on the management of common bile duct stones (CBDS). Gut 2008; 57: 1004–1021. doi:10.1136/gut.2007.121657

17. D. The Health Protection Team should be notified

Campylobacter is the most common cause of food poisoning in the UK. Undercooked meat (often poultry), unpasteurized milk, and untreated water are common causes. It is a gram-positive organism, the incubation period is 1–11 days (usually 2–5 days), and it is contagious. It is a notifiable disease.

Public Health England. https://www.gov.uk/government/collections/campylobacter-guidance-data-and-analysis

18. C. Flexible sigmoidoscopy

Infective causes for his diarrhoea have been excluded, and the symptoms are ongoing, so further investigation is warranted to investigate for inflammatory bowel disease. Colonoscopy with multiple biopsies is the first-line procedure in diagnosing colitis and allows classification of disease, but in acute severe colitis, as in this case, it is rarely needed and may be contraindicated due to the risk of perforation. Flexible sigmoidoscopy is considered safe (except if there is colonic dilatation) and allows direct visualization and biopsies, so is preferred to non-invasive investigations if it can be tolerated. Further imaging and endoscopy may be needed depending on the results.

Mowat C, Cole A, Windsor A et al. British Society of Gastroenterology. Guidelines for the management of inflammatory bowel disease in adults. Gut 2011. doi:10.1136/gut.2010.224154.

19. A. pH

Acute liver failure (ALF) is defined as the acute onset of liver failure with symptoms of encephalopathy which has developed rapidly. Lactic acid is predominantly metabolized in the liver. Lactic acidosis can occur due to severely impaired hepatic metabolism of lactate or excessive tissue lactate production. Lactic acidosis predominantly occurs in paracetamol overdose and reflects deteriorating metabolic liver function.

The King's College hospital liver transplant criteria for paracetamol-induced liver failure are as follows:
- pH <7.3

or all of:
- grade III/IV encephalopathy
- creatinine >300 µmol/L
- prothrombin time >100 s (INR >6.5)

For non-paracetamol acute liver failure transplant criteria are:
- prothrombin time >100 s

Or any three of:
- Age <10 years or >40 years
- prothrombin time >50 s
- bilirubin >300 µmol/L
- Time from jaundice to encephalopathy >two days
- NonA, nonB hepatitis, halothane, or drug-induced acute liver failure

Reproduced from Gut, 45, O'Grady, J et al., 'Indications for referral and assessment in adult liver transplantation: a clinical guideline', copyright (1999) with permission from BMJ Publishing Group Ltd.

Discussion with a liver unit should occur before these criteria are met ideally, so transfer can be arranged safely if appropriate.

Devlin J, O'Grady J. British Society of gastroenterology. Indications for referral and assessment in adult liver transplantation: a clinical guideline. Gut 2000; 45: VI1–VI22.

Sleisenger & Fordtran's gastrointestinal and liver disease pathophysiology, diagnosis, management. Sleisenger, edited by Mark Feldman, Lawrence S Friedman, Lawrence J Brandt; consulting editor, Marvin H (2009) (9th edn ed.). St. Louis.

20. B. Alcoholic cardiomyopathy is a major determinant of outcome

The majority of liver transplants are done for chronic liver disease, not acute presentations. In alcoholic liver disease abstinence is mandatory, as a period of abstinence may allow the liver to recover to a sufficient degree so that transplant is no longer needed. The period of abstinence required is controversial, but any improvement in liver function is seen within three months of abstinence; therefore, three months is the recommendation from NICE. Age is not a barrier to transplant, and physiological age is more important than chronological age. One-year survival is around 90%. Adequate cardiac output is a major determinant of early transplant outcome, so alcoholic cardiomyopathy should be looked for. However, alcoholic cardiomyopathy usually improves with abstinence, and is not a contraindication to transplant. Patients with decompensated liver disease should be referred for consideration of transplant if they still have decompensated liver disease after best management and a period of three months of abstinence, and they are otherwise suitable for a transplant.

Devlin J, O'Grady J. British Society of Gastroenterology. Indications for referral and assessment in adult liver transplantation: a clinical guideline. Gut 2000; 45: VI1–VI22.

National Institute for Health and Care Excellence. Clinical Guideline 100. Alcohol use disorders: diagnosis and management of complications. June 2010.

21. C. Liver biopsy

This patient has primary biliary cirrhosis (PBC). PBC is most commonly diagnosed in middle-aged women. Anti-mitochondrial antibodies are the hallmark of the disease. Staging is based on histology: in stage 1 there is portal inflammation, bile duct abnormalities, or both; in stage 2 there is periportal fibrosis; stage 3 shows septal fibrosis; and stage 4 is cirrhosis.

Treatment aims to slow the progression of the disease, with ursodeoxycholic acid and immunosuppressants, but liver transplantation is the only life-saving procedure.

Drebber U, Mueller J, Klein E et al. Liver biopsy in primary biliary cirrhosis: clinicopathological data and stage. Pathol Int. August 2009; 59(8): 546–554.

22. E. Steroids

This patient has alcoholic hepatitis. Patients with acute severe alcoholic hepatitis are at risk of death, mortality is greater than 35% at 30 days.

Maddrey's discriminant function is a scoring system to predict prognosis and is used to decide if a patient is suitable for treatment with corticosteroids. The formula to calculate the discriminant function is:

$$4.6 \times [PT - \text{control PT (seconds)}] + \text{bilirubin (mg/dL)}$$

To calculate the DF using bilirubin in micromol/L, divide the bilirubin value by 17.

Data from *Gastroenterology*, Maddrey WC et al., 'Corticosteroid therapy of alcoholic hepatitis', 1978, 75.2, pp. 193–199.

A discriminant function of more than 32 indicates severe disease; in this case steroid therapy should be considered. Trial results for using corticosteroids in alcoholic hepatitis have been inconsistent, most showing improved short- and long-term survival, but some showing increased rates of gastrointestinal bleeding and infection. One problem with the current evidence is differing inclusion and exclusion criteria in the different studies. Other treatments such as pentoxyphylline have some evidence base in small trials but the recent STOPAH (steroids and pentoxyphylline for alcoholic hepatitis) trial showed no mortality benefit with pentoxyphylline, and only a small 28-day mortality benefit with prednisolone that did not reach statistical significance. There was no improvement in outcomes at 90 days or one year. The steroid group had higher rates of infection.

National Institute for Health and Care Excellence. Clinical Guideline 100. Alcohol use disorders: diagnosis and management of physical complications. June 2010.

Forrest E, Mellor J, Stanton L et al. Steroids or pentoxifylline for alcoholic hepatitis (STOPAH): study protocol for a randomised controlled trial. Trials 2013; 14: 262.

Thursz MR, Richardcon P, Allison M et al. Prednisolone or Pentoxyphylline for alcoholic hepatitis. NEJM 2015; 372:1619–28. DOI 10.1056/NEJMoa1412278.

23. D. Steroids

This patient has decompensated alcoholic liver disease with hepatorenal syndrome (HRS). HRS occurs in patients with cirrhosis and portal hypertension, and can only be diagnosed in the absence of other causes of renal failure (shock, infection, nephrotoxins, obstruction) and after no improvement in renal function after at least 1.5 L intravenous volume replacement—usually 0.9% sodium chloride. HRS is a life-threatening complication of advanced liver failure which results from renal dysfunction related to changes of circulation related to increasing liver dysfunction/failure. It is subdivided into two types; type 1 HRS is rapid, with a doubling of serum creatinine over two weeks or less, and is associated with a mortality of 50% at one month. Type 2 HRS is slower, associated with diuretic resistant ascites, and has a median survival of six months without transplant.

Large-volume ascitic drainage without albumin cover can precipitate HRS; however, in the presence of tense ascites, this could be obstructing the renal tract and should be drained with appropriate albumin replacement to prevent fluid shifts. Spontaneous bacterial peritonitis should always be excluded via an ascitic tap and is a common precipitant for type 1 HRS.

Treatment with terlipressin for vasoconstriction (as the initial event in HRS is vasodilatation of the splanchnic circulation) and intravenous albumin for volume replacement has resulted in improved outcomes and is therefore recommended. Transjuglular intrahepatic portosystemic shunting (TIPPS) can be considered for patients with type 2 HRS and refractory ascites. Transplant should be considered if appropriate.

There is no evidence of severe alcoholic hepatitis in this case so there is no role for steroids.

Nadim M, Kellum J, Davenport A et al. Hepatorenal syndrome: the 8th international consensus conference of the Acute Dialysis Quality Initiative (ADQI) Group. Crit Care. 2012; 16(1): R23.

24. D. Intravenous fluids and surgical exploration

The transition point is the area where bowel loops change in calibre from normal to dilated, and indicates the area of obstruction. An obstructing lesion, e.g. a hernia or tumour, is often seen on CT. The most likely cause of obstruction in this patient is adhesions from his previous abdominal surgery. A surgical opinion should be sought for this patient. The presence of free fluid in the abdomen may indicate vascular compromise of the obstructed bowel and surgery will be needed. If there is no transition point and the obstruction is thought to be due to paralytic ileus, a traditional 'drip and suck' approach can be used, with careful monitoring and correction of electrolytes.

Wilson M, Ellis H, Menzies D et al. A review of the management of small bowel obstruction. Members of the Surgical and Clinical Adhesions Research Study (SCAR). Annals of the Royal College of Surgeons of England 1999; 81(5): 320–328.

25. D. Faecal calprotectin

The differential diagnosis here is between irritable bowel syndrome, a very common, benign, condition; and inflammatory bowel disease, a much more serious but less common diagnosis requiring appropriate treatment and follow-up. The presence of a slightly raised CRP in the context of no infection raises the possibility that this is more than simple irritable bowel syndrome. However, you wouldn't want to subject this patient to invasive endoscopic tests with the associated risks given the low chance of significant disease. Faecal caloprotectin is detected in bowel inflammation and is a non-invasive, simple test which has been approved by NICE as an option to distinguish between inflammatory and non-inflammatory bowel conditions when cancer is not suspected.

National Institute for Health and Care Excellence. Diagnostics Guidance 11. Faecal calprotectin diagnostic tests for inflammatory diseases of the bowel. October 2013.

26. B. Offer full course of proton pump inhibitor treatment for 4 weeks

Dyspepsia is very common. Red flag signs and symptoms should be ruled out, including: chronic gastrointestinal bleeding, progressive unintentional weight loss, progressive difficulty swallowing, persistent vomiting, iron deficiency anaemia, or an epigastric mass. Drugs which may cause dyspepsia should be reviewed and lifestyle advice given. If there are no alarm symptoms then a therapeutic trial with regular standard dose proton pump inhibitor for one month should be offered. Helicobacter pylori testing should be considered. Leave a 2-week washout period after proton pump inhibitor (PPI) use before testing for Helicobacter pylori with a breath test or a stool antigen test. In patients aged over 55 with unexplained and persistent dyspepsia, an urgent referral for endoscopy should be made.

National Institute for Health and Care Excellence. Clinical Guideline 17. Gastro-oesophageal reflux disease and dyspepsia in adults: investigation and management. September 2014.

27. B. Intravenous hydrocortisone

This is an acute flare of her ulcerative colitis. Truelove and Witts defined criteria for acute colitis requiring steroids in 1955 and they are still useful today. To fulfil the criteria the patient must be passing at least six stools per day, plus have one of:

- Erythrocyte Sedimentation Rate >30 mm/hr
- Haemoglobin <105 g/L
- Pulse rate >90 beats per minute
- Temperature >37.5°C.

Data from BMJ, Truelove SC and Witts LI, 'Cortisone in ulcerative colitis; preliminary report on a therapeutic trial', 1954, 2, 4884, pp. 375–378.

Steroids in this group have dramatically reduced mortality from more than 50% to 1–2%. However, 30% will have an incomplete response to steroids, and 40% will require a colectomy within 12 months. Patients need to be carefully monitored and their response to steroids assessed on day three. If they are not responding appropriately, other therapies—for example, infliximab, ciclosporin, or surgical intervention—need to be considered. These patients are at high risk for requiring a colectomy. Delayed surgery for patients who do not respond to medical therapy is associated with worse post-operative outcomes.

Truelove SC, Witts LJ. Cortisone in ulcerative colitis: final report on a therapeutic trial. BMJ 1955; ii: 1041–1048.

Carter M, Lobo A, Travis I. Guidelines for the management of inflammatory bowel disease in adults. Gut 2004; 53: v1–v16.

28. A. Continuous positive airways pressure

This is acute, severe pancreatitis. Many severity scoring systems exist, including variables such as increasing age, white cell count, low partial pressure of oxygen, low calcium, high urea, low albumin, high LDH and AST, and high glucose. In severe disease, mortality is up to 30%, secondary to multi-organ failure. Treatment is supportive, based on cardiovascular and respiratory support and nutrition.

This patient needs to be managed on an intensive care unit; she needs respiratory support which can be continuous positive airways pressure initially, but she may need invasive ventilation.

She will need a CT of the pancreas to assess for pancreatic necrosis, but this does not need to be immediate and she needs to be stable enough to go to the CT scanner.

Antibiotics are only needed if infection is present.

Albumin and intravenous vitamin B + C are not standard treatments but may be used in certain circumstances.

Gallstones and alcohol are major causes of pancreatitis; other causes include drugs, ERCP, and infections.

United Kingdom guidelines for the management of acute pancreatitis. Prepared by a Working Party of the British Society of Gastroenterology, Association of Surgeons of Great Britain and Ireland, Pancreatic Society of Great Britain and Ireland, and Association of Upper GI Surgeons of Great Britain and Ireland. Gut 2005;54(Suppl III):iii1–iii9. doi: 10.1136/gut.2004.057026.

29. B. Chest X-ray

This patient has a systemic inflammatory response. Because of her history and recent endoscopy, the most likely cause is oesophageal rupture. A chest X-ray would be the most likely investigation to give you the diagnosis as you could see a widened mediastinum, pneumomediastinum, pneumopericardum, subcutaneous emphysema, and pleural effusions. The other investigations listed may be performed but are unlikely to give you a diagnosis. If needed, she could proceed to CT. She is likely to need surgical correction.

Costamagna G, Michele Marchese M. Management of esophageal perforation after therapeutic endoscopy. Gastroenterol Hepatol (NY) 2010; 6(6): 391–392.

Green J. Complications of Gastrointestinal Endoscopy. British Society of Gastroenterology Guidelines in endoscopy. 2006.

30. D. Food containing less than 20 parts per million of gluten can be labelled as gluten-free

Coeliac disease is an inflammatory condition of the small bowel, characterized by villous atrophy and intra-epithelial lymphocytosis caused by an immunological response to proteins found in wheat, barley, and rye (collectively termed gluten for simplicity, although gluten is strictly the protein found in wheat).

Food containing less than 20 parts per million of gluten can be labelled as gluten-free.

Antibodies to tissue transglutaminase are found in patients with coeliac disease who are consuming gluten but will become negative on a gluten-free diet. Similarly, duodenal villous atrophy and intra-epithelial inflammation commonly found in coeliac disease improves on a gluten-free diet.

Oats remain controversial in coeliac disease; they are taxonomically different from wheat, barley, and rye and do not contain the same proteins, yet some people with coeliac disease get symptoms and signs of disease after consuming oats. This may be largely due to contamination with wheat (either in the field or in processing). The recommendation is that oats labelled as gluten-free are safe to consume, but excluding oats all together for the first 6–12 months after diagnosis is pragmatic to enable patients to settle on gluten-free diets without any possible symptoms from oats.

Approximately 95% of patients with coeliac disease express HLA-DQ2; the remainder express DQ8.

People with coeliac disease are at higher risk for osteoporosis, but bone mineral density significantly increases on a gluten-free diet. DEXA scanning should be offered in those patients where concerns have been raised during an annual review. Everyone with coeliac disease should be advised to consume 1500 mg calcium per day. Only those with relevant oesteopenia/osteoperosis diagnosed on DEXA scan or those who have acquired a fracture should be offered bisphosphonates.

Ciclitira P, Dewar D, McLaughlin S et al. British Society of Gastroenterology. The Management of Adults with Coeliac Disease. 2010.

National Institute for Health and Care Excellence. Coeliac disease: recognition, assessment and management. NICE Guideline 20. September 2015.

31. B. He should be prescribed prophylactic dose low molecular weight heparin

Patients with inflammatory bowel disease are at high risk of venous thromboembolism (VTE) and should be prescribed appropriate chemical prophylaxis. There is no need for treatment doses unless VTE is suspected. The small amount of bleeding per rectum is not a contraindication to low molecular weight heparin, but should be closely monitored.

National Institute for Health and Care Excellence. Clinical Guideline 92. Venous thromboembolism: reducing the risk for patients in hospital. January 2010.

32. B. Colonoscopy

This patient has suspected colorectal malignancy and flexible sigmoidoscopy is not enough to rule this out as half of his colon has not been visualized. NICE guidelines recommend colonoscopy as the first line for patients with suspected colorectal malignancy without significant comorbidities. For patients with significant comorbidities who would not tolerate colonoscopy, investigation should be either CT colonography or flexible sigmoidoscopy then barium enema.

National Institute for Health and Care Excellence. Clinical Guideline 131. Colorectal cancer: diagnosis and management. November 2011 (updated December 2014).

33. A. She should be allowed home with symptomatic management

This patient has end-stage malignancy and should have regular contact with the palliative care team to help to manage her symptoms and plan for what she wants as her cancer progresses.

Further endoscopies are unlikely to benefit her, and the benefits and risks of each intervention should be discussed with her. She doesn't have symptomatic anaemia so a blood transfusion would not benefit her. If she is eating and drinking then the stent is not blocked and doesn't need assessment with a barium swallow. The oncology team should be involved if radiotherapy is considered, and will advise if further treatment would be advantageous. Palliative radiotherapy may be considered if bleeding is a predominant feature of the patient's presentation. Small amounts of coffee-ground vomit do not justify such an invasive approach, i.e. palliative radiotherapy.

Allum W, Blazeby J, Griffin S et al. Guidelines for the management of oesophageal and gastric cancer. Gut 2011; 60: 1449–1472. doi:10.1136/gut.2010.228254.

34. C. Colonoscopy every three years

Colonoscopic surveillance should be offered to people with inflammatory bowel disease whose symptoms started ten years ago and who have ulcerative colitis (but not proctitis alone) or Crohn's disease involving more than one section of the colon.

Patients can be divided into low, intermediate, or high risk of developing colorectal cancer.

Low risk: extensive but quiescent ulcerative colitis (UC) or Crohn's, or left-sided UC or Crohn's of a similar extent.

Intermediate risk: extensive UC or Crohn's with mild active inflammation that has been confirmed endoscopically or histologically; or post inflammatory polyps; or family history of colorectal cancer in a first-degree relative aged over 50 years.

High risk: extensive UC or Crohn's with moderate or severe inflammation that has been confirmed histologically or endoscopically; or primary sclerosing cholangitis; or colonic stricture in the last five years; or any grade of dysplasia in the last five years; or family history of colorectal cancer in a first-degree relative under 50 years.

Patients at low risk should have a surveillance colonoscopy every five years, those at intermediate risk every three years, and those at high risk every year.

National Institute for Health and Care Excellence. Clinical Guideline 118. Colonoscopic surveillance for prevention of colorectal cancer in people with ulcerative colitis, Crohn's disease or adenomas. March 2011.

35. E. Parenteral vitamins B + C (Pabrinex®) two pairs three times daily

This patient has features which suggest Wernicke's encephalopathy. The classic triad of confusion, ataxia, and ophthalmoplegia is rarely seen, but Wernicke's is very common and should be treated aggressively to prevent progression to Korsakoff's psychosis.

The treatment dose of thiamine for Wernicke's is two pairs (four ampoules) of high-potency B complex vitamins (pabrinex®) three times daily for five days. Patients who are at risk of Wernicke's but not showing signs or symptoms should be prescribed intravenous B complex vitamins one pair once a day (od) for three to five days. Patients at risk include harmful or dependent drinkers who are malnourished, have decompensated liver disease, or are in acute alcohol withdrawal. For those patients who are admitted to hospital (whether alcohol related or not), they should be given intravenous thiamine followed by oral thiamine. For those patients in the community, they should be given oral thiamine.

National Institute for Health and Care Excellence. Clinical Guideline 100. Alcohol use disorders: diagnosis and management of physical complications. June 2010.

36. C. Lorazepam

The most likely cause for his seizures is alcohol withdrawal. Assessment using the ABCD approach is necessary to ensure patient safety. The management of his seizures should be with intravenous short-acting benzodiazepines such as lorazepam. He will not tolerate oral medication such as chlordiazepoxide while fitting. Haloperidol can be used for delirium tremens but is not a treatment for alcohol withdrawal seizures. Phenytoin should be avoided in alcohol withdrawal seizures as it was shown to be no more effective than placebo at preventing recurrent seizures.

If a patient fits while undertaking an alcohol withdrawal regime, their regime needs to be assessed, as it is likely that they have been under-dosed.

National Institute for Health and Care Excellence. Clinical Guideline 100. Alcohol use disorders: diagnosis and management of physical complications. June 2010.

37. E. Hypophosphataemia

The risks here are of re-feeding syndrome. Re-feeding syndrome is caused by rapid fluid and electrolyte shifts in malnourished patients who receive an increased calorific intake, and patients with anorexia nervosa are at risk. The hallmark feature is hypophosphataemia, but magnesium, potassium, calcium, and glucose can also be deranged. With the sudden introduction of food into a long-term catabolic state, serum glucose rises and insulin secretion stimulates the cellular uptake of phosphate, magnesium, calcium, and potassium, so plasma levels fall. Hypophosphataemia can be particularly rapid and can induce arrhythmias, sudden death, heart failure, seizures, renal failure, marrow suppression, and delirium.

To reduce the risk of re-feeding syndrome, nasogastric feeding should be started slowly, initially 5–10 mL/hr of I kCal/mL feed, and electrolytes monitored and replaced daily.

National Institute for Health and Care Excellence. Clinical Guideline 32. Nutrition support for adults: oral nutrition support, enteral tube feeding and parenteral nutrition. February 2006.

38. E. Oral vancomycin 125 mg four times daily

This is severe clostridium difficile infection (CDI). Severity features include: white cell count >15 × 10^9/L, acutely rising creatinine to >50% of baseline, temperature >38.5°C, or radiological or clinical evidence of severe colitis.

In patients with severe CDI, oral vancomycin 125 mg qds for 10–14 days is preferred to metronidazole as it is superior. Oral fidoximicin (200 mg bd) should be considered in patients with a high risk of recurrence, including elderly patients with multiple comorbidities on concomitant antibiotics, or if there is no response to vancomycin. An alternative, if there is no response to vancomycin, is to increase the dose to 500 mg qds and add intravenous metronidazole. Oral rifampicin or intravenous immunoglobulin may be tried but there is no robust data to support these strategies. Colectomy should be considered, especially if the caecal dilatation is greater than 10 cm. If serum lactate is more than 5 mmol/L before colectomy is performed, survival is very poor.

Oral metronidazole is used in mild to moderate cases.

Intravenous vancomycin is not effective.

Relapse of CDI occurs in 10–25% of patients treated with metronidazole or vancomycin. Recent case series have shown faecal microbiota transplantation (FMT) or faecal donor instillation therapy (FDIT) to be successful in 81–94% of patients who suffer from repeated relapses.

Brandt L, Aroniadis O, Mellow M et al. Long-term follow-up for colonoscopic faecal microbiota transplant for recurrent Clostridium difficile infection. American Journal of Gastroenterology 2012; 107(7): 1079.

Public Health England. Clostridium difficile: guidance, data and analysis. July 2014.

39. C. Macrogol

Macrogol has an osmotic effect. Docusate sodium is a softener and stimulant. Ispaghula husk has a bulking effect. Senna is a stimulant and sodium picosulphate is a softener and stimulant.

A multifaceted approach may be needed depending on the cause of the constipation.

Peppas G, Alexiou V, Mourtzoukou E et al. Epidemiology of constipation in Europe and Oceania: a systematic review. BMC Gastroenterology 2008; 8: 5 (ISSN: 1471–230X).

40. D. Oesphagectomy

All patients with a new diagnosis of cancer should be referred to the relevant multidisciplinary team for staging and treatment planning. Oesophagectomy (open or minimally invasive) is a curative treatment option for appropriate patients.

Stage 1 disease (confined to the lamina propria, submucosa, or muscularis propria) is usually amenable to endoscopic therapy. Stage 2–3 disease is usually considered for chemoradiation then surgery, and stage 4 disease (metastatic) is normally treated by chemotherapy or supportive and palliative care.

Stage 2a is still confined to the oesophagus (T3 N0 M0) and is amenable to surgery.

Allum W, Blazeby J, Griffin S et al. Guidelines for the management of oesophageal and gastric cancer. Gut 2011; 60: 1449–1472. doi:10.1136/gut.2010.228254.

chapter 3

RESPIRATORY

QUESTIONS

1. A 28-year-old male bartender presented to the acute medical unit with pleuritic chest pain and breathlessness, which came on at rest. He had no significant past medical history. He had a 14-pack year smoking history, and continued to smoke. He took no recreational drugs and was taking no medication. He consumed 20 units of alcohol per week.

   His temperature, pulse, and blood pressure were all normal. His respiratory rate was 22 breaths per minute and oxygen saturation 95% on air. Clinical examination demonstrated decreased breath sounds over the right side of his chest.

   Investigations:

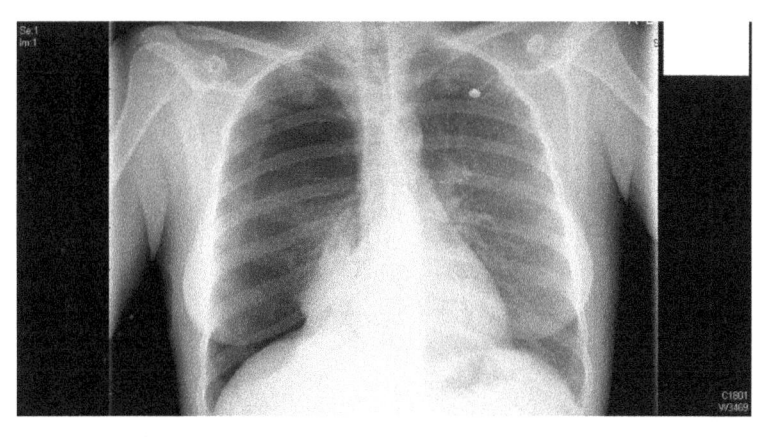

   Figure 3.1 Chest X-ray.

   What is the most appropriate management?
   A. Aspiration via an 18 G cannula in the safe triangle
   B. Aspiration via an 18 G cannula in the 2nd intercostal space, mid-clavicular line
   C. Conservative management with high flow oxygen and observation
   D. Insertion of a 14 F drain into the safe triangle
   E. Insertion of a 28 F drain into the safe triangle

2. A 28-year-old woman presented to the acute medical unit with pleuritic chest pain and breathlessness, which came on at rest. She had a history of menorrhagia. She had a ten-pack year smoking history, and continued to smoke. She smoked cannabis occasionally as a recreational drug and was taking the combined oral contraceptive pill. She consumed 16 units of alcohol per week.

Her temperature, pulse, and blood pressure were all normal. Her respiratory rate was 24 breaths per minute and oxygen saturation 96% on air. Clinical examination demonstrated decreased breath sounds over the right side of her chest.

Chest X-ray showed a moderate right pneumothorax.

What is the most appropriate follow-up advice?

A. Air travel can normally be undertaken on discharge if a small pneumothorax remains on chest X-ray
B. SCUBA diving may be undertaken after three months
C. Smoking is associated with an increased incidence of pneumothorax in men compared with women
D. There is good evidence that contact sports should be avoided for three months
E. Waiting at least three months after full resolution before flying is recommended

3. **A 62-year-old man presented to the acute medical unit with a three-day history of mild breathlessness on exertion, occasional right-sided chest pain, and sweats. He looked well and was not breathless at rest. He had no significant past medical history. His temperature was 37.7°C. He had a few crackles at the right base, dullness to percussion, and decreased vocal resonance at the right base.**

   Investigations:

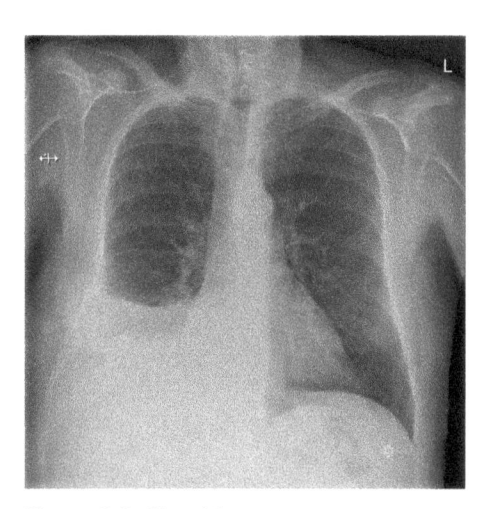

   Figure 3.2 Chest X-ray.

haemoglobin	140 g/L	(130–180)
white cell count	18 × 10⁹/L	(4.0–11.0)
serum sodium	135 mmol/L	(137–144)
serum potassium	3.6 mmol/L	(3.5–4.9)
serum urea	5.3 mmol/L	(2.5–7.0)
serum creatinine	100 µmol/L	(60–110)
serum C-reactive protein	30 mg/L	(<10)
serum total protein	70 g/L	(61–76)
serum albumin	32 g/L	(37–49)
serum total bilirubin	20 µmol/L	(1–22)
serum alanine aminotransferase	30 U/L	(5–35)
serum alkaline phosphatase	50 U/L	(45–105)
serum troponin T	9 mg/L	(<14)

   What is the next step in management?
   A. CT scan of chest with contrast timed for pleural enhancement
   B. Diuretics and monitoring of response with a chest X-ray
   C. Empirical antibiotics and monitoring of response with a chest X-ray
   D. Insertion of a therapeutic drain
   E. Pleural ultrasound and diagnostic aspiration

4. An 82-year-old woman was admitted to the acute medical unit with a three-week history of breathlessness on exertion. Her exercise tolerance had fallen from approximately 1 mile to 0.25 miles limited by breathlessness. She had no chest pain or other symptoms. She had no significant past medical history. She took no medication.

She had dullness to percussion and decreased vocal resonance at the left base. Cardiovascular, abdominal, and neurological examination was normal. Her temperature was normal.

Her ECG was normal.

Chest X-ray: moderate left-sided pleural effusion

A diagnostic aspiration of 50 millilitres of straw coloured fluid was performed.

```
Investigations:
    haemoglobin                         115 g/L              (130-180)
    white cell count                    7.1 × 10⁹/L          (4.0-11.0)
    platelet count                      222 × 10⁹/L          (150-400)
    serum sodium                        137 mmol/L           (137-144)
    serum potassium                     4.1 mmol/L           (3.5-4.9)
    serum urea                          3.3 mmol/L           (2.5-7.0)
    serum creatinine                    95 µmol/L            (60-110)
    serum total bilirubin               8 µmol/L             (1-22)
    serum alanine aminotransferase      56 U/L               (5-35)
    serum alkaline phosphatase          46 U/L (45-105)
    serum total protein                 31 g/L (61-76)
    serum C-reactive protein            15 mg/L              (<10)
    serum lactate dehydrogenase         218 U/L              (10-250)

    pleural fluid protein               25 g/L
    pleural fluid lactate               180
       dehydrogenase
    pleural fluid cytology: 'No malignant cells seen'
    pleural fluid microbiology: 'Gram stain negative; few
       white cells; no organisms seen'
    pleural fluid pH                    7.22
```

What is the next step in management?

A. Check a troponin and commence diuretic therapy
B. CT scan of the chest with contrast timed for pleural enhancement
C. Fibre-optic bronchoscopy
D. Insert a chest drain under ultrasound guidance
E. Repeat the pleural aspirate for amylase and triglycerides

5. An 83-year-old woman was admitted to the acute medical unit with a three-week history of increasing breathlessness. She had a past medical history of myocardial infarction two years ago and a single coronary stent.

   Clinical examination revealed dullness to percussion at both bases. Temperature was 36.6°C; pulse was 60 beats per minute. Blood pressure was 130/80 mmHg. Respiratory rate was 18 breaths per minute and oxygen saturation 94% on air.

   Full blood count, urea and electrolytes, and liver function tests were all normal.

   Chest X-ray: bilateral basal effusions with the right slightly larger than the left.

   How should she be managed?
   A. CT chest with contrast timed for pleural enhancement
   B. Blind diagnostic aspiration of the right pleural effusion
   C. Empirical diuretics and arrange an echocardiogram
   D. Ultrasound guided diagnostic aspiration of left and right pleural effusions
   E. Ultrasound of the pleural cavities to look for abnormalities

6. A 70-year-old man had three exacerbations of his chronic obstructive pulmonary disease (COPD) in the last year, and complained of persistent breathlessness. He used a short-acting beta agonist inhaler four times per day. His usual forced expiratory volume in 1 second (FEV_1) was 60% of the predicted value. He was currently stable.

   What inhaler therapy should now be offered?
   A. Start a long-acting beta agonist and a long-acting muscarinic antagonist
   B. Start a long-acting beta agonist and an inhaled corticosteroid in a combination inhaler
   C. Start a long-acting beta agonist or a long-acting muscarinic antagonist
   D. Start a methylxanthine
   E. Start an inhaled corticosteroid

7. A 62-year-old woman was admitted to the acute medical unit with an exacerbation of COPD. She normally took a combined inhaled corticosteroid and long-acting beta agonist.

   What is the most appropriate next step in management?
   A. Five-day course of prednisolone 20 mg daily
   B. Five-day course of prednisolone 30 mg daily
   C. 7–14 day course of prednisolone 20 mg daily
   D. 7–14 day course of prednisolone 30 mg daily
   E. Prednisolone 40 mg daily until 48 hours after nebulizers have been stopped

8. **A patient was referred to the acute medical unit from the emergency department with an exacerbation of COPD. Due to a shortage of beds the duty manager asked you if the patient could be sent home with appropriate treatment.**

   Which would you consider a reason to admit the patient for inpatient treatment?
   A. Arterial PaO$_2$ <9.0 kPa
   B. Cough productive of green phlegm
   C. Current smoker
   D. Normal chest X-ray
   E. Oxygen saturation of 89%

9. **A 70-year-old patient with COPD had chronic bronchitis and frequent exacerbations requiring hospital admission. His FEV$_1$ was 38% predicted when well. His was on long-term oxygen therapy (LTOT). He took a combined long-acting beta agonist and inhaled corticosteroid inhaler, a long-acting muscarinic antagonist inhaler, and oral theophylline.**

   What degree of airflow limitation does this man have?
   A. Stage 0 (none) airflow limitation (and may be a candidate for azithromycin)
   B. Stage 1 (mild) airflow limitation (and may be a candidate for erlotinib)
   C. Stage 2 (moderate) airflow limitation (and may be a candidate for carbocisteine)
   D. Stage 3 (severe) airflow limitation (and may be a candidate for roflumilast)
   E. Stage 4 (very severe) airflow limitation (and may be a candidate for omalizumab)

10. **A 65-year-old man with confirmed COPD had been started on long-term oxygen therapy (LTOT). A new respiratory nurse asked for up-to-date information on LTOT.**

    What should you tell her?
    A. LTOT is indicated for patients with COPD who have a PaO$_2$ <7.0 kPa when stable
    B. LTOT is indicated for patients with COPD who have a PaO$_2$ <8.0 kPa and secondary polycythaemia when stable
    C. LTOT provides symptomatic relief but not a mortality benefit
    D. LTOT should be taken for ten hours per day
    E. LTOT should not be given in hypercapnic respiratory failure

11. **A 25-year-old woman presented to the emergency department with an acute exacerbation of asthma. She used a salbutamol inhaler infrequently. She had never been admitted before with an exacerbation of asthma. She had recently moved house.**

    Her temperature was 37.2°C with a pulse rate of 120 beats per minute. Her respiratory rate was 30 breaths per minute and oxygen saturation 93% on air. Her peak expiratory flow rate was 40% of her predicted.

    ```
    Investigations:
      Arterial blood gas on air:
      pH       7.35        (7.35-7.45)
      pO2      10.5 kPa    (11.3-12.6)
      pCO2     5.6 kPa     (4.7-6.0)
    ```

    What level of asthma exacerbation severity is this?
    A. Acute severe asthma
    B. Life-threatening asthma
    C. Mild asthma
    D. Moderate asthma
    E. Near-fatal asthma

12. **A 40-year-old man was admitted to the acute medical unit with an acute severe exacerbation of asthma. His oxygen saturation was 96% on air. Initial response to a bolus dose of nebulized salbutamol 5 mg was poor.**

    Which would _not_ be appropriate in his management?
    A. Adding nebulized ipratropium to salbutamol to increase bronchodilation
    B. Continuous nebulization of salbutamol at 5–10 mg/hour
    C. Further nebulized salbutamol driven by oxygen
    D. Nebulized adrenaline (epinephrine) if nebulized salbutamol is ineffective
    E. Nebulized terbutaline, which is equally efficacious to nebulized salbutamol

13. **A 38-year-old woman presented to the acute medical unit with an acute severe asthma attack. She was 29 weeks pregnant. Her pre-pregnancy weight was 60 kg. She was given repeated doses of nebulized beta 2 agonists, and started on prednisolone 40 mg daily, but she failed to improve.**

    What is the next step in her management?
    A. Intravenous aminophylline 180 mg over 20 minutes
    B. Intravenous aminophylline 300 mg over 20 minutes
    C. Intravenous magnesium and aminophylline should not be given
    D. Intravenous magnesium sulphate 2 g over 20 minutes
    E. Intravenous magnesium sulphate 20 mg over 20 minutes

RESPIRATORY | QUESTIONS

14. A 32-year-old man was admitted to the acute medical unit with an exacerbation of asthma. After three days he had improved considerably and he wanted to go home.

    Which condition should be met prior to discharge?
    A. Diurnal variation in peak flow <15%
    B. Follow-up in respiratory clinic within four weeks
    C. GP follow-up arranged for two weeks
    D. He should have been on discharge medication for 48 hours
    E. Peak expiratory flow rate is >80% of best/predicted

15. A 72-year-old man was admitted to the acute medical unit via the emergency department with an acute exacerbation of COPD. He was alert and orientated. There were no focal abnormalities on his chest X-ray.

    On examination his heart rate was 100 beats per minute, and his blood pressure was 120/85 mmHg. His respiratory rate was 24 breaths per minute. His oxygen saturation was 96% on room air.

    After one hour of nebulized bronchodilators, intravenous steroids, and a loading dose of aminophylline, his blood gas showed the following results.

    Investigations:

    ```
    FiO2            60%
    pH              7.31        (7.35-7.45)
    pO2             13.1 kPa    (11.3-12.6)
    pCO2            7.1 kPa     (4.7-6.0)
    bicarbonate     36 mmol/L   (21-29)
    base excess     4 mmol/L    (±2)
    ```

    What is the most appropriate next step in his management?
    A. Continuous positive airway pressure, CPAP (5 cm H_2O)
    B. Invasive ventilation
    C. Magnesium sulphate infusion
    D. Non-Invasive ventilation (IPAP 10 cm H_2O/EPAP 4 cm H_2O)
    E. Reduce the inspired oxygen to 28%

16. A patient was admitted to the acute medical unit with acute on chronic type 2 respiratory failure due to an exacerbation of COPD, and after an hour of optimal treatment he failed to improve and was commenced on non-invasive ventilation (NIV).

    What is the management of a patient on non-invasive ventilation?
    A. Blood gases should be measured after two hours of initiation of NIV
    B. Blood gases should be measured 30 minutes after any setting changes
    C. Continuous electrocardiogram measurement is not necessary after the first hour
    D. Observations should be made every 15 minutes for the first hour
    E. Once on NIV, target oxygen saturations should be >94%

17. **A 65-year-old man was admitted to the acute medical unit with community-acquired pneumonia, which was confirmed on chest X-ray.**

    His pulse rate was 100 beats per minute and blood pressure was 120/65. He was apyrexial. His respiratory rate was 28 breaths per minute. His abbreviated mental test was 9/10. His serum urea was 9 mmol/L.

    What is his predicted mortality?
    A. 30-day mortality of less than 3%
    B. 30-day mortality of around 6%
    C. 30-day mortality of around 9%
    D. 30-day mortality of around 12%
    E. 30-day mortality of around 15%

18. **A 55-year-old man was admitted with a six-day history of fevers, headaches, breathlessness, and myalgia after returning from a package holiday in Spain. His chest X-ray showed consolidation and a urine test for legionella antigen was positive. His CURB-65 score was 1. He had no allergies and took no medication. His renal and liver function were normal.**

    What antibiotic should he be treated with?
    A. Ceftriaxone
    B. Co-amoxiclav plus clarithromycin
    C. Co-trimoxazole
    D. Erythromycin
    E. Levofloxacin

19. **A 64-year-old woman was admitted to the acute medical unit with a first episode of pulmonary embolus after a one-day history of pleuritic chest pain and breathlessness. She had no past medical history, was on no medications, and had no other symptoms.**

    Physical examination was normal.

    Which set of tests should be performed first?
    A. Chest X-ray, full blood count, serum calcium, liver function tests, and D-dimer
    B. Chest X-ray, full blood count, serum calcium, liver function tests, and urinalysis
    C. Chest X-ray, full blood count, serum calcium, liver function tests, urinalysis, and an abdominal and pelvic CT
    D. Chest X-ray, full blood count, serum calcium, liver function tests, urinalysis, and a colonoscopy
    E. Chest X-ray, full blood count, serum calcium, liver function tests, urinalysis, and a mammogram

20. **A 58-year-old woman receiving adjuvant chemotherapy for breast cancer presented with a first episode of pulmonary embolus. She had a WHO performance status of 1, normal renal and liver function, and has had no problems with bleeding.**

    Which anticoagulation strategy is correct?
    A. Low molecular weight heparin for five days, then three months' vitamin K antagonist
    B. Low molecular weight heparin for five days, then six months' vitamin K antagonist
    C. Low molecular weight heparin for five days, then lifelong vitamin K antagonist
    D. Low molecular weight heparin for six months, then reassess risks/benefits of anticoagulation
    E. Low molecular weight heparin lifelong reassessing benefit every five years

21. **A 44-year-old man was admitted to the acute medical unit with a productive cough and signs and symptoms consistent with pulmonary tuberculosis. His partner had multi-drug resistant tuberculosis (MDR TB).**

    What is the management for a patient with MDR TB?
    A. The patient should be admitted to a negative pressure room immediately and before discharge the patient should be discussed with the Department of Health Chief Medical Officer
    B. The patient should be admitted to a negative pressure room immediately and should not be allowed to leave for any reason
    C. The patient should be admitted to a negative pressure room immediately and staff and visitors should wear FFP3 masks for brief visits/consultations
    D. The patient should be admitted to a negative pressure room immediately and the patient should use disposable cutlery
    E. The patient should be admitted to a negative pressure room immediately and staff and visitors should wear surgical masks for brief visits/consultations

22. **A 55-year-old woman was admitted to the acute medical unit via the emergency department with a first episode of haemoptysis (approximately 500 mL over 24 hours).**

    What would you tell the junior doctor asking for advice?
    A. The bleeding is most likely from a bronchial vein
    B. Infection is an unlikely cause of haemoptysis
    C. Nebulized adrenaline 5–10 mL of 1:10,000 may be used
    D. The patient should be managed in the recovery position with the bleeding side (if known) uppermost
    E. Surgery in the setting of massive haemoptysis has a mortality rate of >70%

23. An anxious 68-year-old man with COPD had taken an accidental overdose of diazepam, and presented with acute type 2 respiratory failure and reduced conscious level.

    What is the best dosage strategy of flumazenil?
    A. 5 micrograms over 15 seconds with bolus 1 microgram doses up to 10 micrograms total
    B. 10 micrograms over 15 seconds with bolus 5 micrograms doses up to 50 micrograms total
    C. 200 micrograms over 15 seconds with further 100 microgram doses up to 1 mg total
    D. 2 mg over 15 seconds with bolus doses up to 10 mg total
    E. 200 mg over 15 seconds with further 200 mg doses up to 1 g total

24. A 66-year-old man was discharged from the respiratory ward following an episode of severe community-acquired pneumonia. He asked about risks and possible preventative measures for developing pneumonia in the future.

    What would you tell him?
    A. Influenza vaccination of patients over 65 years is ineffective in preventing death
    B. Pneumococcal polysaccharide vaccination of patients over 65 does prevent invasive pneumococcal disease
    C. Pneumococcal polysaccharide vaccine cannot be given at the same time as influenza vaccination
    D. Pneumococcal polysaccharide vaccine may safely be given a second time one year after the first
    E. Smoking is associated with an increased risk of community-acquired tuberculosis

25. A 45-year-old man was seen on the acute medical unit with right lower lobe community-acquired pneumonia. His CURB-65 score was 1.

    What could you tell him?
    A. If he has Legionella pneumonia radiological resolution is likely to be slower than average
    B. Lower lobe involvement is characteristic of Klebsiella pneumonia
    C. Mycoplasma pneumoniae usually affects older patients
    D. The likelihood that this is due to a virus is 2–4%
    E. The yield from combined sputum and blood culture is expected to be approximately 30%

26. **A 52-year-old man presented to the acute medical unit with gradual onset of breathlessness, wheeze, and chronic cough. He had a reduced peak flow. His chest X-ray and a representative slice of his CT scan of chest is shown (Figures 3.3 and 3.4).**

Investigations:

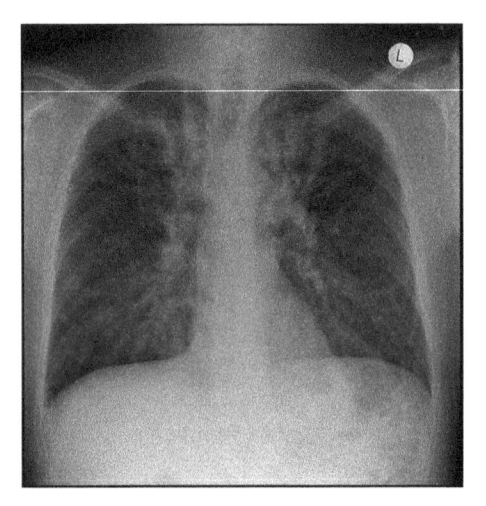

Figure 3.3 Chest X-ray.

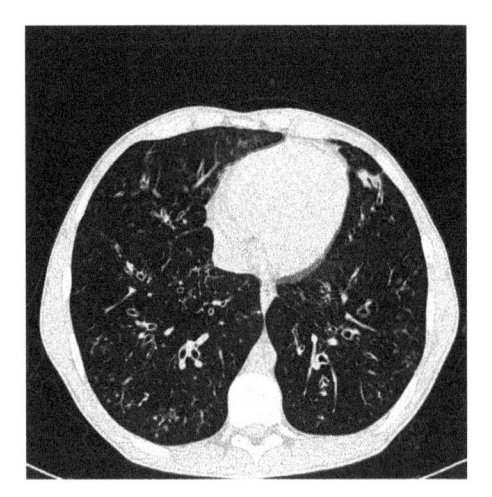

Figure 3.4 CT scan of thorax.

What is likely to be helpful in managing his condition?
A. Advice on stopping smoking
B. IgE RAST to aspergillus
C. Rheumatoid factor
D. Sputum culture
E. Urinary Bence Jones protein

RESPIRATORY | QUESTIONS

27. A 39-year-old woman presented to the acute medical unit with a one-week history of feeling generally unwell with a sore throat and high temperature. On examination she had a temperature of 38.7°C, pleuritic chest pain, and tenderness over the area of her right jugular vein. A CT scan of her neck and chest revealed a thrombosed jugular vein, several pulmonary cavitations, and a small right pleural effusion.

What is the most likely organism?
- A. Aspergillus fumigatus
- B. Bacteroides fragilis
- C. Burkholderia cepacia
- D. Fusobacterium necrophorum
- E. Pseudomonas aeruginosa

28. A 52-year-old man with bronchiectasis was admitted to the acute medical unit with malaise and an increase in both sputum volume and thickness. This was his third exacerbation over the last year. His sputum culture had twice grown Pseudomonas aeruginosa in the last six months.

Which of the following is not useful in managing patients with this condition?
- A. An acapella device
- B. Antibiotics that treat Pseudomonas started without waiting for a new sputum culture
- C. Chest physiotherapy to clear sputum
- D. Maintenance therapy with colomycin nebulizers
- E. Nebulized recombinant human DNase

29. A 69-year-old man with moderate-severe COPD was admitted to the acute medical unit with an exacerbation.

When explaining his case to a medical student what teaching point would you emphasize?
- A. Respiratory viruses are rarely isolated when tested for
- B. Sputum purulence is a reliable indicator of the presence of bacteria
- C. A tapering course of prednisolone over seven days would be appropriate
- D. There is a 10% chance that pathogenic bacteria will be isolated from his sputum
- E. Twice-daily measurement of his peak flow will be helpful to guide discharge

30. **A 33-year-old woman with a three-year history of extremely difficult to control asthma and allergic rhinitis was admitted to the intensive care unit having been deteriorating at home for several weeks.**

    Investigations:

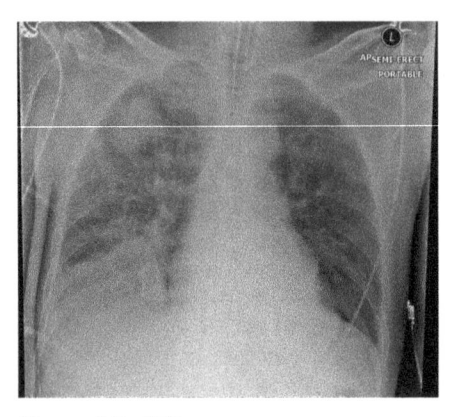

    Figure 3.5 CXR.

    Blood tests from a GP consultation last week were available:

    ```
    haemoglobin                         121 g/L              (115–165)
    white cell count                    11.8 × 10⁹/L         (4.0–11.0)
    neutrophil count                    7.6 × 10⁹/L          (1.5–7.0)
    lymphocyte count                    0.9 × 10⁹/L          (1.5–4.0)
    monocyte count                      0.4 × 10⁹/L          (<0.8)
    eosinophil count                    3.03 × 10⁹/L         (0.04–0.40)
    basophil count                      0.02 × 10⁹/L         (<0.1)
    platelet count                      135 × 10⁹/L          (150–400)
    serum C-reactive protein            103 mg/L             (<10)
    Liver and renal function tests:     normal

    Anti-neutrophil cytoplasmic antibodies:
    c-ANCA     negative
    p-ANCA     positive
    PR3        5 U/mL         (<10)
    MPO        100 U/mL       (<10)
    ```

    What is the most likely diagnosis?
    A. Anti-glomerular basement antibody (anti-GBM) disease (Goodpasture's syndrome)
    B. Eosinophilic granulomatosis with polyangiitis (Churg Strauss syndrome)
    C. Granulomatosis with polyangiitis (Wegener's syndrome)
    D. Legionnaires' disease
    E. Microscopic polyangiitis

31. A 50-year-old woman had a three-month history of cough. She had never smoked and took no medication. Her chest X-ray was normal.

    Which is <u>least likely</u> to be the cause of her cough?
    A. Cough variant asthma
    B. Eosinophillic bronchitis
    C. Gastro-oesophageal reflux disease
    D. Non-specific interstitial pneumonia
    E. Rhinitis

32. A 32-year-old male surfboarder was admitted after a near-drowning incident.

    Investigations:

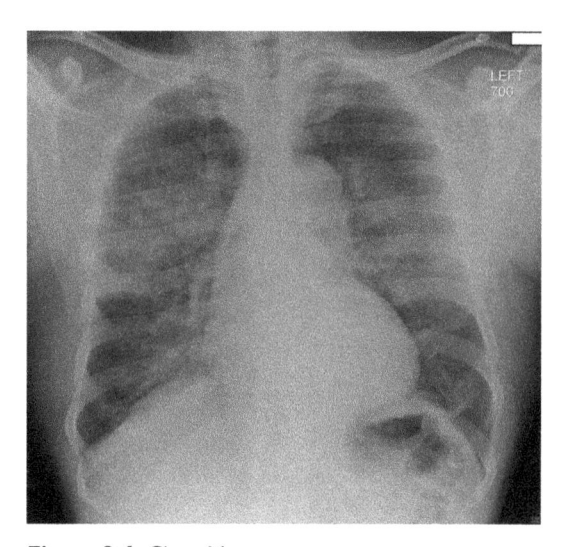

    Figure 3.6 Chest X-ray.

    PaO$_2$/FiO$_2$ is 20 kPa.

    Which of the following would be essential information when talking to the intensive care unit team?
    A. He has acute lung injury but not acute respiratory distress syndrome
    B. He has acute respiratory distress syndrome
    C. High tidal volume ventilation strategy has proved beneficial
    D. His mortality rate is likely to be approximately 20%
    E. Inhaled nitric oxide improves mortality in this situation

33. **A 45-year-old female smoker presented to the acute medical unit with a three-day history of haemoptysis. She was haemodynamically stable, and the volume of haemoptysis was small, mostly streaking of sputum.**

    She had a normal CRP, full blood count, renal and liver function, and calcium.

    Her chest X-ray was normal.

    What would you explain to her?
    A. The chance that this is due to lung cancer is approximately 6%
    B. The chance that this is due to lung cancer is approximately 30%
    C. She does not need invasive investigation if the symptoms settle within one week
    D. She should have a staging CT scan of chest and proceed to bronchoscopy only if the scan is abnormal
    E. She should undergo bronchoscopy and proceed to a staging CT scan of chest if an abnormality is found

34. **A 66-year-old woman with a background of heart failure and rheumatoid arthritis was admitted to the acute medical unit with a 1–2 month history of breathlessness. She took rituximab for her arthritis.**

    Her chest X-ray showed a moderate left pleural effusion. A diagnostic pleural aspirate was performed.

    What would you discuss with the junior doctor who performed the aspiration?
    A. High glucose concentration in the sample suggests rheumatoid disease as the aetiology
    B. Lidocaine contamination within the sample will raise the pH
    C. A lymphocyte predominant effusion would be unusual for malignancy
    D. A lymphocyte predominant effusion would be unusual for tuberculosis
    E. Pleural fluid adenosine deaminase (ADA) levels are usually raised in tuberculous pleurisy

35. **A 27-year-old woman with cystic fibrosis was admitted to the acute medical unit with a two-day history of colicky abdominal pain, constipation, nausea, and a palpable right lower quadrant mass. There were no signs of peritoneal irritation.**

    Investigations:

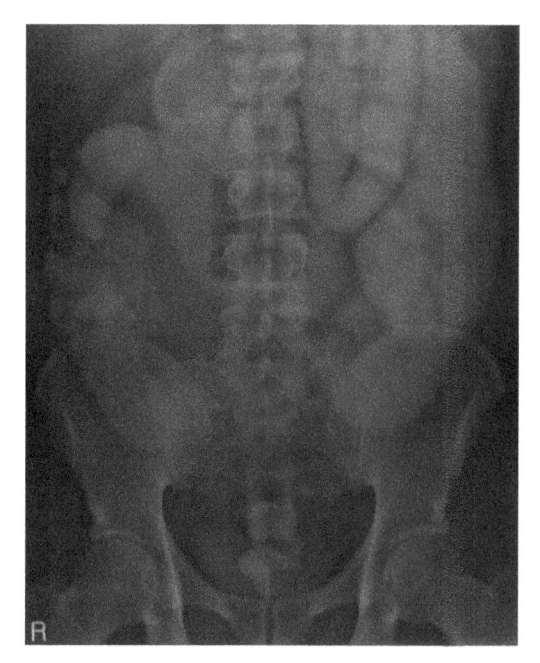

    Figure 3.7 Abdominal X-ray.

    Which of the following is <u>incorrect</u>?
    A. High dose macrogol may be used
    B. It is unlikely that abdominal surgery will be required
    C. Klean-Prep® (an osmotic laxative) may be used
    D. Oral gastrografin is not recommended
    E. Sub-optimal pancreatic enzyme therapy may contribute to the problem

36. **A 48-year-old woman presented to the acute medical unit with a one-month history of progressive breathlessness. She had recently been diagnosed with Grave's disease, and had an obvious goitre.**

    If her breathlessness was due to the compressive effects of her goitre, which of the following is true?
    A. Coughing and hoarseness are unlikely to accompany the breathlessness
    B. The Empey Index would be less than 10
    C. Her gas transfer would be normal on pulmonary function testing
    D. She will not have excessive daytime sleepiness
    E. There would be a proportionally larger reduction in forced expiratory volume in 1 second than peak expiratory flow rate

37. A 49-year-old man was admitted to the emergency department after a road traffic collision. His body mass index (BMI) was 42. His wife, who was a passenger in the car at the time, thinks he may have fallen asleep at the wheel. The possibility of obstructive sleep apnoea/hypopnoea syndrome (OSAHS) is raised.

Which is true regarding OSAHS?
A. An Epworth sleepiness score of 5 implies significant sleepiness
B. Nocturia is a not a feature of OSAHS
C. A normal overnight oximetry will effectively exclude OSAHS
D. Smoking and alcohol consumption are associated with OSAHS
E. Uvulopalatopharyngoplasty (UPPP) is recommended for the treatment of OSAHS

38. A 33-year-old woman, who was a Somalian refugee, was referred to the acute medical unit by her GP. She had a two-month history of worsening cough, fevers, night sweats, poor appetite, and malaise.

Her GP sent a sputum sample last week and checked her HIV status. The lab informed you that she was smear positive for acid and alcohol fast bacilli (AAFB) and was HIV positive.

What is true regarding her management?
A. Anti-tuberculosis treatment should be started before anti-retrovirals
B. She should be considered infectious until four weeks of anti-tuberculous treatment have been taken
C. She should be started on a three-drug regimen of rifampicin, isoniazid, and ethambutol
D. She should stay in a side room until two sputum samples are negative for AAFB
E. A side room is only required if multi-drug resistant tuberculosis is suspected

39. A 61-year-old man with a recent diagnosis of mesothelioma was admitted to the acute medical unit with worsening breathlessness and severe chest pain. He lived alone. His exercise tolerance was approximately 100 metres. His daughter did his shopping for him, but he was otherwise independent.

His medication included morphine sulphate modified release 100 mg twice daily with morphine sulphate oral solution for breakthrough pain, diclofenac 50 mg three times daily, and paracetamol 1 g four times daily.

He had a moderate pleural effusion on his chest X-ray, and signs of ascites on examination.

Which is true?
A. Combination radiotherapy plus chemotherapy would have a slim chance of curing him
B. His ascites is not due to peritoneal metastases
C. An indwelling pleural catheter is not helpful to manage his effusion
D. Percutaneous cervical cordotomy at C1/C2 level is an option for pain management
E. Severe pain due to mesothelioma is uncommon

40. Researchers assessed the efficacy of varenicline, a licensed cigarette smoking cessation aid, in helping adult users of smokeless tobacco to quit. A randomized double-blind, placebo-controlled trial study design was used. Varenicline was administered at a dose of 1 mg twice daily for 12 weeks. A total of 431 participants were recruited and randomized to varenicline (n = 213) or placebo (n = 218). All participants were offered brief behavioural support or counselling at the discretion of the investigators.

The primary endpoint was continuous abstinence from using smokeless tobacco for four weeks at the end of treatment (weeks 9–12). The rate of continuous abstinence was significantly higher in the varenicline group than for placebo (59% v 39%; relative risk 1.6, 95% confidence interval 1.32 to 1.87; P<0.001; number needed to treat five).*

What is the best interpretation of number needed to treat (NNT) of five for continuous abstinence at end of treatment in users of smokeless tobacco for varenicline compared with placebo?

A. Five users need to be treated with varenicline for one to experience an adverse side effect following treatment

B. Five users need to be treated with placebo for one to experience an adverse side effect following treatment

C. On average, five users need to be treated with varenicline for one person to be abstinent at the end of treatment

D. On average, for every five users treated with varenicline one more would be abstinent at the end of treatment than if those same people received placebo

E. On average, if five users were treated with varenicline then all of them would be abstinent at the end of treatment whereas none of them would be if treated with placebo

---

* Data included in this question is from K Fagerström et al., 'Stopping smokeless tobacco with varenicline: randomised double blind placebo controlled trial', *BMJ*, 2010; 341: c6549

chapter 3

RESPIRATORY

ANSWERS

1. B. Aspiration via an 18 G cannula in the 2nd intercostal space, mid-clavicular line

This patient has a primary spontaneous pneumothorax (PSP) as shown in the chest X-ray (Figure 3.1). The pathophysiology of PSP is not fully understood, but is thought to relate to the rupture of small sub-pleural blebs, which can sometimes be seen on CT scanning patients with PSP. Additionally, smoking causes inflammation and obstruction in the distal small airways and may thereby increase the pressure in the distal lung parenchyma.

Management of a spontaneous pneumothorax depends first on whether there are life-threatening features. If there are bilateral pneumothoraces or haemodynamic instability (sometimes due to a tensioning pneumothorax compressing the mediastinum and reducing venous return), then a chest drain should be inserted.

If there are no life-threatening features then management depends on whether the patient has a primary or a secondary pneumothorax, the size of the pneumothorax, and symptoms of breathlessness. Defining whether a primary pneumothorax is small or large is useful when deciding if the patient needs to undergo a therapeutic aspiration or may be considered for discharge. In the British Thoracic Society (BTS) (2010) guidelines, a rim of air >2 cm when measured at the level of the hilum is the definition of a 'large' pneumothorax.

Primary spontaneous pneumothorax (PSP)

Size >2cm and/or breathless: Aspirate (up to 2.5 L) via 16–18 G cannula.

- if improvement (<2 cm rim and not breathless) then consider outpatient review 2–4 weeks.
- if not improved then insert 8–14 F chest drain.

Size < 2cm and not breathless: consider discharge and review in 2–4 weeks.

Secondary spontaneous pneumothorax (SSP)

Due to, for example, COPD, acute asthma, interstitial lung disease, etc.

Size >2 cm or breathless: insert 8–14 F chest drain.

Size 1–2 cm: aspirate (up to 2.5 L) via 16–18 G cannula.

- if improvement (<1 cm rim) then observe, high flow O_2 (if not oxygen-sensitive).
- if not improved then insert 8–14 F chest drain.

Size <1 cm: admit, observe, high flow O_2 (if not oxygen-sensitive).

All patients with SSP should be admitted for at least 24 hours and be given oxygen. The majority of these patients will need a chest drain, and all should be referred to a chest physician. Patients with persistent air leak should have an early thoracic surgical opinion (day 3–5) with a view to either open thoracotomy with pleurectomy (1% recurrence rate) or video-assisted thoracic surgery

(VATS) (5% recurrence rate). If the patient is unwilling or unable to undergo a surgical solution then eventually a (less effective) chemical pleurodesis may be performed by a respiratory specialist.

MacDuff A, Arnold A, Harvey J on behalf of the British Thoracic Society Pleural Disease Guideline Group. Management of Spontaneous Pneumothorax, BTS Pleural Disease guideline 2010. Thorax 2010; 65(2). http://www.brit-thoracic.org.uk

2. C. Smoking is associated with an increased incidence of pneumothorax in men compared with women

Primary spontaneous pneumothorax (PSP) is more common in men than women. Additionally, smoking is associated with a 22-fold increase in relative risk of PSP in men, and a ninefold increase in women.

Patients should SCUBA dive only after bilateral pleurectomy and pleural abrasion, and satisfactory post-operative lung function tests (+/− CT scanning) have been performed.

Patients should not fly until full chest X-ray resolution has occurred. There is no good evidence on which to guide advice about flying once a pneumothorax has resolved. The latest (2011) British Thoracic Society (BTS) Air Travel Guidelines note that many physicians feel that waiting one week after a pneumothorax has resolved is prudent, and that ideally for a traumatic pneumothorax a two-week delay is suggested.

There is also no good evidence on which to base advice regarding resuming contact sports, but many physicians advise a six-week delay after pneumothorax resolution.

MacDuff A, Arnold T, Harvey J. Management of Spontaneous Pneumothorax. British Thoracic Society Pleural Disease Guideline. Thorax 2010; 65(2). http://www.brit-thoracic.org.uk

3. E. Pleural ultrasound and diagnostic aspiration

The chest X-ray (Figure 3.2) shows a right-sided pleural effusion. The next step is to perform a 50 mL diagnostic aspirate with a fine bore (21 G) needle under bedside ultrasound guidance.

The most likely diagnosis given the short history and sweats is of pneumonia with a parapneumonic effusion or empyema. A therapeutic drain is not *necessarily* required for a parapneumonic effusion. In a presumed parapneumonic effusion, the diagnostic aspirate will help to decide if a drain is needed. Diagnostic aspirates should be sent for cytology, protein, lactate dehydrogenase, gram stain, and microbiological culture (including inoculation of blood culture bottles with pleural fluid if infection is particularly suspected). Straw-coloured parapneumonic effusions should have a pH measurement, and a drain inserted if the pH is less than 7.2. A drain should also be inserted if the fluid is gram stain or culture positive.

If the patient was breathless at rest or on minimal exertion, then a drain would be indicated.

A CT scan of the chest may be needed at a later stage if the patient has an exudative effusion that remained unexplained or in cases of complex pleural infection where surgery may be indicated.

Hooper C, Lee Y, Maskell N. Investigation of a Unilateral Pleural Effusion in Adults. British Thoracic Society Pleural Disease Guideline. Thorax 2010; 65(2). http://www.brit-thoracic.org.uk

4. B. CT scan of the chest with contrast timed for pleural enhancement

This woman has an exudative effusion by Light's criteria. There have been a number of studies looking at criteria which are useful in distinguishing between an exudate and a transudate when the pleural fluid protein levels are between 25 g/L and 35 g/L. For example Paramothyan and Barron (2002) showed that "if both the fluid LDH is > 130 U/Litre or the fluid to serum total protein ratio is > 0.4, the fluid should be regarded as an exudate". In this case the pleural fluid protein/serum protein ratio is 0.8.

There are no clues as to the cause from the cytology or microbiology, and history and serology is not suggestive of infection. The next step is a CT scan of her chest. In the absence of symptoms suggestive of a pulmonary embolism then a CT scan with contrast timed for pleural enhancement will provide the most diagnostic information. If the CT scan is also non-diagnostic then pleural biopsy under direct vision is the next step (either via VATS or medical thoracoscopy).

Pleural fluid amylase is normally only performed in suspected cases of oesophageal rupture or pancreatitis. Triglycerides are not sent routinely, but only in cases of suspected chylothorax (usually milky white in nature resulting from leakage of fluid from the thoracic duct or one of the large lymphatics draining into it, often secondary to surgical trauma or lymphoma).

Bronchoscopy should not be done when investigating an exudative pleural effusion unless there is a specific lesion suspected on the chest X-ray or CT scan.

Pleural fluid may be acidic in malignant effusions as well as in para-pneumonic effusions, and does not indicate by itself the need for a chest drain. The pleura is best imaged by CT when there is still some fluid in the pleural cavity.

Hooper C, Lee Y, Maskell N. Investigation of a Unilateral Pleural Effusion in Adults. British Thoracic Society Pleural Disease Guideline. Thorax 2010; 65(2). http://www.brit-thoracic.org.uk

Light RW, Macgreggor MI, Luchsinger PC, et al. Pleural effusions: the diagnostic separation of transudates and exudates. Annals of Internal Medicine 1972;77:508–13.

Vives M, Porcel JM, Vicente de Vera C, et al. A study of Light's criteria and possible modifications for distinguishing exudative from transudative pleural effusions. Chest 1996;109:1503–7.

Romero S, Candela A, Martin C, et al. Evaluation of different criteria for the separation of pleural transudates from exudates. Chest 1993;104:399–404.

Parathomyan NS and Barron J. New criteria for the differentiation between transudates and exudates. Journal of Clinical Pathology 2002;55:69–71.

5. C. Empirical diuretics and arrange an echocardiogram

Most cases of bilateral pleural effusions will be transudative effusions due to heart failure, and if the history, clinical, and serological findings are consistent with this diagnosis then the patient should ordinarily be managed empirically with diuretics. If the effusion on one side is significantly larger than the other side then a diagnostic aspiration is indicated. Likewise, if the effusions fail to resolve or there are features which cast doubt onto the diagnosis of heart failure (such as normal heart size, fevers, suspicion of pulmonary embolus, or a systemic disease) then a diagnostic aspiration is indicated.

Other causes of transudative pleural effusions include: liver cirrhosis, nephrotic syndrome, peritoneal dialysis, constrictive pericarditis, post-operative atelectasis, and hypothyroidism.

Hooper C, Lee Y, Maskell N. Investigation of a Unilateral Pleural Effusion in Adults. British Thoracic Society Pleural Disease Guideline. Thorax 2010; 65(2). http://www.brit-thoracic.org.uk

6. C. Start a long-acting beta agonist or a long-acting muscarinic antagonist

For patients with stable COPD, National Institute for Health and Care Excellence (NICE) guidelines advise a step up in treatment from a short-acting beta agonist (SABA) if the patient has persistent breathlessness or exacerbations. The options depend on whether the patient's FEV_1 is greater or less than 50%. If it is 50% or more than predicted then either a long-acting beta agonist (LABA) or a long-acting muscarinic antagonist (LAMA) is appropriate. If the FEV_1 is less than 50% predicted then either a LABA + inhaled corticosteroid (ICS) or LAMA should be offered.

National Institute for Health and Care Excellence. Clinical Guideline 101. Chronic obstructive pulmonary disease in over 16s: diagnosis and management. June 2010.

RESPIRATORY | ANSWERS

7. D. 7–14 day course of prednisolone 30 mg daily

Prednisolone 30 mg daily for 7–14 days should be given to all patients requiring admission to hospital (unless contraindicated).

National Institute for Health and Care Excellence. Clinical Guideline 101. Chronic obstructive pulmonary disease in over 16s: diagnosis and management. June 2010.

8. E. Oxygen saturation of 89%

NICE clinical guideline 101 lists 16 factors that should be considered when deciding where to manage a patient. Some factors that favour treatment in hospital include: changes on the chest radiograph, receiving long-term oxygen therapy, oxygen saturations of <90%, rapid rate of symptom onset, and significant co-morbidity (particularly cardiac disease and insulin-dependent diabetes).

National Institute for Health and Care Excellence. Clinical Guideline 101. Chronic obstructive pulmonary disease in over 16s: diagnosis and management. June 2010.

9. D. Stage 3 (severe) airflow limitation (and may be a candidate for roflumilast)

Both the NICE COPD clinical guideline 101 (2010) and the GOLD guideline (2011) define severity of airflow limitation as an FEV_1 of:

- ≥80% Stage 1—Mild (symptoms must be present for diagnosis of COPD)
- 50–79% Stage 2—Moderate
- 30–49% Stage 3—Severe
- < 30% Stage 4—Very severe (or FEV_1 <50% with respiratory failure)

Note that assessing the severity of the disease itself should also take into account symptoms, risk of exacerbations, and co-morbidities (osteoporosis, depression, anxiety, lung cancer, skeletal muscle dysfunction, and cardiovascular disease). The GOLD guidance states that the (relatively new) phosphodiesterase-4 inhibitor roflumilast may be used to reduce exacerbations for patients with chronic bronchitis, severe and very severe airflow limitation, and frequent exacerbations that are not adequately controlled on long-acting bronchodilators.

The 2011 GOLD guideline also provides a scoring matrix which places patients into one of four categories depending on their symptoms, the degree of airflow limitation, and number of exacerbations.

Erlotinib (tarceva) is a tyrosine kinase inhibitor that may be used to treat non-small cell lung cancer. Omalizumab (xolair) is a monoclonal antibody to IgE that may be used to treat allergic asthma.

There is some evidence that azithromycin taken daily for a year can decrease the frequency of COPD exacerbations and improve quality of life in selected patients. In studies, a small percentage of patients suffered a reduction in their hearing.

Global Initiative for Chronic Obstructive Lung Disease. COPD Diagnosis and Management At-A-Glance Desk Reference, 2015. http://www.goldcopd.org

10. B. LTOT is indicated for patients with COPD who have a PaO_2 <8.0 kPa and secondary polycythaemia when stable

Long term oxygen therapy (LTOT) is indicated in patients with COPD who have a PaO_2 less than 7.3 kPa when stable or a PaO_2 of less than 8 kPa when stable *and* one of: secondary polycythaemia, nocturnal hypoxaemia (oxygen saturation less than 90% for more than 30% of the night), peripheral oedema, or pulmonary hypertension.

The need for LTOT should be assessed in all patients with very severe airflow obstruction (forced expiratory volume in 1 second (FEV_1) <30% predicted) cyanosis or polycythaemia. The LTOT assessment is to confirm hypoxaemia and to ascertain the oxygen flow rate that will safely improve the hypoxaemia. Arterial blood gases are measured when the patient is stable—at least six weeks after an exacerbation, and once the patient has been medically optimized.

At the LTOT assessment sequential blood gas analysis determines the amount of oxygen that can safely be delivered. Hypercapnic respiratory failure due to COPD is not a contraindication to LTOT.

There is a mortality benefit when LTOT is taken for at least 15 hours (including overnight). Greater benefits are seen in patients receiving oxygen for 20 hours per day.

National Institute for Health and Care Excellence. Clinical Guideline 101. Chronic obstructive pulmonary disease in over 16s: diagnosis and management. June 2010.

11. B. Life-threatening asthma

This is defined as life-threatening asthma because the patient has a normal pCO_2 along with features of severe asthma.

Life-threatening asthma is 'severe asthma' *plus* any one of: altered conscious level, exhaustion, silent chest, poor respiratory effort, cyanosis, arrhythmia, hypotension, peak expiratory flow <33% best or predicted, SpO_2 <92%, pO_2 <8 kPa, pCO_2 4.7–6.0 kPa (35–45 mmHg).

Near-fatal asthma is defined as patients with a raised pCO_2 and/or requiring mechanical ventilation with raised inflation pressures.

Acute severe asthma is when any one of the following are present: peak expiratory flow 33–50% best or predicted, respiratory rate ≥25 per minute, heart rate ≥110 beats per minute, inability to complete sentences in one breath.

Moderate asthma exacerbation is defined as: increasing symptoms, peak expiratory flow >50–75% best or predicted, no features of acute severe asthma.

Predicted peak expiratory flow values should be used only if the recent best peak expiratory flow (within two years) is unknown.

British Thoracic Society/Scottish Intercollegiate Guidelines Network. Guideline 141, British Guideline on the Management of Asthma, October 2014. http://www.brit-thoracic.org.uk; http://www.sign.ac.uk

12. D. Nebulized adrenaline (epinephrine) if nebulized salbutamol is ineffective

Nebulized adrenaline (epinephrine) is a non-selective beta 2 agonist and does not provide significant benefit over salbutamol or terbutaline (both of which are equally efficacious). Adding ipratropium increases bronchodilation and should be given to those with severe or life-threatening asthma, or to those that do not respond adequately to initial treatment. Nebulized beta 2 agonist bronchodilators should preferably be driven by oxygen in acute asthma.

If the patient is not responding adequately to an initial bolus dose of beta 2 agonist then either repeat the initial dose at 15–30 minute intervals or give continuous nebulization of salbutamol at 5–10 mg/hour. Continuous nebulization requires a specific nebulizer. 'Continuous nebulization' does not mean 'consecutive bolus doses without pause'—this increases the chance of significant side effects.

British Thoracic Society/Scottish Intercollegiate Guidelines Network. Guideline 141, British Guideline on the Management of Asthma, October 2014. http://www.brit-thoracic.org.uk; http://www.sign.ac.uk

13. D. Intravenous magnesium sulphate 2 g over 20 minutes

Drug therapy for acute severe asthma in pregnancy is the same as it is for non-pregnant patients. Intravenous magnesium, aminophylline, beta 2 agonists, and steroids can all be used. Oxygen should be given to maintain saturations above 94%. In pregnancy, progesterone drives an increase in minute ventilation, which can lead to relative hypocapnia and respiratory alkalosis and higher PaO_2. However, oxygen saturations are unaltered. Continuous foetal monitoring is recommended in severe acute asthma.

RESPIRATORY | ANSWERS

A single dose of intravenous magnesium sulphate (1.2–2 g over 20 minutes) should be considered for patients with acute severe asthma who have not had a good initial response to nebulized bronchodilator therapy, and for patients with life-threatening or near-fatal asthma. It is safe and may improve lung function.

The safety and efficacy of repeated intravenous doses of magnesium sulphate has not been assessed. Repeated doses could cause hypermagnesaemia with muscle weakness and respiratory failure. More studies are needed to determine the optimal dose, frequency, and route of magnesium therapy.

In acute severe asthma intravenous aminophylline is not likely to result in additional bronchodilation compared with inhaled bronchodilators and steroids. Some patients with life-threatening or near-fatal asthma may gain benefit (5 mg/kg loading dose over 20 minutes). These patients are probably rare and have not been identified in meta-analyses of trials.

British Thoracic Society/Scottish Intercollegiate Guidelines Network. Guideline 141, British Guideline on the Management of Asthma, October 2014. http://www.brit-thoracic.org.uk; http://www.sign.ac.uk

14. B. Follow-up in respiratory clinic within four weeks

Patients should be seen in a respiratory clinic within four weeks, and by their GP within two working days.

At discharge from hospital patients should have been on discharge medication for 12–24 hours and have had inhaler technique checked and recorded. They should have oral and inhaled steroids in addition to bronchodilators. They should have a peak flow meter and a written asthma action plan (these can decrease hospitalization and deaths from asthma).

Peak expiratory flow should be >75% of best/predicted and diurnal peak flow variability should be <25%. Variability is taken to be the highest peak expiratory flow value minus the lowest value divided by *either* the highest or average value. A respiratory physician may agree discharge before these criteria are met, and may accept peak flow stability in lieu of achieving these peak flow targets.

Some patients should have longer-term specialist respiratory follow-up. Patients admitted with severe asthma should have specialist follow up for a least one year, and those admitted with near-fatal or brittle asthma should remain under specialist supervision indefinitely.

British Thoracic Society/Scottish Intercollegiate Guidelines Network. Guideline 141, British Guideline on the Management of Asthma, October 2014. http://www.brit-thoracic.org.uk; http://www.sign.ac.uk

15. E. Reduce the inspired oxygen to 28%

The patient has acute on chronic type 2 respiratory failure, and should be given controlled oxygen therapy (24–28% FiO_2), while continuing with nebulized bronchodilators. If the pCO_2 fails to improve despite appropriate oxygen administration then non-invasive ventilation (NIV) would be appropriate.

His respiratory drive is adequate; the rise seen in the pCO_2 when excessive oxygen is administered is due to attenuation of the (useful) hypoxic pulmonary vasoconstriction which diverts blood from damaged emphysematous areas to less damaged parts of the lungs. The aim should be to maintain oxygen saturations between 88–92%.

Roberts M, Young K, Plant P et al. The use of non-invasive ventilation in the management of patients with chronic obstructive pulmonary disease admitted to hospital with acute type II respiratory failure. British Thoracic Society/Royal College of Physicians of London/Intensive Care Society Guidelines 2008.

16. D. Observations should be made every 15 minutes for the first hour

Observations should be performed every 15 minutes for the first hour, then every 30 minutes between 1–4 hours, then hourly between 4–12 hours. They should include patient comfort, chest wall movement, accessory muscle use, and ventilator synchrony, as well as standard observations.

Arterial blood gases should be performed one hour after commencement of NIV, and one hour after any adjustment. If improving then repeat blood gases should be taken at four hours.

The patient should have continuous pulse oximetry and electrocardiography for the first 12 hours.

Hypoxia on NIV is ideally improved by optimizing pressure support rather than increasing FiO_2. Aim for oxygen saturations on NIV of 88–92%.

NIV should be started at IPAP 10 cm H_2O, EPAP 4–5 cm H_2O. The IPAP should be increased by 2–5 cm H_2O at a rate of around 5 cm H_2O over ten minutes with a target pressure of 20 cm H_2O.

Roberts M, Young K, Plant P et al. The use of non-invasive ventilation in the management of patients with chronic obstructive pulmonary disease admitted to hospital with acute type II respiratory failure. British Thoracic Society/Royal College of Physicians of London/Intensive Care Society Guidelines 2008. http://www.brit-thoracic.org.uk

17. C. 30-day mortality of around 9%

His CURB-65 score is 2.
- Confusion (AMT 8 or less) = 0
- Urea (> 7 mmol/L) = 1
- Respiratory rate (≥30) = 0
- SBP (<90mmHg), DBP (60 mmHg) = 0
- Age (≥65) = 1

All patients admitted with community-acquired pneumonia should have their CURB-65 score calculated on admission. The score predicts (on average) the 30-day mortality rate:

- Score 0–1   (low severity)   <3% mortality at 30 days
- Score 2   (moderate severity)   9% mortality at 30 days
- Score 3–5   (high severity)   15–40% mortality at 30 days

Patients scoring 0 or 1 may be suitable for oral antibiotic treatment at home. Patients scoring 4 or 5 should be considered for admission to a high dependency or intensive care unit.

Adapted from *Thorax*, WS Lim et al., 'Defining community acquired pneumonia severity on presentation to hospital: an international derivation and validation study', 58, 5, pp. 377–382, Copyright 2003, with permission from BMJ Publishing Group Ltd.

Lim W, Baudouin S, George R et al. British Thoracic Society Guidelines for the Management of Community Acquired Pneumonia in Adults: 2009 Update. Thorax 2009; 64(3): iii1–55. doi: 10.1136/thx.2009.121434. http://www.brit-thoracic.org.uk

Lim W, Smith D, Wise M et al. British Thoracic Society community acquired pneumonia guideline and the NICE pneumonia guideline: how they fit together. Thorax 2015; 0: 1–3. doi:10.1136/thoraxjnl-2015-206881.

18. E. Levofloxacin

Fluroquinolones (such as levofloxacin) are recommended first-line treatment for low and moderate severity legionella pneumonia. In high-severity or life-threatening legionella pneumonia (Legionnaire's disease) a macrolide (such as azithromycin) can be added for the first few days. There is a risk of cardiac electrophysiological abnormalities with quinolone-macrolide combinations.

Erythromycin was historically used to treat legionella pneumonia; however, newer macrolides and fluroquinolones appear more active, with fluroquinolones being favoured in the latest BTS guidelines.

If legionella is confirmed by urine antigen testing then the Health Protection Agency should be notified and sputum samples should be sent for culture specifically looking for legionella to provide isolates for epidemiological typing.

Pontiac fever is due to legionella infection and causes fever, headaches, and muscle aches but not pneumonia. It usually resolves spontaneously within a few days and antibiotics are not required.

There are no documented cases of Legionnaires' disease associated with person-to-person transmission.

Lim W, Baudouin S, George R et al. British Thoracic Society Guidelines for the Management of Community Acquired Pneumonia in Adults: 2009 Update. Thorax 2009; 64(3): iii1–55. doi: 10.1136/thx.2009.121434. http://www.brit-thoracic.org.uk

Lim W, Smith D, Wise M et al. British Thoracic Society community acquired pneumonia guideline and the NICE pneumonia guideline: how they fit together. Thorax 2015; 0: 1–3. doi:10.1136/thoraxjnl-2015-206881.

19. B. Chest X-ray, full blood count, serum calcium, liver function tests, and urinalysis

The latest NICE guideline suggests that all patients diagnosed with unprovoked DVT or PE who are not already known to have cancer should routinely receive a chest X-ray, full blood count, serum calcium, liver function tests, and urinalysis. These tests detect cancer in 9–10% of patients with a first episode of unprovoked VTE with no prior cancer diagnosis. Over the next two years an additional 11–12% of patients are diagnosed with cancer.

An abdomino-pelvic CT scan (and a mammogram for women) should be considered in all patients aged over 40 years with a first unprovoked DVT or PE who do not have signs or symptoms of cancer based on initial routine tests. Sensitivity for picking up cancer was >90%.

Optimum anticoagulation form and duration for patients whose VTE is provoked by cancer is different than for patients that don't have cancer. It is based largely on this fact that the latest guidelines suggest that more intensive investigation for an underlying cancer is worthwhile and leads to a significant reduction in VTE recurrence rates. Early diagnosis of underlying cancer may also lead to diagnosis at an earlier curative stage and improvement in cancer-related mortality.

National Institute for Health and Care Excellence. Clinical Guideline 144. Venous thromboembolic diseases: diagnosis, management and thrombophilia testing. June 2012.

20. D. Low molecular weight heparin for six months then reassess risks/benefits of anticoagulation

Low molecular weight heparin (LMWH) should be offered to all patients with active cancer and confirmed proximal DVT or PE, and continued for six months. At six months the risks and benefits of continuing anticoagulation should be reassessed. In patients with cancer, the evidence suggests that anticoagulation for six months with LMWH leads to better outcomes compared with using a vitamin K antagonist (VKA) after initial LMWH treatment. It is unknown whether continuing with LMWH beyond six months is superior to VKA or not.

'Active cancer' means receiving active anti-mitotic treatment; being diagnosed within last six months; recurrent or metastatic cancer; or where the cancer is inoperable.

National Institute for Health and Care Excellence. Clinical Guideline 144. Venous thromboembolic diseases: diagnosis, management and thrombophilia testing. June 2012.

21. C. The patient should be admitted to a negative pressure room immediately and staff and visitors should wear FFP3 masks for brief visits/consultations

Tuberculosis (TB) is not spread through utensils, handshakes, or toilet seats. MDR TB (Multidrug-resistant TB) means that the TB is resistant to both isoniazid and rifampicin.

Before discharging a patient with MDR TB, their case should be discussed with the infection control team, the local microbiologist, the TB service, and the consultant in communicable disease control.

National Institute for Health and Care Excellence. Clinical Guideline 117. Tuberculosis: Clinical diagnosis and management for tuberculosis, and measures for its prevention and control. March 2011.

22. C. Nebulized adrenaline 5–10 mL of 1:10,000 may be used

Definitions of massive haemoptysis vary between >100 mL to >600 mL in 24 hours.

Nebulized adrenaline 5–10 mL of 1:10,000 can be used, or delivered directly at bronchoscopy to the bleeding area. The bleeding is usually from a bronchial artery.

Common causes of massive haemoptysis include bronchiectasis, aspergilloma, TB, endobronchial cancer, and trauma. Death from haemoptysis is usually due to asphyxia rather than exsanguination. The patient should be managed on their side with bleeding lung in the dependent position to keep the unaffected lung clear. A single lumen endotracheal tube may be introduced into either main bronchus to protect the unaffected side. Double lumen tubes may be used where local expertise is available—these lumens are smaller and may block with blood. Surgery in the setting of massive haemoptysis has a reported mortality of 20–30%.

Du Rand I, Blaikley J, Booton R et al. British Thoracic Society guideline for diagnostic flexible bronchoscopy in adults. Thorax 2013; 68: i1–i44. doi:10.1136/thoraxjnl-2013–203618. http://www.brit-thoracic.org.uk

23. C. 200 micrograms over 15 seconds with further 100 microgram doses up to 1 mg total

200 micrograms over 15 seconds with further 100 microgram doses every minute up to 1 mg total is the correct dosing. A total of up to 2 mg may be given if on an intensive care unit.

UK National Poisons Information Service. Guideline for benzodiazepine poisoning. Commissioned by Public Health England. http://www.toxbase.org

24. B. Pneumococcal polysaccharide vaccination of patients over 65 does prevent invasive pneumococcal disease

Pneumococcal polysaccharide vaccination of patients over 65 is effective in preventing invasive pneumococcal disease. The efficacy is approximately 40–70% but decreases with age.

Smoking is associated with developing community-acquired pneumonia. All patients should be offered smoking cessation advice.

National Institute for Health and Care Excellence. Clinical Guideline 101. Chronic obstructive pulmonary disease in over 16s: diagnosis and management. June 2010.

25. A. If he has Legionella pneumonia radiological resolution is likely to be slower than average

The yield from routine microbiological tests including sputum and blood cultures is less than 15% for patients with non-severe community acquired pneumonia. In the UK, 11–13% of patients with CAP have viral pneumonia (mostly influenza A).

Klebsiella pneumoniae characteristically affects the upper lobes, can cause cavitation, and may present with thick, blood-stained sputum—so-called currant jelly sputum. Mycoplasma pneumoniae typically affects patients younger than 40 years.

Lim W, Baudouin S, George R et al. British Thoracic Society Guideline for the Management of Community Acquired Pneumonia in Adults: 2009 Update. Thorax 2009; 64(3): iii1–55. doi: 10.1136/thx.2009.121434. http://www.brit-thoracic.org.uk

Lim W, Smith D, Wise M et al. British Thoracic Society community acquired pneumonia guideline and the NICE pneumonia guideline: how they fit together. Thorax 2015; 0: 1–3. doi:10.1136/thoraxjnl-2015-206881.

RESPIRATORY | ANSWERS

26. B. IgE RAST to aspergillus

The chest X-ray and CT scan (Figures 3.3 and 3.4) demonstrate bronchiectasis. Autoimmune studies are not helpful in the investigation or management of bronchiectasis. Serum immunoglobulins to exclude hypogammaglobulinaemia should be checked.

Allergic bronchopulmonary aspergillosis (ABPA) should be considered. Patients with ABPA typically have symptoms of asthma, bronchiectasis, blood eosinophilia more than 10%, a total serum IgE >1000 ng/mL, positive skin prick testing to Aspergillus fumigatus, and a positive aspergillus-specific IgE RAST test. Management focuses on suppressing the immune reaction to the fungus with oral prednisolone and sometimes using itraconazole.

Pasteur C, Bilton D, Hill A. British Thoracic Society Guideline for non-CF Bronchiectasis. Thorax 2010; 65(1). http://www.brit-thoracic.org.uk

27. D. Fusobacterium necrophorum

This patient has most of the signs and symptoms of Lemierre's disease. Eighty percent of cases are caused by Fusobacterium necrophorum, and a further 10% by other Fusobacterium species. The infection typically starts in the pharynx and spreads through to the jugular vein where an infected thrombus forms, causing local pain and inflammation. Septic emboli break off from this thrombus and can cause lung abscesses and septic infarctions, as well as sometimes causing joint, liver, renal, and nervous system infections. Fusobacterium necrophorum is usually sensitive to penicillin-derived antibiotics combined with a beta-lactamase inhibitor.

Eilbert W, Singla N. Lemierre's syndrome. International Journal of Emergency Medicine 2013; 6: 40. doi: 10.1186/1865-1380-6-40

28. E. Nebulized recombinant human DNase

Nebulized recombinant human DNase has not shown any benefit in patients with non-cystic fibrosis bronchiectasis. It appeared to worsen the decline in lung function and exacerbations in studies.

An outpatient trial of nebulized Colomycin -2 mega units twice daily, may be helpful for patients chronically infected with Pseudomonas who experience exacerbations to see if it improves their symptoms and exacerbation frequency. Once chronically infected with Pseudomonas, management focuses on controlling the infection rather than eradication, which is practically impossible.

Pasteur C, Bilton D, Hill A. British Thoracic Society guideline for non-CF Bronchiectasis. Thorax 2010; 65(1). http://www.brit-thoracic.org.uk

29. B. Sputum purulence is a reliable indicator of the presence of bacteria

Pathogenic bacteria will be isolated from approximately 50% of patients with moderate–severe COPD during an exacerbation. Many patients have the same species isolated from their sputum when they are well. The bacteria have colonized their lungs but may very well not be causing the exacerbation. When studied, viruses are also commonly isolated at the time of an exacerbation. For both these reasons antibiotics are often ineffective.

Peak flow measurements will be consistently low and of no real help in assessing progress.

Most guidelines recommend 10–14 days of 30–40 mg prednisolone without tapering.

National Institute for Health and Care Excellence. Clinical Guideline 101. Chronic obstructive pulmonary disease in over 16s: diagnosis and management. June 2010.

30. B. Eosinophilic granulomatosis with polyangiitis (Churg Strauss syndrome)

The chest X-ray (Figure 3.5) shows 2 areas of opacification on the right side and loss of the right hemi diaphragm border (and an endo-tracheal tube). The most likely diagnosis is eosinophilic granulomatosis with polyangiitis (eosinophilic granulomatosis with polyangiitis-EGPA), which tends to progress through three phases: atopy (asthma, rhinitis, sinusitis), eosinophilia >10% (often with pulmonary infiltrates), and necrotizing multi-system small vessel vasculitis. Neurological examination, urine dipstick and 24-hour protein collection, ECG, and echocardiogram as an initial screen for vasculitic involvement at this point is indicated.

pANCA (MPO predominant) is positive in 40–70% of patients with EGPA.

pANCA (MPO predominant) is positive in up to 90% of patients with microscopic polyangiitis; these patients tend to have diffuse alveolar haemorrhage rather than ENT or asthma symptoms.

cANCA (PR-3 predominant) is positive in up to 90% of patients with granulomatosis with polyangiitis (Wegener's syndrome); asthma does not tend to feature.

High-resolution CT of chest typically shows multiple non-segmental consolidation. Ground glass changes and interlobular septal thickening and nodules may be seen.

National Institute for Health and Care Excellence. Clinical Guideline 163. Idiopathic Pulmonary Fibrosis. June 2013.

31. D. Non-specific interstitial pneumonia

For patients who have a 'chronic cough' (i.e. lasting >eight weeks) without any obvious cause and a normal chest X-ray, then the most common causes are: gastro-oesophageal reflux disease (acid or non-acid), 'asthma syndromes' (cough variant asthma and eosinophillic bronchitis), and rhinitis.

Cough variant asthma is a subgroup of asthma in which spirometry may also be normal but bronchial hyper-responsiveness can be demonstrated (e.g. using methacholine challenge). Approximately half of these patients also have eosinophillic bronchitis.

Eosinophilic bronchitis can occur without the bronchial hyper-reactivity seen in asthma.

Non-specific interstitial pneumonia (NSIP) is one of the interstitial idiopathic pneumonias (IIPs) and is relatively rare with prevalence ranging from 1–3/100,000. It can cause cough and breathlessness often with only a mild basal opacification on plain chest X-ray; crackles are often heard on auscultation.

Morice A, McGarvey L, Pavord I. British Thoracic Society recommendations for the management of cough in adults. Thorax 2006;61(Suppl I):i1–i24. doi: 10.1136/thx.2006.065144. http://www.brit-thoracic.org.uk

National Institute for Health and Care Excellence. Clinical Guideline 163. Idiopathic Pulmonary Fibrosis. June 2013.

32. B. He has acute respiratory distress syndrome

The chest X-ray (Figure 3.6) shows diffuse bilateral coalescent opacities in a typical pulmonary oedema pattern. Acute respiratory distress syndrome was redefined in 2012 using the Berlin criteria.

Changes from the previous 1994 AECC (American European Consensus Conference) definition are that the term acute lung injury has been abandoned in favour of the new severity categorization, radiographic criteria were changed and pulmonary capillary wedge pressure criteria were removed.

ARDS can be mild (PaO2/FiO2 26.7–40 kPa, mortality 27%), moderate (paO2/FiO2 13.3–26.7 kPa, mortality 32%) or severe (PaO2/FiO2 <13.3 kPa, mortality 45%) A low tidal volume ventilation strategy which minimizes lung injury appears to be beneficial (ARDS Network Trial). Inhaled nitric oxide improves oxygenation but there is no evidence of mortality benefit.

The ARDS Definition Task Force. Acute respiratory distress syndrome: the Berlin definition. Journal of the American Medical Association 2012; 307(23): 2526–2533.

33. A. The chance that this is due to lung cancer is approximately 6%

Smokers over the age of 40 with haemoptysis and a normal chest X-ray should be investigated with a CT scan of chest and bronchoscopy, usually as an outpatient. Approximately 6% of this group will have lung cancer.

Overall, lung cancer accounts for 30% of patients with haemoptysis; the majority of these have an abnormal chest X-ray.

National Institute for Health and Care Excellence. Clinical Guideline 121. Lung cancer: diagnosis and management. April 2011.

34. E. Pleural fluid adenosine deaminase (ADA) levels are usually raised in tuberculous pleurisy

Lidocaine is acidic, so contamination will lower the pH of the sample.

Rheumatoid effusions typically have low pH and glucose levels, and frequently resolve spontaneously; often 2–3 months of non-steroidal anti-inflammatories are used. A pleural fluid glucose of >1.6 mmol/L makes rheumatoid disease unlikely as the aetiology. Empyema and rheumatoid disease cause low pleural glucose levels.

Malignancy and tuberculosis commonly cause lymphocyte predominant effusions. Although not tested routinely pleural fluid adenosine deaminase levels are raised (>40 IU/L) in pleural tuberculosis; low levels virtually excluding tuberculosis as a cause.

Hooper C, Lee Y, Maskell N. Investigation of a Unilateral Pleural Effusion in Adults. British Thoracic Society Pleural Disease Guideline. Thorax 2010; 65(2). http://www.brit-thoracic.org.uk

35. D. Oral Gastrografin is not recommended

The abdominal X-ray (Figure 3.7) is consistent with small bowel obstruction. The patient has distal intestinal obstruction syndrome (DIOS), which only occurs in patients with cystic fibrosis (CF), and is relatively common (10–20% prevalence). It can often be successfully treated with oral gastrografin. The incidence increases with age, and is more common in adults than children. Mucofaeculant material impacts in the terminal ileum, caecum, and ascending colon causing colicky abdominal pain, nausea, signs of small bowel obstruction, and a tender mass in the right iliac fossa. Inadequate pancreatic enzyme replacement leads to fat malabsorption which contributes, but is not the only factor, in developing the condition.

Laxatives as mentioned in the question can be used; additionally, oral N-acetylcysteine (as a mucolytic) may be beneficial.

Local or systemic inflammation should prompt investigations to exclude appendicitis or extra-uterine pregnancy. Surgery is a last resort, which carries high post-operative mortality.

Somaraju UR, Solis-Moya A. Pancreatic enzyme replacement therapy for people with cystic fibrosis. Cochrane Database of Systematic Reviews 2014, Issue 10. Art. No.: CD008227. DOI: 10.1002/14651858.CD008227.pub2.

36. C. Her gas transfer would be normal on pulmonary function testing

Coughing, hoarseness, breathlessness, and difficulty swallowing can all be symptoms due a large goitre. On pulmonary function testing, peak expiratory flow rate (PEFR) best reflects large airway calibre. There should be a proportionally larger reduction in PEFR than forced expiratory volume in 1 second (FEV_1) when there is upper airway obstruction. The Empey Index is the FEV_1 (in mL)/PEFR (in L/min). A normal value is <10. A value of >10 implies upper-airway obstruction. Obstructive sleep apnoea can occur with a large goitre resulting in excessive daytime sleepiness. Gas transfer will be normal assuming there are no other diseases and she is able to inspire to her normal vital capacity.

West, J. Respiratory physiology, the essentials. Eighth edn. Lippincott Williams and Wilkins, 2008.

37. D. Smoking and alcohol consumption are associated with OSAHS

The Epworth Sleepiness Scale consists of eight questions regarding the subjective likelihood of falling asleep in a given situation. A score of 10 or more implies excessive sleepiness.

Uvulopalatopharyngoplasty (UPPP) is not recommended as a treatment for obstructive sleep apnoea/hypopnoea syndrome (OSAHS).

Typically in patients with OSAHS the throat muscles relax as normal during stage 3–4 sleep (deep, refreshing sleep); the airway narrows to the point of either complete collapse (causing an apnoea) or becomes severely narrowed (causing an effortful hypopnoea); the effort to breathe against a closed or narrow airway eventually causes an arousal waking the patient up to stage 1–2 sleep (light, unrefreshing sleep); the muscle tone (and airway calibre) improves so air flow recommences with a loud gasp; the patient soon slips back into deep sleep, and the cycle continues. Disruption of deep sleep usually causes excessive daytime sleepiness.

When the patient's airway is compromised their oxygen saturation (often) slowly falls by more than 4%, then rises suddenly back to baseline once arousal lightens sleep and muscle tone improves opening the airway. This change in saturation is not always seen (particularly in young, thin patients), so a normal oximetry study does not rule out OSAHS.

Usually, OSAHS is due to the normal throat muscle relaxation combined with excessive neck weight; sometimes, however, the throat muscles simply become excessively relaxed during deep sleep in a patient of normal weight. Alcohol exacerbates the reduction in throat muscle tone. Smoking can cause throat inflammation contributing to the narrowed airway. Nocturia, decreased libido, and irritability can all be features of OSAHS.

National Institute for Health and Care Excellence. Technology Appraisal 139. Continuous positive airway pressure for the treatment of obstructive sleep apnoea/hypopnoea syndrome. March 2008. http://www.sleep-apnoea-trust.org.

38. A. Anti-tuberculosis treatment should be started before anti-retrovirals

In this scenario it is very likely that the patient has tuberculosis (TB) (rather than an alternative mycobacteria); she comes from a high-risk demographic and has both symptoms and X-ray appearances consistent with TB. Further confirmatory early morning sputum samples should be sent off, and she should start on empirical TB treatment pending culture results (which may take up to eight weeks).

Standard treatment is a four-drug regimen: rifampicin, isoniazid, pyrazinamide, and ethambutol for 2 months, followed by a continuation phase of rifampicin and isoniazid for a further four months. These should be given as combination tablets to improve compliance and prevent resistance to individual drugs developing.

$$\text{Rifater} = \text{Rifampicin} + \text{Isoniazid} + \text{Pyrazinamide}$$
$$\text{Rifinah} = \text{Rifampicin} + \text{Isoniazid}$$

Patients who cough are considered infectious until completing two weeks of treatment.

If admitted, patients should be nursed in a side room with good ventilation and not allowed onto the open ward until three sputum samples are smear negative.

Starting anti-TB treatment takes precedence over anti-retrovirals. Pyridoxine 10 mg once daily may be added to her treatment regimen due to the increased risk of peripheral neuropathy with HIV and anti-TB medication. Starting anti-retrovirals first would increase the risk of immune reconstitution inflammatory syndrome.

Ideally, patients with TB should be managed as an outpatient. Having TB is not a reason to admit. TB should be treated by a specialist physician (usually respiratory physician) with experience in managing TB.

Pozniak AL, Coyne KM, Mille RF et al. British HIV Association guidelines for the treatment of TB/HIV co-infection 2011. HIV Medicine 2011; 12: 517–524. doi: 10.1111/j.1468–1293.2011.00954.x

39. D. Percutaneous cervical cordotomy at C1/C2 is an option for pain management

Primary peritoneal mesothelioma commonly causes ascites, abdominal metastases from pleural mesothelioma is a less common, but still seen, cause of ascites.

Unfortunately, severe chest pain is common. Mesothelioma commonly presents with chest pain and breathlessness either due to an associated (usually blood-stained) pleural effusion or due to encasement of the lung. An indwelling pleural catheter can be used to manage to the recurrent effusion. If the diagnosis is made by biopsy at thoracoscopy or Video-assisted thoracoscopic surgery (VATS) then a surgical pleurodesis or talc podrage may be undertaken at the same time.

For refractory pain a percutaneous cervical cordotomy at C1/C2 level which causes contralateral loss of pain sensation can be very effective.

No therapies currently offer a cure. Radiotherapy may be helpful for localized pain (e.g. from bone invasion). Combination chemotherapy may provide approximately three months' survival advantage.

British Thoracic Society Standards of Care Committee. BTS statement on malignant mesothelioma in the UK. Thorax 2007; 62: ii1–ii19. doi: 10.1136/thx.2007.087619

40. D. On average, for every five users treated with varenicline one more would be abstinent at end of treatment than if those same people were treated with placebo

Number needed to treat (NNT) is constructed as a measure of the benefit from treatment with the intervention compared to the control for a clinical trial. NNT is sometimes referred to as number needed to treat to benefit (NNTB). In the trial above, the rate of abstinence was higher in the varenicline group than for the placebo group. The NNT of five reflects the benefit of treatment with varenicline compared with placebo. On average if five patients were treated with varenicline then one *additional* patient will benefit (i.e. be abstinent) at the end of treatment than if those same people had been treated with placebo (see Sedgwick & Joekes, 2014; Sedgwick, 2015a).

At the end of treatment, 59% of the varenicline treatment group achieved abstinence compared to 39% of the placebo group. Therefore, the varenicline group demonstrated an increase of 20% in abstinence compared to placebo. Hence, if 100 users of smokeless tobacco were treated with varenicline there would be 20 more achieving abstinence than if those same users had been treated with placebo. Hence, on average, five users need to be treated with varenicline for one more user to benefit than if those same five users had been treated with placebo. More generally, NNT is calculated as the reciprocal of the absolute risk difference between the treatment groups in the outcome of complete abstinence. In statistics, risk is an alternative name for probability or proportion. The risk difference between treatments was 0.20. Hence, NNT=$1 \div 0.20 = 5$.

When using NNT to describe the benefit of varenicline compared with placebo, it is important that the absolute rates of continuous abstinence for the varenicline and placebo groups are presented. In particular, an NNT of five could have been achieved with different trial results but so long as the difference between treatment groups in percentage continuous abstinence was 20% in favour of varenicline. However, if the rate of abstinence was 99% for the varenicline treatment group and 79% for the placebo group, it would no doubt have a different significance for the clinician and patient if the rate of abstinence was, for example, 29% for the varenicline treatment group and 9% for the placebo group.

NNT is a measure of the benefit of treatment with the intervention (varenicline) compared to control (placebo). If the intervention caused harm—for example, resulted in more side effects than placebo, or an inferior rate of abstinence—then the measure number needed to harm (NNH) would be used to reflect the harm caused by treatment (see Sedgwick, 2015b).

As a measure of the benefit of treatment, NNT is a comparative statement of the effectiveness of intervention (varenicline) with control (placebo) as described above. However, the comparator treatment is often not stated when interpreting NNT resulting in a misleading statement about the effectiveness of intervention. For example, the statement that 'five users need to be treated with varenicline for one person to be abstinent at end of treatment' implies for every five users treated with varenicline, one will benefit (achieve abstinence) and four will not. This is obviously an incorrect interpretation of NNT and the benefit of treatment with varenicline since at the end of the treatment, 59% of the varenicline treatment group had achieved abstinence; hence, approximately three out of five users of varenicline achieved abstinence.

Sedgwick P, Joekes K. Randomised controlled trials: evaluating and communicating treatment effects. *BMJ* 2014; 348: g1905.

Sedgwick P. Measuring the benefit of treatment: number needed to treat. *BMJ* 2015a; 350: h2206.

Sedgwick P. Measuring the detriment of treatment: number needed to harm. *BMJ* 2015b: 350: h2763.

chapter 4

CARDIOLOGY

QUESTIONS

1. A 66-year-old man with a 20-pack year history of smoking was admitted with a two-hour history of central chest pain. He had never had this pain before. His 12-lead ECG showed ST depression of 2 mm in the anterior leads. He was not taking any medications and had not been to his GP for ten years. He was adopted when he was three years old.

    Based on this information, what is his TIMI risk of death and further ischaemic events at 14 days?
    A. 4.7% risk
    B. 8.3% risk
    C. 13.2% risk
    D. 19.9% risk
    E. 26.2% risk

2. A 72-year-old woman was admitted to the acute medical unit with central chest pain. She described the pain as similar to her previous myocardial infarction five weeks ago. On further questioning she stated that she had a stent in the 'right side of her heart'. The ECG confirmed ST elevation in II, III, and aVF. She was taking aspirin, clopidogrel, ramipril, and simvastatin.

    What would you prescribe for the patient prior to coronary angiography?
    A. Aspirin 300 mg and clopidogrel 300 mg
    B. Aspirin 300 mg and prasugrel 10 mg
    C. Aspirin 300 mg and prasugrel 60 mg
    D. Aspirin 300 mg only
    E. No loading required

3. An 82-year-old man was admitted to the acute medical unit with a five-day history of intermittent chest pain consistent with unstable angina. His ECG demonstrated T wave inversion in the lateral leads with worsening ST depression when compared with his initial ECG.

On examination, his heart rate was 80 beats per minute and regular and his blood pressure was 135/70 mmHg. He still had chest pain. He was admitted to the coronary care unit after being given aspirin 300 mg, clopidogrel 600 mg, bisoprolol 2.5 mg, and fondaparinux 2.5 mg subcutaneously.

What would be the best drug option to assist in the management of this patient?

A. Simvastatin
B. Tenecteplase
C. Ticagrelor
D. Tirofiban
E. Unfractionated heparin

4. A 58-year-old woman was admitted to the acute medical unit with fever, malaise, and anorexia for the last 48 hours. On examination, she had a temperature of 39.0°C, was haemodynamically stable, and had a pansystolic murmur. The rest of her examination was unremarkable. Her blood tests demonstrated a normochromic normocytic anaemia, leucocytosis, and raised inflammatory markers. Blood cultures were positive. An echocardiogram was arranged.

What is the most likely organism causing this infection?

A. Diptheroids
B. Enterococci
C. Gram negative bacilli
D. Staphylococci
E. Streptococci

5. A 52-year-old man was admitted to the acute medical unit after feeling unwell for 12 hours and complaining of palpitations. An ECG confirmed atrial fibrillation (AF) with a rate of 135 beats per minute. His blood pressure was 115/70 mmHg. His cardiovascular and respiratory examinations were otherwise normal. He did not smoke and was on no medications. On further questioning, he admitted to excessive alcohol consumption two nights previously at his wife's 50th birthday party.

What is your first line of approach?

A. Amiodarone
B. DC cardioversion
C. Flecainide
D. Metoprolol
E. Sotalol

6. **A 51-year-old man attended the ambulatory care clinic for review of the results of his CT calcium scoring. He had been investigated for numerous episodes of recurrent ischaemic-sounding chest pain on exerting himself. His ECG was unremarkable. His CT calcium score was 520.**

   What would be the next investigation?
   A. Coronary angiography
   B. Exercise tolerance test
   C. Myocardial perfusion imaging
   D. Reassurance, no further investigation warranted
   E. Sixty-four slice CT coronary angiogram

7. **A worried foundation doctor showed you an ECG that she was concerned about. The patient had been admitted with episodes of dizziness but was otherwise well. He was haemodynamically stable.**

   Investigations:

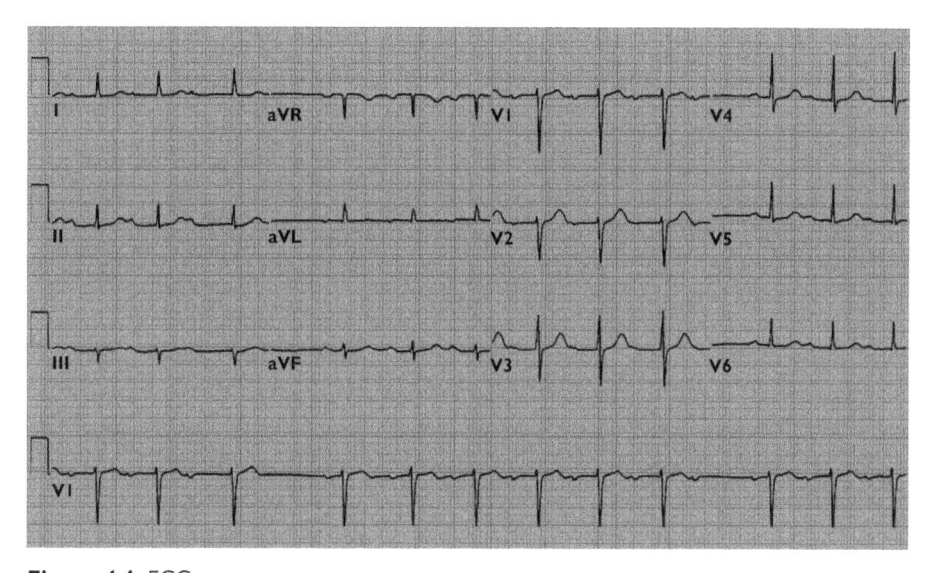

   Figure 4.1 ECG.

   What is the most likely diagnosis?
   A. Atrial fibrillation
   B. First-degree heart block
   C. Second-degree heart block—Mobitz type 1
   D. Second-degree heart block—Mobitz type 2
   E. Third-degree heart block

8. A 35-year-old man admitted to the acute medical unit with collapse was concerned when telling you his history on the post take ward round that he had recently started a new medication for palpitations. He had read on the Internet that some drugs can cause a prolonged QT and this ran in his family. So far he had not been diagnosed with prolonged QT syndrome.

   Which of the following drugs does not cause a prolonged QT interval?
   A. Amiodarone
   B. Dipyridamole
   C. Disopyramide
   D. Quinindine
   E. Sotalol

9. A 62-year-old man was admitted from the community with an anterior STEMI to the local district general hospital. He complained of severe chest pain before his wife rang for help. She noted he was clammy and sweaty. About five minutes after being transferred into the emergency department a student nurse pointed out that the patient looked unwell and appeared grey. The cardiac monitor showed a broad complex tachycardia. His femoral pulse was palpable and his blood pressure was 76/36 mmHg.

   What would be your next approach?
   A. Adrenaline
   B. Amiodarone
   C. DC cardioversion
   D. Start CPR
   E. Transfer to tertiary centre for immediate PCI

10. A 70-year-old woman was admitted to the acute medical unit after a collapse. The admitting junior doctor suspected an arrhythmia and showed you her ECG.

    Which of the following is not an indication when considering temporary transvenous pacing?
    A. Mobitz type 1
    B. Mobitz type 2
    C. Third-degree heart block with a broad QRS complex
    D. Ventricular standstill of 6 s
    E. Ventricular standstill of 10 s

11. A 66-year-old woman presented to the emergency department with a 36-hour history of increasing breathlessness and palpitations. She had recently completed a course of antibiotics for a chest infection. She denied any chest pain. She was a current smoker and had a 40-pack year smoking history.

On examination, her pulse was 136 beats per minute and irregularly irregular, blood pressure was 90/50 mmHg, respiratory rate was 20, and oxygen saturation was 92% on air. She had a hyper-expanded chest with wheeze throughout both lung fields. She appeared euthyroid.

```
Investigations:
```

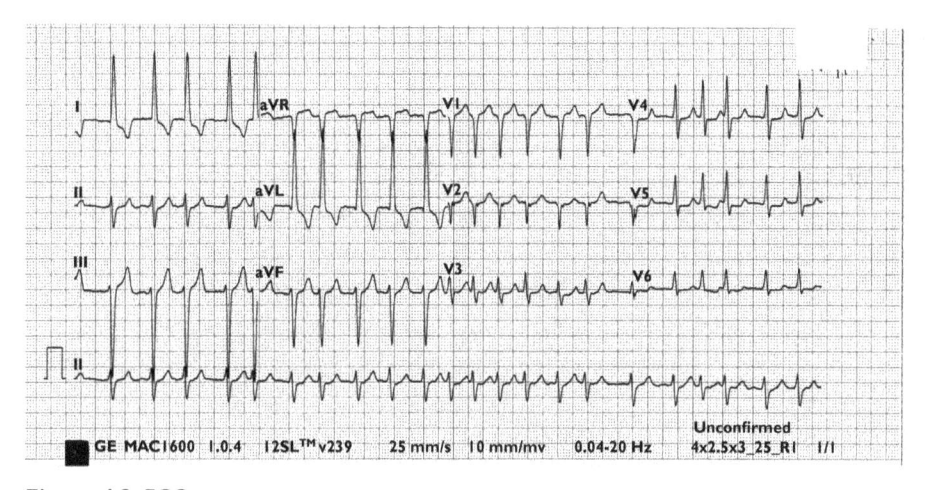

Figure 4.2 ECG.

```
chest X-ray: hyper-expanded lung fields, no focal
  consolidation
```

What is the best management strategy?
A. Antibiotics for community-acquired pneumonia
B. Anticoagulation and delay rhythm control for three weeks
C. Rate control with a ß-adrenoceptor blocker
D. Rate control with a rate-limiting calcium channel blocker
E. Rhythm control with heparin cover

CARDIOLOGY | QUESTIONS

12. A 37-year-old man was admitted to the acute medical unit with fever and malaise. He had a patent ductus arteriosus closed as a child. He was a veterinary surgeon. On examination, he looked flushed. He was pyrexial at 38.1°C, his pulse was 95 beats per minute and regular, and blood pressure was 110/60 mmHg. He had generalized muscle tenderness, red painless spots on his palms and soles, and signs of recent weight loss. No cardiac murmurs were heard.

```
Investigations:
    serum C-reactive protein:   238 mg/L   (<10)
    blood culture: coxiella burnetii
```

What is the most appropriate next step in management?
A. Further blood cultures should be taken prior to starting antibiotics
B. If the transthoracic echocardiogram is normal then transoesophageal echocardiography is needed
C. Transthoracic echocardiogram should be performed prior to starting antibiotics
D. Treatment for infective endocarditis should not be started until there are two positive blood cultures 12 hours apart
E. Treatment for infective endocarditis should start immediately as the diagnostic criteria have been met

13. An 84-year-old woman was on the coronary care unit having had a temporary pacing wire inserted for complete heart block two days ago. The nursing staff had checked the temporary wire and the threshold was 3 V.

What is the best course of action?
A. Reposition the temporary wire immediately
B. Set the output to 1.5 V
C. Set the output to 3 V
D. Set the output to 6 V
E. Set the sensitivity to 3 V

14. A 56-year-old woman presented to the acute medical unit with chest pain. She had been experiencing episodes of chest pain over the last few weeks; they were typically brought on by exercise and relieved by rest. She described the pain as tightness across the front of her chest. She had no significant past medical history and was a non-smoker. Her risk of having coronary artery disease was estimated at 38%.

What is the best test to evaluate the possibility of coronary artery disease?
A. CT calcium scoring
B. CT coronary angiography
C. Exercise tolerance test
D. Invasive coronary angiography
E. Myocardial perfusion scan

15. A 54-year-old woman was referred to the acute medical unit with severe chest pain. The pain was central and radiated through to the back. She had a history of hypertension and a 20-pack year smoking history. On examination, she had a pulse rate of 92 beats per minute and blood pressure of 170/90 mmHg. Cardiovascular and respiratory examination was normal.

Investigations:

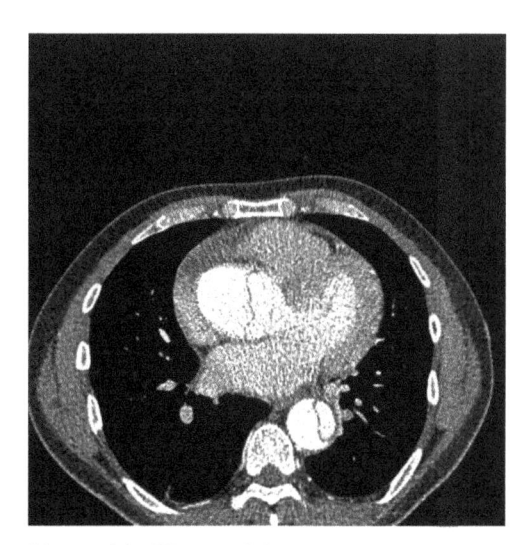

Figure 4.3 CT scan of chest.

```
D-dimer      500 mg/L    (<0.5)
troponin T   50 ng/L     (<14)

chest X-ray: normal

ECG: sinus rhythm, no ischaemia
```

What treatment is needed?
A. ACE inhibitor
B. Clopidogrel
C. Low molecular weight heparin
D. Percutaneous coronary intervention
E. Urgent surgery

CARDIOLOGY | QUESTIONS

16. A 45-year-old man was referred to the acute medical unit from his optician. He had gone to have his eyes tested because he was getting headaches. The optician had found bilateral papilloedema.

On examination, his pulse rate was 70 beats per minute and blood pressure was 240/130 mmHg. His heart sounds were normal and he had bilateral crepitations on chest examination. Abdominal examination was normal.

```
Investigations:
    haemoglobin:          140 g/L            (130-180)
    white cell count:     6.7 × 10⁹/L        (4.0-11.0)
    platelets:            245 × 10⁹/L        (150-400)
    serum sodium:         140 mmol/L         (137-144)
    serum potassium:      5.5 mmol/L         (3.5-4.9)
    serum urea:           16.3 mmol/L        (2.5-7.0)
    serum creatinine:     210 µmol/L         (60-110)

    ECG: left ventricular hypertrophy

    chest X-ray: mild pulmonary oedema
```

What is the best management?

A. Intravenous labetalol
B. Intravenous sodium chloride 0.9%
C. Oral amlodipine
D. Oral ramipril
E. Sublingual nifedipine

17. A 58-year-old woman was referred to the acute medical unit with headaches and hypertension. Her pulse rate was 70 beats per minute and blood pressure was 240/130 mmHg. Her heart sounds, chest examination, and abdominal examination were normal. Fundoscopy was normal.

```
Investigations:
    haemoglobin:          140 g/L            (115-165)
    white cell count:     6.7 × 10⁹/L        (4.0-11.0)
    platelets:            245 × 10⁹/L        (150-400)
    serum sodium:         140 mmol/L         (137-144)
    serum potassium:      4.6 mmol/L         (3.5-4.9)
    serum urea:           5.3 mmol/L         (2.5-7.0)
    serum creatinine:     89 µmol/L          (60-110)

    ECG: normal

    chest X-ray: normal
```

What is the best management?

A. Intravenous labetalol
B. Intravenous sodium chloride 0.9%
C. Oral amlodipine
D. Oral ramipril
E. Sublingual nifedipine

18. **A 96-year-old woman was admitted to the acute medical unit with chest pain. The staff at her care home called the ambulance because she complained of chest pain and looked pale. She had a history of dementia and couldn't remember having the pain. She also had a past medical history of ischaemic heart disease, having had four previous myocardial infarctions, AF, a previous stroke, hypertension, type 2 diabetes, osteoporosis, and osteoarthritis. Her medications included warfarin, bisoprolol, ramipril, isosorbide mononitrate, and simvastatin. She lived in a nursing home and required help with all activities of daily living. She mobilized from the bed to chair only.**

```
Investigations:
  ECG: Lateral ST depression
  Troponin was 76 ng/L (<14)
```

What is the best management for her acute coronary syndrome?

A. Aspirin, clopidogrel, and fondaparinux
B. Continue current medication and treat symptomatically
C. Percutaneous coronary intervention
D. Stop warfarin and start aspirin
E. Withhold warfarin and give fondaparinux when the INR is <2

19. A 76-year-old man was admitted to the acute medical unit with loss of consciousness. There was no warning prior to his collapse, an ambulance was called, and he spontaneously regained consciousness after less than a minute. He now felt well. He had a history of hypertension and his only medication was amlodipine 5 mg once daily.

On examination, his heart rate was 35 beats per minute and blood pressure was 160/80 mmHg.

Investigations:

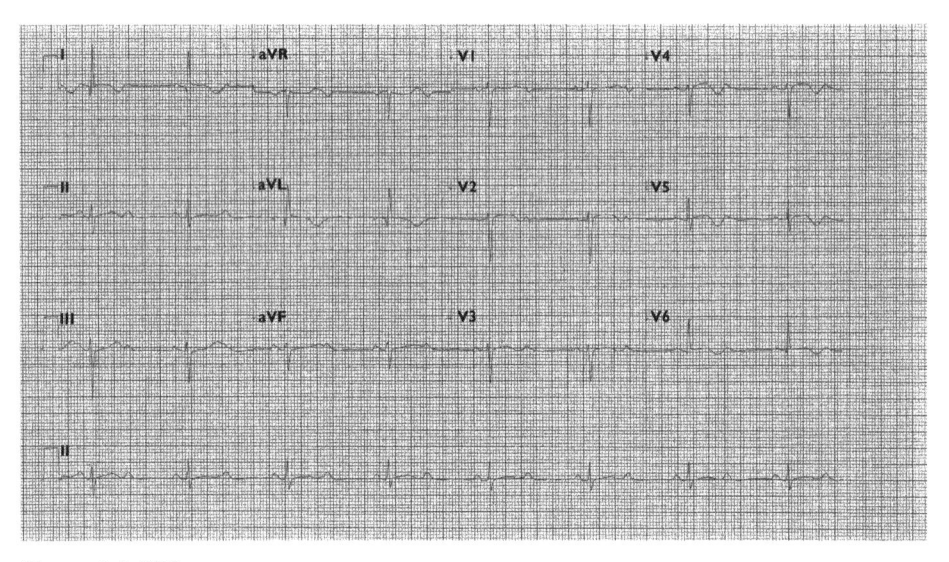

Figure 4.4 ECG.

What is the best management for this patient?
A Inpatient permanent pacemaker
B. Isoprenaline infusion
C. Stop amlodipine and arrange an outpatient 24-hour Holter monitor ECG
D. Stop amlodipine and arrange inpatient cardiac monitoring for 24 hours
E. Temporary pacing wire

20. A 76-year-old woman was seen in the acute medicine follow-up clinic. She had been admitted with palpitations but at the time of admission her 12-lead ECG showed normal sinus rhythm. She had had these episodes a few times before and they always reverted spontaneously. She had no past medical history. An outpatient 24-hour ECG was performed which showed a 10-minute run of AF. The patient did not feel palpitations at this time.

    What is first-line management?
    A. No treatment necessary as the AF is short and self-terminating
    B. Pill-in-the-pocket flecainide
    C. Regular amiodarone
    D. Regular beta-adrenergic blocker
    E. Regular digoxin

21. A 66-year-old man presented to the emergency department with palpitations and dizziness. He had a past medical history of hypertension and ischaemic heart disease, and had had a myocardial infarction six months previously for which he had percutaneous coronary intervention to the left anterior descending artery.

    On examination, his heart rate was 190 beats per minute and the 12-lead ECG showed ventricular tachycardia. His blood pressure was 60/30 mmHg, his respiratory rate was 16 breaths per minute, and oxygen saturation was 96% on air. He denied chest pain and his lungs were clear on examination. He underwent emergency DC cardioversion to sinus rhythm in the emergency department. His sinus rhythm ECG showed evidence of an old anterior infarction and nil else.

    Troponin T was 25 ng/L (<14) at presentation and 40 ng/L (<14) at 12 hours after the onset of symptoms.

    An echocardiogram on the following day showed left ventricular anterior wall hypokinesia/akinesia and an ejection fraction of 35%.

    What is the best long-term management strategy?
    A. Refer for an in-patient implantable cardioverter defibrillator
    B. Refer for in-patient electrophysiology testing and ablation of VT
    C. Refer for in-patient percutanous coronary intervention
    D. Refer to the cardiology outpatient department for assessment
    E. Start him on long-term amiodarone

22. A 34-year-old woman presented with palpitations. She had recently been assessed by a cardiac electrophysiologist and was awaiting an electrophysiological study with a view to ablation. She had tried the Valsalva manoeuvre at home but it hadn't worked. Vagal manoeuvres in the emergency department had no effect. Her heart rate was 200 beats per minute and blood pressure was 140/80 mmHg.

Investigations:

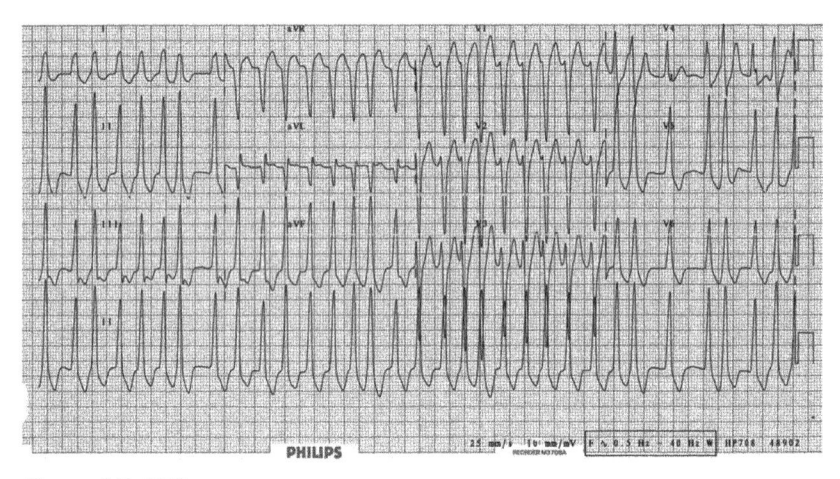

Figure 4.5 ECG.

What is the best treatment?

A. Intravenous adenosine
B. Intravenous amiodarone
C. Intravenous digoxin
D. Intravenous metoprolol
E. Intravenous verapamil

23. The obstetric team asked for a medical opinion. A 32-year-old woman was being treated for gestational hypertension with labetalol. She had delivered a baby boy three days previously. She was not breast-feeding. Her blood pressure was 155/105 mmHg. Her obstetric team was concerned that her blood pressure had not reverted to normal levels following delivery.

What would you advise?

A. Continue labetalol and reassess blood pressure in two weeks
B. Serum renin and aldosterone levels
C. Switch to methlydopa
D. Twenty-four hour urine collection for catecholamines
E. Ultrasound renal tract with Doppler flow

CARDIOLOGY | QUESTIONS

24. A 25-year-old Somali woman, who was 38 weeks pregnant, was admitted to the acute medical unit with lethargy and breathlessness. She had been well throughout her pregnancy and was taking no regular medication.

    On examination, her temperature was 36.0°C and pulse 100 beats per minute. Blood pressure was 110/70 mmHg. Respiratory rate was 25 breaths per minute and oxygen saturation 94% on air. Cardiovascular examination revealed a laterally displaced apex beat and gallop rhythm. On auscultation of her chest, there were crepitations to the mid-zones bilaterally. Abdominal examination was consistent with pregnancy.

    What medication regimen would be safe for this patient?
    A. Bisoprolol, hydralazine, and enalapril
    B. Candesartan, isosorbide mononitrate, and digoxin
    C. Furosemide, digoxin, and bisoprolol
    D. Hydralazine, irbesartan, and bisoprolol
    E. Isosorbide mononitrate, hydralazine, and ramipril

25. A 75-year-old man with a history of ischaemic heart disease was admitted to the acute medical unit with chest pain and collapse. He had a myocardial infarction ten years previously and a single drug eluting stent to the left anterior descending artery.

    On examination, his pulse was 60 beats per minute and regular. His blood pressure was 100/70 mmHg. He had a loud ejection systolic murmur that radiated to the carotids.

    ```
    Investigations:
        ECG: sinus rhythm 60 beats per minute with left ventricular
          hypertrophy.
        Echocardiogram: left ventricular hypertrophy, thickened
          and immobile aortic valve, and dilated aortic root. Mean
          gradient 50 mmHg and valve area 0.8 cm².
    ```

    What would prompt you to refer for an aortic valve replacement?
    A. Angina and syncope
    B. Evidence of left ventricular hypertrophy on echocardiography
    C. Harshness of systolic murmur
    D. Mean gradient of over 20 mmHg
    E. Valve area of less than 1 cm^2

26. **A 75-year-old woman with permanent AF presented to the acute medical unit with blackouts. She was taking bisoprolol 5 mg daily and warfarin. Her history included an AF ablation procedure two years ago but her AF had recurred. The heart rate on the monitor varied from 90 to 120 beats per minute in AF.**

   The patient's GP had arranged a 24-hour ECG and it showed a 5 second pause at 02:35 hours and another 6.2 second pause at 09:00 hours. The symptom diary reported a collapse in shower at 09:00 hours.

   What would be the best management?
   A. Permanent pacemaker set to DDD
   B. Permanent pacemaker set to VVIR
   C. Repeat ablation
   D. Stop bisoprolol and repeat 24-hour ECG
   E. Stop bisoprolol and start digoxin

27. Researchers investigated if there was an association between chronic Helicobacter pylori infection and coronary heart disease in young patients. A case–control study design was used. The cases were 1,122 survivors of suspected acute myocardial infarction aged between 30 and 49 years. For each case, a control matched for age and sex with no history of coronary heart disease was recruited. For the cases and controls, the risk factor of chronic infection with H pylori was confirmed serologically. Participants were categorized as seropositive or seronegative for H pylori infection antibodies. The participants provided information on other risk factors for coronary heart disease, including smoking behaviour, indicators of socioeconomic status, obesity, and blood lipid concentrations. Cases were asked about their habits and history just before their myocardial infarction, whereas controls were asked about their current habits and history. Blood samples were obtained from cases within 24 hours of the onset of symptoms, and from controls after the collection of the information for the other risk factors.

Of the 1,122 cases with early onset myocardial infarction, 472 (42%) were seropositive for H pylori antibodies compared with 272 (24%) of the 1,122 controls. The unadjusted odds ratio of early onset myocardial infarction if seropositive compared to seronegative for H pylori infection antibodies was 2.27 (95% confidence interval 1.89–2.72).*

Table 4.1 Cross tabulation of the frequencies of chronic infection with H pylori confirmed serologically for the cases and controls. (BMJ 1999;319:1157)

	H pylori infection antibodies		Total
	Seropositive	Seronegative	
Case	472	650	1,122
Control	272	850	1,122
Total	744	1,500	

Adapted from The BMJ, J Danesh et al., 'Helicobacter pylori infection and early onset myocardial infarction: case-control and sibling pairs study', 319, Copyright (1999), with permission from BMJ Publishing Group Ltd

What is the best interpretation of the unadjusted odds ratio of early onset myocardial infarction if seropositive to seronegative for H pylori infection antibodies?

A. If seronegative for H pylori infection antibodies, the odds of early onset myocardial infarction were decreased significantly and by 2.27 times compared to seronegative for H pylori antibodies
B. If seropositive for H pylori infection antibodies, the odds of early onset myocardial infarction were increased significantly and by 1.27 times compared to seronegative for H pylori antibodies
C. No significant difference between seropositive and seronegative for H pylori infection antibodies in the odds of early onset myocardial infarction
D. The odds of early onset myocardial infarction if seropositive for H pylori infection antibodies were increased, but not significantly, by 2.27 times compared to seronegative for H pylori antibodies
E. The odds of early onset myocardial infarction if seropositive for H pylori infection antibodies were reduced but not significantly, compared to seronegative for H pylori infection antibodies

* Data included in this question is from J Danesh et al., "Helicobacter pylori infection and early onset myocardial infarction: case-control and sibling pairs study', BMJ, 1999; 341:6549

CARDIOLOGY | QUESTIONS

28. A 67-year-old man presented to the acute medical unit with a three-day history of palpitations. His ECG confirmed AF with a fast ventricular response at 130 beats per minute. He had no chest pain. He had a history of hypertension and diet-controlled diabetes and was taking ramipril 2.5 mg daily. The admitting doctor in the emergency department administered 2.5 mg of bisoprolol and aspirin 75 mg for the AF.

    On examination, his pulse rate was 85–95 beats per minute irregularly irregular. His BP was 130/60 mmHg. The patient asked if he would need to continue the aspirin long term to prevent a stroke.

    What do you tell him?
    A. His annual stroke risk is around 3% and he should commence an oral anticoagulant
    B. His annual stroke risk is around 6% and he should commence an oral anticoagulant
    C. No, he can stop the aspirin as his heart rate has now slowed and he has a low annual stroke risk
    D. Yes, he needs the aspirin long term
    E. You are not sure but will ensure he has a cardiology outpatient appointment in two weeks

29. A 77-year-old man was admitted to the coronary care unit with a non-ST elevation myocardial infarction. His ECG showed lateral ST depression.

    On examination, his heart rate was 70 beats per minute and blood pressure 180/90 mmHg.

    Chest X-ray showed acute pulmonary oedema. His serum troponin T was 750 ng/L (<14).

    What further information do you need to calculate the GRACE 2.0 score?
    A. Aspirin usage
    B. ß-blocker usage
    C. Diuretic usage
    D. Oxygen saturation
    E. Serum creatinine

30. **An 85-year-old woman attended the acute medicine follow-up clinic. She had been on the acute medical unit one week previously with AF. She had a history of gout. Her current medication included dabigatran 110 mg twice daily, bisoprolol 2.5 mg once daily, and quinine sulphate 300 mg at night.**

    Her blood tests were all normal. Her ECG showed AF at a rate of 90 beats per minute. She had been told by a friend to stop the dabigatran as she was at 'high' risk of bleeding.

    What should you tell her?
    A. Her friend is correct and she should stop the dabigatran
    B. She should stop the dabigatran and switch to aspirin
    C. She should stop the dabigatran and switch to warfarin
    D. She should stop the quinine as it interacts with dabigatran
    E. You should reassure her and ask her to continue with her current medication

31. **A 25-year-old man presented to the emergency department complaining of feeling unwell with diffuse, dull, aching, central chest pain that was preceded by some localized retrosternal sharp pains (these had subsided). He was known to have arrhythmogenic right ventricular cardiomyopathy and had an implantable cardioverter defibrillator implanted five days ago after presenting with syncopal ventricular tachycardia.**

    On examination, he had a resting pulse of 101 beats per minute and a blood pressure of 100/60 mmHg. His JVP was slightly elevated otherwise physical examination was normal.

    His ECG showed T wave inversion in the right-sided precordial leads.

    What is the best step in his management?
    A. Aspirin, clopidogrel, and fondaparinux
    B. Chest X-ray
    C. Echocardiography
    D. Implantable cardioverter defibrillator check and data download
    E. Serum troponin

32. A 67-year-old man with a history of diabetes presented to the acute medical unit 24 hours after the onset of severe retrosternal chest pain radiating to the left arm. At presentation the chest pain had subsided almost completely but he was feeling breathless and unwell.

On examination, he had a pulse rate of 100 beats per minute and a blood pressure of 110/70 mmHg. Oxygen saturation was 94% on air. His JVP was elevated at 12 cm. Auscultation of the chest revealed bilateral crepitations in the lower two-thirds of the lung fields. Cardiac auscultation revealed an S3 gallop.

Chest X-ray showed acute pulmonary oedema.

Investigations:

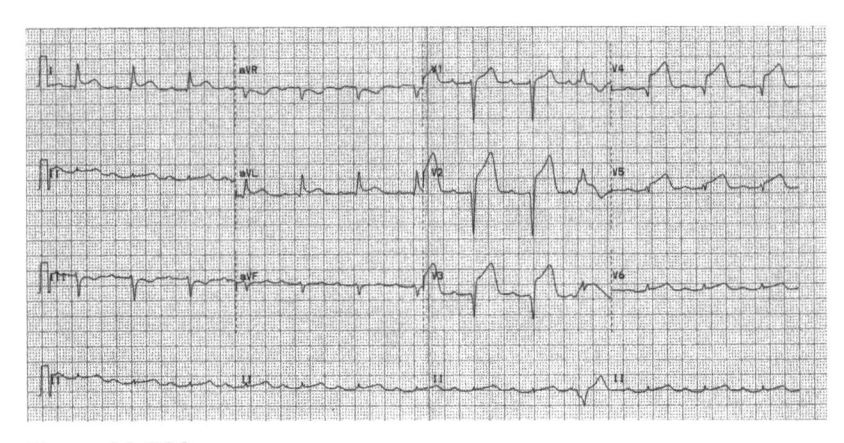

Figure 4.6 ECG.

Which of the following is least useful in the initial treatment of this patient?

A. Intravenous dobutamine infusion
B. Intravenous furosemide bolus
C. Intravenous isosorbide dinitrate infusion
D. Invasive pulmonary artery catheter
E. Supplemental oxygen

chapter 4

CARDIOLOGY

ANSWERS

1. C. 13.2% risk

With regard to the TIMI risk score calculation, one point is given for each of the following:
- Age ≥65
- Aspirin use in the last seven days (or patient experiences chest pain despite aspirin use in past seven days)
- At least two angina episodes within the last 24 hours
- ST changes of at least 0.5 mm on admission ECG
- Elevated serum cardiac biomarkers
- Known coronary artery disease (CAD) (coronary stenosis ≥50%)
- At least three risk factors for CAD, such as hypertension—140/90 mmHg or on antihypertensives, cigarette smoking, HDL <1.03 mmol/L, diabetes, family history of premature CAD (CAD in any male first-degree relative, or father less than 55, or any female first-degree relative or mother less than 65).

The percentage risk at 14 days of all-cause mortality, new or recurrent MI, or severe recurrent ischaemia requiring urgent revascularization:
- Score of 0–1 = 4.7% risk
- Score of 2 = 8.3% risk
- Score of 3 = 13.2% risk
- Score of 4 = 19.9% risk
- Score of 5 = 26.2% risk
- Score of 6–7 = at least 40.9% risk

Data from *Heart*, Conway MA et al., 'TIMI risk score accurately risk stratifies patients with undifferentiated chest pain presenting to an emergency department', 2006, 92, 9, pp.1333–1334.

Conway MA et al. TIMI risk score accurately risk stratifies patients with undifferentiated chest pain presenting to an emergency department. Heart 2006; 92(9): 1333–1334.

2. C. Aspirin 300 mg and prasugrel 60 mg

The patient is most likely experiencing acute stent thrombosis. As she is already on clopidogrel, there may be some degree of clopidogrel resistance/failure. Another antiplatelet may therefore be used and there is enough data to support prasugrel use in this situation. As with clopidogrel, the use of prasugrel requires a loading dose followed by maintenance. The loading dose of prasugrel is 60 mg and the maintenance dose is 10 mg.

The clinical indications for the use of prasugrel are:

1. Patients with acute STEMI undergoing PCI
2. Patients with definite stent thrombosis during clopidogrel treatment
3. Patients with presumed stent thrombosis during clopidgrel treatment
4. Patients at high risk of developing stent thrombosis
5. Those presenting with acute coronary syndrome with diabetes mellitus

National Institute for Health and Care Excellence. Technology Appraisal 317. Prasugrel with percutaneous coronary intervention for treating acute coronary syndromes. July 2014.

3. D. Tirofiban

Tirofiban is a synthetic, non-peptide inhibitor acting at glycoprotein (GP) IIb/IIIa receptors in human platelets. Its half-life is approximately two hours. The main value of GPIIb/IIIa antagonists is their use as adjunctive treatment in patients who then go on to have a PCI. However, evidence also points to benefits when tirofiban is used as primary early treatment for unstable angina/NSTEMI where pooled trial data have revealed a 34% reduction in mortality and reinfarction with early tirofiban (and other GPIIb/IIIa antagonists) treatment that appears to be independent of its benefits in PCI. This early benefit appears to be more prominent in high-risk patients (e.g. diabetics, troponin positive patients, and those with persistent pain and ECG changes).

Boersma E, Harringtone R et al. Platelet glycoprotein IIb/IIIa inhibitors in acute coronary syndromes: a meta-analysis of all major randomized clinical trials. Lancet 2002; 359: 189–198.

4. E. Streptococci

The most likely diagnosis is infective endocarditis given the unexplained fever, positive blood cultures, and the evidence of structural mitral valve disease. The common organisms in native valve infective endocarditis are:

- 50–60% Streptococci
- 10% Entercocci
- 25% Staphlococci
- 5–10% Culture negative
- <1% Gram negative bacilli
- <1% Multiple organisms
- <1% Diptheroids
- <1% Fungi

Ramrakha P, Moore K, Sam A. Oxford Handbook of Acute Medicine (Oxford Medical Handbooks) 2010. Oxford University Press.

5. C. Flecainide

In a patient presenting with new AF it is important to consider rate versus rhythm control. Most patients should be offered rate control. Pharmacological and/or electrical rhythm control should be offered to people with atrial fibrillation whose symptoms continue after heart rate has been controlled or for whom a rate-control strategy has not been successful. Rhythm control should also be considered in those patients:

- who are symptomatic
- whose atrial fibrillation has a reversible cause
- who have heart failure thought to be primarily caused by atrial fibrillation
- with new-onset atrial fibrillation
- with atrial flutter whose condition is considered suitable for an ablation strategy to restore sinus rhythm
- for whom a rhythm control strategy would be more suitable based on clinical judgement.

This man has new onset AF that is probably related to excess alcohol intake (reversible cause) which is known to precipitate AF. Pharmacological or electrical cardioversion is therefore a good option. Long-term antiarrhythmic medication is usually not required and AF does not recur if alcohol intake is reduced.

Pharmacological cardioversion with Flecainide seems reasonable given that this man was previously fit and well and likely to have a structurally normal heart. Another drug to consider for cardioversion is amiodarone. Electrical DC cardioversion would be the answer if this gentleman was haemodynamically unstable or if the AF was longer than 48 hours in duration.

National Institute for Health and Care Excellence. Clinical Guideline 180. Atrial fibrillation: The management of atrial fibrillation. 2014.

6. A. Coronary angiography

The investigation of stable chest pain depends on the clinical assessment, the resting 12-lead ECG, and the estimated likelihood of coronary artery disease (CAD). NICE Clinical Guideline 95 contains detailed information on the percentage of people estimated to have CAD based on age, sex, risk factors and symptoms.

Arrange further diagnostic testing as follows:

- If the estimated likelihood of CAD is more than 90%, manage as angina, further tests are unnecessary.
- If the estimated likelihood of CAD is 61–90%, offer invasive coronary angiography as the first-line diagnostic investigation if appropriate.
- If the estimated likelihood of CAD is 30–60%, offer functional imaging as the first-line diagnostic investigation.
- If the estimated likelihood of CAD is 10–29%, offer CT calcium scoring as the first-line diagnostic investigation.

In this case, if the calcium score is 0, then consider investigating for other causes of chest pain. If the calcium score is 1–400 then do a 64-slice (or above) CT angiogram. If the calcium score is more than 400 then follow the pathway as if the CAD score is 61–90%.

National Institute for Health and Care Excellence. Clinical Guideline 95. Chest pain of recent onset: assessment and diagnosis. March 2010.

7. C. Second-degree heart block—Mobitz type 1

First-degree heart block is prolongation of the PR interval (>0.20 s).

Second-degree heart block:

- Mobitz type 1 (also known as Wenckebach) is progressive increase in the PR interval with occasional failure of the P wave to be conducted.
- Mobitz type 2 is where the PR interval is constant but there is intermittent failure to conduct the P wave.

Third-degree heart block is complete AV dissociation.

Ramrakha P, Moore K, Sam A. Oxford Handbook of Acute Medicine (Oxford Medical Handbooks) 2010. Oxford University Press.

8. B. Dipyridamole

The QT interval is measured from the beginning of the QRS to the end of the T wave and represents depolarization and repolarization of the ventricular myocardium. Any drug that prolongs depolarization or repolarization can cause QT prolongation. A prolonged QT can predispose to polymorphic VT called Torsades de Pointes (TdP) due to its characteristic appearance.

CARDIOLOGY | ANSWERS

Dipyridamole inhibits the phosphodiesterase enzymes that normally break down cAMP and/or cGMP and is therefore used as an antiplatelet to block platelet activity. It is not known to cause prolongation of the QT interval. The rest of the drugs in the answer options are all antiarrhythmics which can prolong the QT.

The following drugs cause prolongation of the QT interval:

- Antiarrythimics
  * Quinidine
  * Procainamide
  * Disopyramide
  * Amiodarone
  * Sotalol
- Antipsychotics
  * Pimozide
  * Thioridazine
- Antihistamines
  * Terfenadine
  * Astemizole
- Antimalarials
  * Halofantrine
- Organophosphate poisoning

Adapted from Ramrakha et al. Oxford handbook of acute medicine, 2010 with permission from Oxford University Press.

Ramrakha P, Moore K, Sam A. Oxford Handbook of Acute Medicine (Oxford Medical Handbooks) 2010. Oxford University Press.

9. C. DC cardioversion

The answer according to European Resuscitation Guidelines guidelines is immediate DC cardioversion given that the patient is haemodynamically compromised and presenting with presumed ventricular tachycardia until proven otherwise. If the patient was stable, amiodarone and magnesium could be considered. It is important to check the electrolytes. Ideally, the patient needs PCI but must be stable before transfer can take place.

There is no role for CPR or adrenaline as this is not a cardiac arrest situation.

Soar J, Nolan J, Böttiger B et al. European Resuscitation Council Guidelines for Resuscitation 2015 Section 3. Adult advanced life support. Resuscitation 95 (2015) 100–147. http://dx.doi.org/10.1016/j.resuscitation.2015.07.016

10. A. Mobitz type 1

Temporary transvenous pacing may be considered when there is documented ventricular standstill (>3 seconds), Mobitz type 2 heart block, and third-degree heart block (especially when the complexes are broad or the heart rate is less than 40 beats per minute).

However, more and more centres in the UK are moving away from temporary pacing and going for immediate (round the clock) permanent pacemaker implantation in these patients where feasible.

Soar J, Nolan J, Böttiger B et al. European Resuscitation Council Guidelines for Resuscitation 2015 Section 3. Adult advanced life support. Resuscitation 95 (2015) 100–147. http://dx.doi.org/10.1016/j.resuscitation.2015.07.016

CARDIOLOGY | ANSWERS

11. E. Rhythm control with heparin cover

The ECG shows AF with a fast and uncontrolled ventricular response. The patient is clinically unstable and needs urgent rhythm control. The duration of AF is less than 48 hours, so formal anticoagulation prior to any attempt at cardioversion is not required.

Beta-adrenoceptor blockers are relatively contraindicated in the presence of COPD and wheeze (although not normally contraindicated in COPD, this patient has widespread wheeze, however, indicating bronchospasm). The rate-limiting calcium channel blockers have some negative inotropic effect.

Cardioversion with either amiodarone or a DC shock is probably the best option. If she had a recent echo showing a normal heart, then class 1C agents (e.g. flecainide) could be used. The episode of AF has a clear precipitant (chest infection) and, therefore, continued anticoagulation is not required unless there is previous history suggestive of paroxysmal AF or future recurrence.

Camm A, Lip G, Atar D et al. 2012 Focused update of the European Society of Cardiology Guidelines for the management of atrial fibrillation. European Heart Journal 2012; 33: 2719–2747. http://www.escardio.org/guidelines

National Institute for Health and Care Excellence. Clinical Guideline 180. Atrial fibrillation: management. June 2014.

12. E. Treatment for infective endocarditis should start immediately as the diagnostic criteria have been met

This patient has one major (blood culture positive for Coxiella Burnetii—only one positive culture needed for this organism) and three minor criteria (pyrexia >38.0°C, predisposing factor with previous closure of patent ductus arteriosus and Janeway lesions) making the diagnosis of infective endocarditis.

Box 4.1 Duke's Criteria

Major criteria

1. Positive blood culture with a typical organism from two separate blood cultures taken 12 hours apart or in all of three bottles drawn one hour apart.
   Typical organisms are: Viridans group streptococci, Streptococcus bovis, HACEK group (Haemophilus, Actinobacillus, Cardiobacterium, Eikenella, Kingella), Staphylococcus aureus, Enterococci.
2. A single positive blood culture for Coxiella Burnetii.
3. Transthoracic or transoesophageal echocardiograph positive for vegetations (a TOE is recommended with prosthetic valves).

Minor criteria

1. Intravenous drug use or predisposing heart condition.
2. Fever >38.0°C.
3. Vascular phenomena: major arterial emboli, conjunctival haemorrhage, Janeway lesions, splinter haemorrhages, intracranial haemorrhage, septic pulmonary infarcts, and mycotic aneurysms.
4. Immunological phenomena: glomerulonephritis, Osler's nodes, Roth's spots, and positive rheumatoid factor.
5. Positive blood cultures not meeting the major criteria above.

Data from *The American Journal of Medicine*, 96.3, 1994, Durack DT et al., 'New criteria for diagnosis of infective endocarditis: utilization of specific echocardiographic findings', pp. 200–209; *Clinical Infectious Diseases*, 30.4, 2000, Li J et al., 'Proposed Modifications to the Duke Criteria for the Diagnosis of Infective Endocarditis'.

The diagnosis of infective endocarditis is made using Duke's criteria (Box 4.1). The diagnosis is confirmed if there are two major criteria, one major and three minor, or five minor criteria.

Durack D, Lukes A, Bright D. New criteria for diagnosis of infective endocarditis: utilization of specific echocardiographic findings. Duke Endocarditis Service. American Journal of Medicine 1994; 96(3): 200–209.

Li J, Sexton D, Mick N et al. Proposed modifications to the Duke Criteria for the diagnosis of infective endocarditis. Clinical Infectious Diseases 2000; 30(4): 633.

Habib G, Lancellotti P, Atunes MJ et al. Guidelines for the management of infective endocarditis. The Task Force for the Management of Infective Endocarditis of the European Society of Cardiology (ESC). European Heart Journal (2015), 3–54. doi:10.1093/eurheartj/ehv319.

13. D. Set the output to 6 V

The aim of temporary pacing is to provide support until a permanent pacemaker is implanted. As long as there is reliable capture there is no need to reposition the wire. It is sufficient to program the output above the threshold (with a safety margin) to ensure capture.

Please note that a sudden rise in pacing threshold may indicate an unstable wire position which may move further leading to failure of capture or it may indicate myocardial perforation. The temporary wire should be used for short periods of time and permanent pacing should be instituted as soon as possible to avoid potential complications, which may include myocardial perforation, tamponade, and sepsis.

Brignole M, Auricchio A, Baron-Esquivias G et al. on behalf of the task force on cardiac pacing and resynchronization therapy of the European Society of Cardiology (ESC). Cardiac Pacing and Cardiac Resynchronization Therapy ESC Clinical Practice Guidelines. European Heart Journal 2013; 34: 2281–2329. doi: 0.1093/eurheartj/eht150. http://www.escardio.org/guidelines

14. E. Myocardial perfusion scan

This woman is less than 65 years old and has symptoms suggestive of stable angina but has no risk factors for coronary artery disease (CAD). Her risk of CAD is, therefore, around 38% and so functional imaging for myocardial ischaemia is indicated.

The 2010 NICE guidelines provide a tool for risk stratifying patients according to the clinical presentation, age, and presence of risk factors for CAD. If risk is less than 30% then CT calcium scoring is the first-line investigation, and if risk is between 30 and 60% then functional imaging is indicated. Invasive coronary angiography is indicated if the risk is 61–90%.

National Institute for Health and Care Excellence. Clinical Guideline 95. Chest pain of recent onset: assessment and diagnosis. March 2010.

15. E. Urgent surgery

This woman has an aortic dissection, which is a life-threatening emergency. Aortic dissection is usually caused by an intimal aortic tear which allows the intraluminal blood pressure to force blood flow through the tear and separate the inner and outer layers of the wall of the aorta causing intense pain.

Aortic dissection is classified as type A, which is any dissection involving the ascending aorta and/or arch (+/− descending aorta) or type B which does not involve the ascending aorta/arch and starts distal to the origin of the left subclavian artery.

The mortality of type A acute aortic dissection is very high due to aortic rupture and is highest at the onset of dissection and reduces with the passage of time. The dissection may cause occlusion of any of the branches of the aorta including one of the coronary or carotid arteries and the presentation may be dominated by the clinical picture of an acute myocardial infarction or acute stroke. It may also compromise the aortic valve ring and cause haemodynamically significant acute aortic regurgitation. The presence of unilaterally weak/absent pulses or an aortic regurgitation murmur in a patient with acute severe chest pain should raise suspicion of an acute dissection.

The treatment of an acute type A dissection is urgent surgical intervention. While awaiting surgery, the blood pressure needs to be significantly lowered to below 120 mmHg systolic and a mean arterial pressure of 60–70 mmHg. Intravenous antihypertensives if needed and beta-blockers are given to reduce the driving force causing further extension of the dissection and aortic rupture. The treatment of type B dissection is usually medical treatment with blood pressure control and beta-blockers, unless there is arterial compromise of the renal or common iliac arteries or in the presence of Marfan syndrome or any other connective tissue disorders where surgery needs to be considered.

Anticoagulants and antiplatelets are absolutely contraindicated in acute dissection and may lead to aortic rupture and patient death.

Erbel R, Aboyans V, Boileau C et al. Guidelines on the diagnosis and treatment of aortic diseases. The Task Force for the Diagnosis and Treatment of Aortic Diseases of the European Society of Cardiology (ESC). European Heart Journal (2014) 35, 2873–2926 doi:10.1093/eurheartj/ehu281. http://www.escardio.org/guidelines

16. A. Intravenous labetalol

This man has a hypertensive emergency, which is a severe increase in blood pressure (>180 mmHg systolic or >110 mmHg diastolic) associated with acute impairment of one or more target organs. He has renal impairment and left ventricular failure as well as papilloedema.

The treatment is to lower the blood pressure within minutes to hours and intravenous antihypertensive medications are recommended. Intravenous nitroprusside is most commonly used due to its rapid onset of action and predictable effect but other intravenous medications such as labetalol can be used. These patients usually have deranged autoregulation of the cerebral circulation and other vital organ circulation. The aim is, therefore, to decrease the systolic blood pressure by no more than 25–30% as soon as possible then gradually to a target of 160/100 mmHg to avoid hypoperfusion of the vital organs if the blood pressure lowering is more precipitous.

Mancia G, Fagard R, Narkiewicz K et al. European Society of Hypertension/European Society of Cardiology Guidelines for the Management of Arterial Hypertension. European Heart Journal 2013; 34: 2159–2219. doi: 10.1093/eurheartj/eht151. http://www.escardio.org/guidelines

17. C. Oral amlodipine

This woman has hypertensive urgency, which is a severe increase in blood pressure (>180 mmHg systolic or >110 mmHg diastolic) not associated with target organ damage. This may be associated with headache, shortness of breath, or nosebleeds. The treatment is to lower the blood pressure within 24–48 hours and oral antihypertensive medications are recommended. Hospitalization is not required. Amlodipine is a dihydropyridine calcium channel antagonist and a potent antihypertensive that can be used in this situation.

Mancia G, Fagard R, Narkiewicz K et al. European Society of Hypertension/European Society of Cardiology Guidelines for the Management of Arterial Hypertension. European Heart Journal 2013; 34: 2159–2219. doi: 10.1093/eurheartj/eht151. http://www.escardio.org/guidelines

18. B. Continue current medication and treat symptomatically

This woman has sustained a non-ST elevation acute coronary syndrome. Her immediate and subsequent management will be determined predominantly by her age and numerous existing co-morbidities. She is already on adequate medical treatment. In view of her age and co-morbidities, a coronary intervention will not improve quality of life and will be associated with significant risk of stroke, bleeding, or further coronary events. She already has a significant risk of bleeding on warfarin (HAS-BLED score of at least 3) and addition of aspirin, clopidogrel, or fondaparinux will markedly increase that risk. She also has a significant risk of thromboembolic complications of AF (CHA_2DS_2-VASc score of 8); therefore, stopping the warfarin is not a good idea.

The best option is, therefore, to continue current medication and treat symptomatically if needed.

The HAS-BLED score was developed to assess the 1-year risk of major bleeding in patients with atrial fibrillation if the patient was anticoagulated. If the patient has, for example, severe hypertension, abnormal liver/renal function test, a stroke history, or a labile INR they would score a point for each. Being over 65 years of age or heavy alcohol use would also increase the bleeding risk according to the score. As the patient's score increases so too does the patient's bleeding risk. A score of 2 or over puts the patient in the moderate risk for major bleeding group and a score of 3 or over should prompt the clinician to consider alternatives to anticoagulation.

Pisters et al. A novel user-friendly score (HAS-BLED) to assess 1-year risk of major bleeding in patients with atrial fibrillation: the Euro Heart Survey. Chest 2010; 138(5): 1093–1100.

19. A. Inpatient permanent pacemaker

The ECG shows second-degree AV block. This elderly man has symptomatic high-grade AV block and needs an inpatient permanent dual chamber pacemaker (class I indication). Ambulatory ECG monitoring will not add any further information.

The calcium channel blocker amlodipine is a dihydropyridine and therefore has no effect on AV node conduction (the phenylalkylamine calcium blockers verapamil and diltiazem have an AV blocking effect). The patient is currently stable haemodynamically and there is, therefore, no indication for isoprenaline or temporary wire insertion. There is increasing tendency currently in the UK to avoid temporary wire insertion and proceed directly with urgent permanent pacemaker implantation in unstable patients with bradycardia where feasible.

Brignole M, Auricchio A, Baron-Esquivias G et al. on behalf of the task force on cardiac pacing and resynchronization therapy of the European Society of Cardiology (ESC). Cardiac Pacing and Cardiac Resynchronization Therapy ESC Clinical Practice Guidelines. European Heart Journal 2013; 34: 2281–2329. doi: 10.1093/eurheartj/eht150. http://www.escardio.org/guidelines

20. D. Regular beta-adrenergic blocker

The diagnosis in this patient is not confirmed as symptom to rhythm correlation was not established but it is likely that she is having paroxysms of AF causing her symptoms. Paroxysmal AF is intermittent AF that occurs suddenly and terminates spontaneously within seven days (most commonly within 48 hours). Persistent AF on the other hand is AF that requires pharmacological or electrical cardioversion to restore sinus rhythm. Permanent AF is a situation in which sinus rhythm cannot be restored for any significant period of time and AF is accepted as a permanent rhythm.

A beta-adrenergic blocker is the first option to treat this patient, although if her symptoms are infrequent then a pill-in-the-pocket strategy may be utilized. Oral flecainide (in a structurally normal heart) or amiodarone or an AF ablation can be used if the paroxysms are still troublesome on a beta-blocker.

More importantly, this woman needs anticoagulation as her CHA_2DS_2VASC score is at least 2.

Camm A, Lip G, Atar D et al. focused update of the European Society of Cardiology Guidelines for the management of atrial fibrillation. European Heart Journal 2012; 33: 2719–2747. http://www.escardio.org/guidelines

National Institute for Health and Care Excellence. Clinical Guideline 180. Atrial fibrillation: management. June 2014.

21. A. Refer for an inpatient implantable cardioverter defibrillator

This man has an ischaemic cardiomyopathy and presented with ventricular tachycardia (VT) with haemodynamic compromise. He is, therefore, stratified to the highest risk category for sudden cardiac death and should receive an implantable cardioverter defibrillator (ICD) for secondary prevention before he goes home. Data from trials have shown that amiodarone on its own is not sufficiently protective and is inferior to ICDs in preventing sudden cardiac death. VT ablation in this patient population is reserved for patients who experience recurrent shocks from their ICD due to VT that is not controlled by antiarrhythmic medication and there is no indication for VT ablation alone in these patients.

There is no evidence that this is an acute ischaemic event. There was no chest pain on presentation and the ECG post cardioversion showed no acute changes. The mild troponin rise seen can be explained by the tachycardia.

Discharging this patient for an outpatient cardiology appointment is inappropriate and unsafe.

Brignole M, Auricchio A, Baron-Esquivias G et al. on behalf of the task force on cardiac pacing and resynchronization therapy of the European Society of Cardiology (ESC). Cardiac Pacing and Cardiac Resynchronization Therapy ESC Clinical Practice Guidelines. European Heart Journal 2013; 34: 2281–2329. doi: 10.1093/eurheartj/eht150. http://www.escardio.org/guidelines

National Institute for Health and Care Excellence. Interventional procedure guidance 454. Insertion of a subcutaneous implantable cardioverter defibrillator for prevention of sudden cardiac death. April 2013.

22. B. Intravenous amiodarone

The ECG shows an irregular tachycardia with bizarre broad complexes. The diagnosis is, therefore, AF with conduction over a manifest accessory pathway (i.e. pre-excited AF).

AF occurs in over 30% of patients with accessory pathways and is a marker for the risk of sudden cardiac death in these patients. The accessory pathway lacks the rate-limiting characteristics of the AV node and the risk of sudden death is related to the refractory period of the accessory pathway (its ability to conduct at very fast rates due to a short recovery time). An idea about the refractory period can be obtained by scanning the pre-excited ECG for the shortest RR interval. In general, pre-excited AF with RR intervals shorter than 260 ms is considered 'unsafe' and warrant inpatient definitive treatment by ablation. This patient's shortest RR interval was 200 ms.

The acute management depends on haemodynamic stability. Haemodynamically unstable patients should be cardioverted electrically. More stable patients can be given medications that slow down pathway conduction (and terminate AF), including class I and III antiarrhythmic drugs. Consideration must be given to the risk of thromboembolism in these patients where relevant before cardioversion. Drugs that only block the AV node (i.e. beta-blockers and calcium channel blockers) increase pre-excitation and are, therefore, not advised. Digoxin has a variable effect on accessory pathway conduction and may reduce its refractory period and increase mortality.

Camm A, Lip G, Atar D et al. 2012 focused update of the European Society of Cardiology Guidelines for the management of atrial fibrillation. European Heart Journal 2012; 33: 2719–2747. http://www.escardio.org/guidelines

National Institute for Health and Care Excellence. Clinical Guideline 180. Atrial fibrillation: management. June 2014.

23. A. Continue labetalol and reassess blood pressure in two weeks

Hypertensive disorders affect around 10% of women in pregnancy and include chronic hypertension, gestational hypertension, and preeclampsia/eclampsia. Gestational hypertension is hypertension developing after week 20 of pregnancy and usually resolves within 6–8 weeks after delivery. NICE guidelines recommend drug treatment of moderate (150/100 to 159/109 mmHg) and severe (160/110 mmHg or higher) gestational hypertension. The first-line drug is labetalol and alternatives include methyldopa and nifedipine. The focus of antenatal follow-up is detection of signs of pre-eclampsia (e.g. proteinuria). Patients who continue to have high blood pressure after delivery should continue on their antenatal medications (methyldopa should be stopped two days after delivery and switched to another antihypertensive medication) and offered a follow-up appointment after two weeks. Specialist referral should take place if the patient is still hypertensive at 6–8 weeks.

Regitz-Zagrosek V, Blomstrom Lundqvist C, Borghi C. European Society of Cardiology guidelines of the management of cardiovascular diseases during pregnancy. European Heart Journal 2011; 32: 3147–3197. doi: 10.1093/eurheartj/ehr218. http://www.escardio.org/guidelines

National Institute for Health and Care Excellence. Clinical Guideline 107. Hypertension in pregnancy: diagnosis and management. June 2010.

24. C. Furosemide, digoxin, and bisoprolol

Peripartum cardiomyopathy is a dilated cardiomyopathy occurring in the last month of pregnancy or within five months after delivery, without pre-existing heart disease or identifiable cause. The diagnosis may be difficult as normal findings in pregnancy may include shortness of breath, fatigue, sinus tachycardia, mildly raised JVP, lower limb oedema, a displaced apex, flow murmurs, and even a physiological S3 over the apex. Around one-half of women recover completely within a few months post-partum, while the other half continue to have varying degrees of systolic dysfunction.

The treatment of peripartum cardiomyopathy follows the same lines of pharmacological treatment as other heart failure conditions, which includes oxygen, digoxin, vasodilators, and diuretics. Note that ACE inhibitors and angiotensin receptor blockers are absolutely contraindicated during pregnancy but should be commenced promptly after delivery.

Regitz-Zagrosek V, Blomstrom Lundqvist C, Borghi C. European Society of Cardiology guidelines of the management of cardiovascular diseases during pregnancy. European Heart Journal 2011; 32: 3147–3197. doi: 10.1093/eurheartj/ehr218. http://www.escardio.org/guidelines

25. A. Angina and syncope

Aortic stenosis is graded as severe when the valve area is <1 cm^2 or the mean gradient across the valve is >40 mmHg by echocardiography. The natural history of aortic stenosis is characterized by a long period of latency in which patients are asymptomatic and have near normal survival. The risk of sudden cardiac death in asymptomatic patients is <2% per year. The onset of severe symptoms results in significant reduction in survival unless aortic valve surgery is performed. Patients with angina pectoris have a 50% survival at five years compared to those with syncope who have a 50% survival at three years, whereas those with heart failure symptoms have a median survival of two years. The development of symptoms with severe aortic stenosis is, therefore, the indication to refer patients for aortic valve surgery irrespective of the level of the gradient across the valve, aortic valve area, or any other physical signs.

Vahanian A, Alfieri O, Andreotti F et al. on behalf of the joint task force on the management of valvular heart disease of the European Society of Cardiology. Guidelines on the Management of Valvular Heart Disease (version 2012). European Heart Journal 2012; 33: 2451–2496. doi: 10.1093/eurheartj/ehs109. http://www.escardio.org/guidelines

26. B. Permanent pacemaker set to VVIR

This patient has permanent AF and the best strategy for her is rate control and anticoagulation. Her heart rate is still not controlled adequately as her resting heart rate in the acute medical unit was up to 120 beats per minute. She therefore needs more rate-limiting medications. However, she also has symptomatic syncopal pauses that indicate a struggling conduction system and an increase in dose of bisoprolol would only aggravate the blackouts.

This lady, therefore, has a class I indication for a single chamber pacemaker set to VVIR.

Brignole M, Auricchio A, Baron-Esquivias G et al. on behalf of the task force on cardiac pacing and resynchronization therapy of the European Society of Cardiology (ESC). Cardiac Pacing and Cardiac Resynchronization Therapy ESC Clinical Practice Guidelines. European Heart Journal 2013; 34: 2281–2329. doi: 10.1093/eurheartj/eht150. http://www.escardio.org/guidelines

CARDIOLOGY | ANSWERS

27. B. If seropositive for H pylori infection antibodies, the odds of early onset myocardial infarction were increased significantly and by 1.27 times compared to seronegative for H pylori antibodies

The purpose of the case–control study was to investigate if H pylori antibody seropositivity was a potential risk factor for acute myocardial infarction in young patients. Two groups of patients were selected on the basis of their disease status: the cases, who were survivors of suspected acute myocardial infarction and aged between 30 and 49 years; and healthy controls matched for age and sex. By definition a case–control study is retrospective in design, with participants providing information about their past exposure to potential risk factors. This is particularly important for the cases whose current exposure to risk factors may have changed as a result of the development of the disease. However, sometimes the controls provide information about their current exposure to risk factors. The cases and controls are then compared to ascertain whether particular risk factors are more common in one group than in the other. In particular, in the above study the cases and controls were compared to ascertain whether H pylori antibody seropositivity was more common in one group than the other. If so, it would be considered a potential risk factor for acute myocardial infarction in young patients.

The association between chronic H pylori infection and coronary heart disease in young patients could not be investigated using a relative risk. This was because it was not possible to estimate the population at risk of early onset myocardial infarction. That is, the proportion of participants who experienced early onset myocardial infarction, whether overall or for those participants who were seropositive for H pylori infection antibodies and for those who were seronegative, did not estimate the proportion in the population. The proportion of participants who had experienced early onset myocardial infarction was dictated by the ratio of cases to controls, which was 1:1, and decided at the design stage. Instead the association between chronic H pylori infection and coronary heart disease in young patients was quantified by an odds ratio, which estimates the population relative risk. The odds ratio will be a good estimate of the population relative risk if the prevalence of the disease outcome in the population is rare, typically considered to be less than 10%.

The cross tabulation of the frequencies of chronic infection with H pylori as confirmed serologically for the cases and controls is shown in Table 4.1. To calculate the odds ratio of early onset myocardial infarction if seropositive compared to seronegative for H pylori infection antibodies, the odds of early onset myocardial infarction if seropositive for H pylori infection antibodies were divided by the odds of early onset myocardial infarction if seronegative for H pylori infection antibodies. The odds of an early onset myocardial infarction if the risk factor was present or absent, i.e. seropositive or seronegative, were not the probability of an early onset myocardial infarction occurring; the odds are an alternative way of expressing probability. For each of the risk factor groups—seropositive and seronegative for H pylori infection antibodies—the odds of an early onset myocardial infarction were derived as the probability of an early onset myocardial infarction occurring divided by the probability of the outcome not occurring. For example, of the 744 participants who were seropositive for H pylori infection antibodies, 472 had experienced an early onset myocardial infarction whereas 272 had not. Therefore, for those participants who were seropositive the odds of an early onset myocardial infarction were $(472 \div 744) \div (272 \div 744) = (472 \div 744) \times (744 \div 272) = 472 \div 272 = 1.74$. Hence, the odds of an early onset myocardial infarction occurring if seropositive for H pylori infection antibodies were the ratio of the number of participants who had experienced an early onset myocardial infarction to those who had not. The odds of an early onset myocardial infarction occurring if seronegative for H pylori infection antibodies were calculated in a similar way—that is, the ratio of the number of participants who had experienced an early onset myocardial infarction to those who had not: $650 \div 850 = 0.76$.

The unadjusted odds ratio of early onset myocardial infarction if seropositive for H pylori infection antibodies compared to seronegative for H pylori infection antibodies was derived as the odds of an early onset myocardial infarction if seropositive divided by the odds if seronegative: $(472 \div 272) \div (650 \div 850) = (472 \div 272) \times (850 \div 650) = (472 \times 850) \div (272 \times 650) = 2.27$. Hence, the odds ratio was the ratio of the cross products of the frequencies in the table. Therefore, the odds of an early onset myocardial infarction if seropositive were 2.27 times those if seronegative—hence the odds was increased by 1.27 times if seropositive compared to seronegative. Early onset myocardial infarction was more likely if seropositive for H pylori infection antibodies than if seronegative. Therefore, being seropositive for H pylori infection antibodies was a potential risk factor for early onset myocardial infarction.

The 95% confidence interval for the population odds ratio was 1.89–2.72; because it excluded unity (1.0) the increased occurrence of an early onset myocardial infarction for the risk factor of seropositive for H pylori infection antibodies compared with seronegative was therefore statistically significant at the 5% level of significance (see Sedgwick, 2012b). The researchers reported that the odds ratio was reduced to 1.87 (1.42–2.47) after adjustment for potential confounding by smoking and indicators of socioeconomic status, and further reduced to 1.75 (1.29–2.36) after additional adjustment for blood lipid concentrations and obesity. Adjustment for confounding was achieved using logistic regression (see Sedgwick, 2013). Hence, a moderate association existed between coronary heart disease and H pylori antibody seropositivity that could not be fully explained by other risk factors. Because the association between chronic H pylori infection and early onset myocardial infarction remained significant after adjustment for confounding, chronic H pylori infection is said to be independently associated with early onset myocardial infarction.

In the above study the cases and controls were matched for age and sex. For each case, an otherwise healthy control of the same age and sex was recruited. The advantage of matching was that it minimized the effects of confounding due to the matching variables (age and sex) when comparing the risk factor groups (seropositive versus seronegative) in the odds of early onset myocardial infarction (see Sedgwick, 2012a). However, when deriving the odds ratio as detailed above the researchers did not take advantage of the matched pairing between the cases and controls. By acknowledging the pairing of cases and controls a more precise odds ratio could have been derived. In order to do so in the above example, it would have been necessary to consider the number of discordant pairs in the risk factor of 'seropositivity' status. A discordant pair would occur if the case was seropositive but their matched control was seronegative, or if the case was seronegative and their matched control was seropositive. Concordant pairs would be those matched pairs of cases and controls that are either both seronegative or both seropositive. For the above example the odds ratio would be derived as the number of pairs where the case was seropositive but the matched control was seronegative, divided by the number of pairs where the case was seronegative but the matched control was seropositive. Those pairs of cases and controls that had the same serological status (i.e. concordant pairs) would have provided no information as to the association between chronic H pylori infection and coronary heart disease in young patients; therefore they would not have been included in the calculation of the odds ratio.

As described above an odds ratio is an estimate of the population relative risk. Often an odds ratio is interpreted as a relative risk. Hence the odds ratio in the above example would indicate that there was an increased risk of 127% of early onset myocardial infarction if seropositive for H pylori infection antibodies compared to being seronegative. In particular the odds ratio will be a good estimate of the population relative risk if the prevalence of the disease outcome in the population is rare, typically considered to be less than 10%. It is anticipated that the disease outcome of early onset myocardial infarction at a young age was rare in the population. Therefore the presented odds ratio would be expected to be a good estimate of the relative risk of early onset myocardial infarction if seropositive compared to seronegative for H pylori infection antibodies.

Danesh J, Youngman L, Clark S, Parish S, Peto R, Collins R for the International Studies of Infarct Survival (ISIS) Collaborative Group. Helicobacter pylori infection and early onset myocardial infarction: case-control and sibling pairs study. *BMJ* 1999;319:1157.

Sedgwick P. Why match in case-control studies? *BMJ* 2012a;344:e691.

Sedgwick P. Confidence intervals and statistical significance: rules of thumb. *BMJ* 2012b;345:e4960

Sedgwick P. Logistic regression. *BMJ* 2013;347:f4488.

28. A. His annual stroke risk is around 3% and he should commence an oral anticoagulant

The presence of AF (paroxysmal or persistent) is associated with risk of formation of thrombi in the left atrium that may subsequently embolize leading to systemic embolic events, the most significant of which is an embolic stroke.

Table 4.3 CHA_2DS_2VASC.

Risk factor	Score
Congestive heart failure	1
Hypertension	1
Age ≥75	2
Age 65–74	1
Diabetes mellitus	1
Stroke/TIA/thrombo-embolism	2
Vascular disease	1
Sex category—female	1

Adapted from *Stroke*, Lip GYH et al., 'Identifying patients at high risk for stroke despite anticoagulation: a comparison of contemporary stroke risk stratification schemes in an anticoagulated atrial fibrillation cohort', 2010, 41, 12, pp. 2731–2738.

As the CHA_2DS_2VASc score increases so too does the associated adjusted stroke rate (% year). For example a CHA_2DS_2VASc score of 0 gives a 0% per year risk, while a score of 1 gives a 1.3% per year risk. A score of 9 gives a 15.2% per year risk'

The risk of stroke is not the same in all patients and is dependent on the clinical characteristics of each patient. Clinical scoring systems are available to aid in risk-stratifying patients and guiding use of anticoagulants. The most commonly used scoring system is the CHA_2DS_2VASc score (Table 4.3). If total score is 1 or higher (2 in females) then oral anticoagulants are indicated. There is no longer a role for aspirin in prevention of thromboembolic complications of AF.

Lip G, Frison L,Halperin J et al. Identifying patients at high risk for stroke despite anticoagulation: a comparison of contemporary stroke risk stratification schemes in an anticoagulated atrial fibrillation cohort. Stroke 2010; 41(12): 2731–2738. doi: 10.1161/STROKEAHA.110.590257. Epub 2010.

Lip G,Nieuwlaat R, Pisters R et al. Refining clinical risk stratification for predicting stroke and thromboembolism in atrial fibrillation using a novel risk factor-based approach: the euro heart survey on atrial fibrillation. Chest 2010; 137: 263–272. http://www.chadsvasc.org

National Institute for Health and Care Excellence. Clinical Guideline 180. Atrial fibrillation: management. June 2014.

29. E. Serum creatinine

The Global Registry of Acute Coronary Events (GRACE) is an international database that is used to track the outcomes of patients presenting with acute coronary syndromes. Based on this database, GRACE acute coronary syndrome (ACS) risk scores and algorithms were devised to predict death or death/myocardial infarction following an initial ACS.

The GRACE 2.0 score takes into consideration the following factors:

- Age
- Systolic blood pressure
- Heart rate
- Killip class

- Serum creatinine
- ST segment deviation
- Cardiac arrest on admission
- Elevated troponin

Reproduced by permission of the GRACE Coordinating Center, Center for Outcomes Research, University of Massachusetts Medical School.

Online calculators and smartphone apps are available for download: http://www.gracescore.org

Fox K, Fitzgerald G, Puymirat E et al. Should patients with acute coronary disease be stratified for management according to their risk? Derivation, external validation and outcomes using the updated GRACE risk score. *BMJ Open* 2014; 4(2): e004425.

30. E. You should reassure her and ask her to continue with her current medication

This woman has non-valvular AF and a CHA_2DS_2-VASc score of 3 (female gender and age). She has an annual stroke risk of 3.2%. She therefore has indications for oral anticoagulation (warfarin or one of the novel oral anticoagulants) for prophylaxis against thromboembolic complications of AF.

Her HAS-BLED score is 1 and she is, therefore, not in a high-risk category for bleeding (1.02–1.50% one-year risk). The balance of risks is, therefore, clearly in favour of oral anticoagulation.

The dose of dabigatran for non-valvular AF is 150 mg bd. However, a lower dose of dabigatran is advised in patients over 80 years of age, in those with mild to moderate renal dysfunction, and in association with some medications that may increase the levels of dabigatran (e.g. verapamil, amiodarone, and, in this case, quinine). This patient is on the lower dose of dabigatran. If quinine is deemed non-essential then it should be stopped.

Lip G, Nieuwlaat R, Pisters R et al. Refining clinical risk stratification for predicting stroke and thromboembolism in atrial fibrillation using a novel risk factor-based approach: the euro heart survey on atrial fibrillation. *Chest* 2010; 137: 263–272. http://www.chadsvasc.org

31. C. Echocardiography

This young man had a recent invasive intra-cardiac device and the first step is to rule out perforation of one of the leads and a pericardial effusion using echocardiography. This is a relatively rare complication and its incidence in device registries is around 1%. Given the sheer number of implanted devices, however, it is not an unusual condition. The incidence is higher with defibrillator leads and in young patients in whom the cardiac muscle is supple and less stiff.

The clinical presentation is not suggestive of an ACS. The ECG changes are most likely caused by the primary cardiac pathology (i.e. arrhythmogenic right ventricular cardiomyopathy). The serum troponin may be raised after the implantable cardioverter defibrillator implant procedure (particularly if a defibrillation test was done) and is, therefore, not useful. Giving anti-thrombotics as part of the usual ACS protocol would cause haemodynamic deterioration due to increasing effusion and tamponade.

There is no suggestion of any arrhythmia that would be detected on a device check and data download. A high 'threshold' would confirm a lead problem and in the presence of an effusion would make the diagnosis of lead perforation extremely likely.

Brignole M, Auricchio A, Baron-Esquivias G et al. on behalf of the task force on cardiac pacing and resynchronization therapy of the European Society of Cardiology (ESC). Cardiac Pacing and Cardiac Resynchronization Therapy ESC Clinical Practice Guidelines. *European Heart Journal* 2013; 34: 2281–2329. doi: 10.1093/eurheartj/eht150. http://www.escardio.org/guidelines

32. D. Invasive pulmonary artery catheter

This is a delayed presentation of an acute anterior myocardial infarction complicated by acute left ventricular failure. The acute treatment of this patient includes supplemental oxygen to improve oxygenation and oxygen delivery to the tissues and intravenous isosorbide dinitrate infusion to reduce preload and, to a lesser extent, afterload, thus reducing pulmonary congestion and improving forward ejection fraction. Intravenous furosemide reduces intravascular volume and also has a systemic vasodilator effect, thus reducing filling pressures and pulmonary congestion by reducing afterload. Dobutamine is a positive inotrope and mild dilator that helps improve forward ejection fraction and cardiac output.

The ESCAPE trial has demonstrated that invasive pulmonary artery catheters did not improve the outcome of these patients but were associated with procedural complications. Its use is reserved for specific cases where there is no response to standard therapies and there is the need to clarify cardiac indices and filling pressures to guide therapy.

The ESCAPE Investigators and ESCAPE Study Coordinators. Evaluation Study of Congestive Heart Failure and Pulmonary Artery Catheterization Effectiveness: The ESCAPE Trial. JAMA 2005; 294(13): 1625–1633. doi: 10.1001/jama.294.13.1625.

chapter 5

DIABETES AND ENDOCRINOLOGY

QUESTIONS

1. **A 36-year-old woman was admitted to the acute medical unit with symptoms of sweatiness, palpitations, and anxiety.** She was normally fit and well and had given birth to twins while in India two years ago. She was not taking any regular medication. Ten days previously she had suffered from a flu-like illness with joint pain, muscle pain and fatigue. Subsequently, she developed pain and swelling in her neck and swallowing was uncomfortable. On examination she had clammy palms and a mild tremor. Her temperature was 38.8°C; her pulse was 110 beats per minute and regular. She had a moderately sized, tender goitre. No lymph nodes were palpable. She had lid lag and lid retraction but no ophthalmoplegia or chemosis.

   ```
   Investigations:
     serum thyroid stimulating      <0.05 mU/L      (0.4-5.0)
       hormone
     serum free T4                  76.1 pmol/L     (10.0-22.0)
     serum free T3                  19.5 pmol/L     (3.0-7.0)
     serum CRP                      30 mg/L         (<10)
   ```

   What is the most appropriate first-line treatment?
   A. Carbimazole 40 mg od
   B. Ibuprofen 300 mg tds
   C. Prednisolone 40 mg od
   D. Propranolol 40 mg tds
   E. Propylthiouracil 200 mg bd

2. A 26-year-old woman had an elective thyroidectomy for hard to control Grave's disease. She was euthyroid at the time of operation. No complications arose from the surgery. The next day she was complaining of tingling in her fingers and around her mouth and spasm of her fingers. An ECG showed a prolonged QT interval. The ward doctor had given three boluses of 10 mL 10% calcium gluconate intravenously and prescribed oral calcium supplements but the patient remained symptomatic.

After the 10% calcium gluconate intravenous boluses blood results were as follows.

```
Investigations:
    serum corrected calcium    1.87 mmol/L    (2.20-2.60)
    serum phosphate            0.9 mmol/L     (0.8-1.4)
    serum magnesium            0.61 mmol/L    (0.75-1.05)
```

What is the most appropriate next step in management?
A. Give 1 alpha-hydroxy-cholecalciferol 500 ng once daily
B. Give magnesium sulphate 8 mmol over six hours intravenously
C. Increase the oral calcium supplement
D. Repeat the bolus of 10 mL 10% calcium gluconate intravenously
E. Start a calcium gluconate infusion intravenously

3. A 36-year-old man presented to the acute medical unit with a severe headache behind the eyes that came on over a day. He felt dizzy and had vomited several times. He was complaining of double vision, photophobia, and neck stiffness. He was normally fit and well but had noticed an increase in shoe size in the past year. On examination, his Glasgow Coma Score (GCS) was 14/15, pulse 98 beats per minute, blood pressure 100/50 mmHg, and capillary blood glucose 9.8 mmol/L. He had prognathism, macroglossia, and an increase in interdental spacing. He had third, fourth, and sixth cranial nerve palsies on the right.

Full blood count, urea, and electrolytes were normal; plasma glucose was 10.2 mmol/L.

What is the most likely diagnosis?
A. Intracerebral haemorrhage
B. Meningitis
C. Pituitary apoplexy
D. Subarachnoid haemorrhage
E. Subdural haematoma

4. A 48-year-old man with lower limb cellulitis attended the ambulatory care unit for assessment for outpatient intravenous antibiotic treatment. This was the second episode of cellulitis requiring antibiotics in the previous six months. There was no history of trauma or insect bites to the skin. He had no other past medical history and was symptomatically well and specifically had no symptoms of thirst, polyuria, polydipsia, or weight loss.

   On examination, he had a body mass index (BMI) of 31 kg/m², temperature 37.7°C, pulse 89 beats per minute, and blood pressure 146/78 mmHg. Cardiovascular, respiratory, and abdominal examination was normal. There was cellulitis of the right calf with dry skin on the heels and tinea pedis. A random capillary blood glucose was 8.4 mmol/L. He had previously had a random plasma glucose of 10.4 mmol/L, but had not had any further investigations. Haemoglobin A1c (HbA1c) was sent on this admission.

   The next step in management is:
   A. Refer to GP to follow-up the result of the HbA1c
   B. Refer to the community diabetes education team
   C. Start gliclazide 40 mg bd
   D. Start metformin 500 mg od increasing up to 1 g bd as tolerated
   E. Start saxagliptin 5 mg od

5. A 23-year-old man was referred by his GP to the acute medical unit at 10:00 a.m. with a two-week history of thirst, polyuria, polydipsia, and weight loss. He had not been vomiting. Random capillary blood glucose at the GP surgery was 23.6 mmol/L. He had previously been fit and well with no past medical history. On examination, he was slim, pulse 78 beats per minute, blood pressure 123/65 mmHg, there was no pigmentation, and he was clinically euthyroid.

   ```
   Investigations:
     Venous blood gas:
     pH                      7.36 (7.35-7.45)
     pCO₂                    5.6 kPa
     pO₂                     6.5 kPa
     bicarbonate             20 mmol/L           (21-29)
     base excess             -2 mmol/L           (±2.0)

     urine ketones           1 +

     plasma glucose          24.6 mmol/L
     urea and electrolytes   normal
   ```

   What is the most appropriate management strategy?
   A. Admit for fixed-rate insulin infusion
   B. Admit for variable-rate insulin infusion
   C. Admit to start subcutaneous insulin
   D. Contact the diabetes team to arrange for the patient to start
   E. Start on oral hypoglycaemic agents and discharge to GP

6. A 37-year-old man who was normally fit and well was referred to the acute medical team from the emergency department with right lower lobe pneumonia. He presented with right-sided chest pain and breathlessness. There was no history of cough or sputum production. On reassessment his pulse was 102 beats per minute, blood pressure 110/67 mmHg, respiratory rate 23 breaths per minute, and oxygen saturation 97% on air. His chest was clear and he had abdominal tenderness.

```
Investigations:
  Arterial blood gas breathing air:
  pH                             7.25           (7.35-7.45)
  pCO₂                           3.6 kPa        (4.7-6.0)
  pO₂                            14.5 kPa       (11.3-12.6)
  bicarbonate                    15.6 mmol/L    (21-29)
  base excess                    -7 mmol/L      (±2)
  lactate                        3.6 mmol/L     (0.5-1.6)

  Blood ketones                  1.3 mmol/L

  serum amylase                  1378 U/L       (60-180)
  serum sodium                   122 mmol/L     (137-144)
  serum creatinine               124 µmol/L     (60-110)
  fasting plasma glucose         23 mmol/L      (3.0-6.0)
  fasting serum triglycerides    23 mmol/L      (0.45-1.69)
  Lipaemic sample, unable to be analysed completely.
```

What is the most appropriate first-line treatment?

A. Amoxicillin 500 mg tds
B. Fluid restriction to 1 L per day
C. Intravenous insulin
D. Plasmapheresis
E. Surgical referral

7. A 43-year-old woman with primary hypothyroidism stopped taking her usual dose of levothyroxine 100 mcg od three months ago because she didn't like taking tablets. She was admitted to the acute medical unit because she collapsed while out shopping. There was no loss of consciousness. She felt dizzy and faint. The ambulance sheet observations were: temperature 34.3°C, pulse 35 beats per minute, blood pressure 80/45 mmHg, GCS 14/15 (E4, V4, M6). On reassessment after 500 mL sodium chloride 0.9% intravenously, her pulse was 40 beats per minute, blood pressure 98/45 mmHg, and GCS 15/15. The rest of the examination was unremarkable.

```
Investigations:
  serum thyroid-stimulating    >95.0 mU/L     (0.4-5.0)
    hormone
  serum free T₄                <5.0 pmol/L    (10.0-22.0)
```

What is the most appropriate first-line treatment?

A. Carbimazole 40 mg od
B. Levothyroxine 50 mcg od
C. Levothyroxine 100 mcg od
D. Liothyronine via a naso-gastric tube
E. Temporary pacing wire

8. A 42-year-old woman presented to ambulatory care clinic with a three-month history of increasing tiredness, lethargy, and poor concentration. She had lost weight because of a reduction in appetite due to non-specific abdominal pain. The pain was not altered by eating, movement, or related to having her bowels open. There was no associated vomiting or diarrhoea. She recently had to return early from holiday in Mexico because she felt so unwell. On examination, she was slim (BMI 20.4 kg/m²) and tanned from her recent holiday. Her temperature was 36.9°C, pulse 89 beats per minute, blood pressure 100/60 mmHg, and respiratory rate 18 breaths per minute. Cardiovascular and respiratory examination was normal. Her abdomen was soft and non-tender.

```
Investigations:
    serum sodium                    128 mmol/L      (137-144)
    serum potassium                 5.6 mmol/L      (3.5-4.9)
    serum urea                      10.8 mmol/L     (2.5-7.0)
    serum creatinine                98 µmol/L       (60-110)
    serum albumin                   38 g/L          (37-49)
    serum alkaline phosphatase      126 U/L         (45-105)
    serum alanine aminotransferase  112 U/L         (5-35)
    serum total bilirubin           12 µmol/L       (1-22)
    serum amylase                   86 U/L          (60-180)
    serum corrected calcium         2.84 mmol/L     (2.20-2.60)
```

What is the next most appropriate investigation?

A. 9:00 a.m. paired cortisol and adrenocorticotrophic hormone (ACTH)
B. Protein electrophoresis
C. Short synacthen test
D. Thyroid function tests
E. Urine and plasma osmolalities

9. A 25-year-old man with type 1 diabetes presented to the acute medical unit with diarrhoea and vomiting over the last three days. He had not been eating and for the previous day had been unable to keep down fluids. He continued taking his glargine but didn't increase the dose despite home blood glucose readings in the 20s. He had type 1 diabetes since the age of four and was on aspart 12 units with meals and glargine 35 units once daily. His most recent HbA1c was 59 mmol/mol and he had some background retinopathy but no other complications from diabetes. He was diagnosed with diabetic ketoacidosis (DKA) and started on intravenous insulin at 6 units per hour and intravenous 0.9% saline over two hours. His glargine was not prescribed.

His initial blood results were as follows.
```
Investigations:
  Arterial blood gas breathing air:
    pH                          6.9             (7.35-7.45)
    pCO2                        3.2 kPa         (4.7-6.0)
    pO2                         15.4 kPa        (11.3-12.6)
    bicarbonate                 7 mmol/L        (21-29)
    base excess                 -12 mmol/L      (±2)

    capillary blood glucose     35.0 mmol/L
    blood ketones               3.6 mmol/L      (<0.6mmol/L)

    serum sodium                145 mmol/L      (137-144)
    serum potassium             5.6 mmol/L      (3.5-4.9)
    serum urea                  12.3 mmol/L     (2.5-7.0)
    serum creatinine            127 µmol/L      (60-110)
    plasma glucose              36.7 mmol/L
```

Six hours after admission he was reassessed. He was alert and orientated but didn't feel any better. His pulse was 98 beats per minute, blood pressure 105/56 mmHg, and respiratory rate 23 breaths per minute. He weighed 100 kg. The rest of the examination was unremarkable.
```
Investigations:
  Venous gas:
    pH                          7.0             (7.35-7.45)
    pCO2                        3.6 kPa         (4.7-6.0)
    bicarbonate                 8 mmol/L        (21-29)
    base excess                 -10 mmol/L      (±2)

    capillary blood glucose     19.2 mmol/L
    capillary blood ketones     3.0 mmol/L      (<0.6 mmol/L)
```

What is your next step?

A. Assume the lack of change in pH is because the second gas sample is venous and continue the infusion at the current rate
B. Give bicarbonate and refer to the Critical Care Team
C. Increase the insulin to 8 units per hour
D. Increase the insulin to 10 units per hour
E. Prescribe the evening glargine dose and continue the current rate of insulin infusion

10. An 84-year-old woman was found collapsed at home by her daughter. She was last seen a week ago. Her daughter noticed that several days' worth of medication had not been taken. She had a history of tablet-treated type 2 diabetes (gliclazide and metformin), hypertension, and angina. Her HbA1c was 64 mmol/mol.

She was unable to give a history. She weighed 43 kg. She was confused and dehydrated. Her pulse was 123 beats per minute and irregularly irregular, blood pressure was 110/67 mmHg, respiratory rate 18 breaths per minute, and oxygen saturation was 97% on 40% oxygen via a venturi mask. GCS was 13/15 (E4, V4, M5). Capillary blood glucose was 'Hi'. There was bronchial breathing at the right base. The rest of her examination was normal.

```
Investigations:
    chest X-ray:            right lower lobe
                            pneumonia
    CT scan of head:        atrophy consistent
                            with age

    serum sodium            155 mmol/L          (137-144)
    serum potassium         5.0 mmol/L          (3.5-4.9)
    serum urea              23.3 mmol/L         (2.5-7.0)
    serum creatinine        245 µmol/L          (60-110)
    plasma glucose          65.6 mmol/L
    haemoglobin             96 g/L              (115-165)
    white cell count        21.0 × 10⁹/L        (4.0-11.0)
    neutrophil count        19.0 × 10⁹/L        (1.5-7.0)
    platelet count          453 × 10⁹/L         (150-400)

    Arterial blood gas
      on 40% FiO₂:
    pH                      7.3                 (7.35-7.45)
    pCO₂                    4.6 kPa             (4.7-6.0)
    pO₂                     12.5 kPa            (11.3-12.6)
    bicarbonate             19 mmol/L           (21-29)

    blood ketones           0.9 mmol/L
```

The diagnosis of diabetic ketoacidosis (DKA) was made and she was commenced on a fixed rate of 4 units/hour of insulin and intravenous sodium chloride 0.9%.

What is the next step in management?

A. Change to a variable-rate insulin infusion and swap the fluids to sodium chloride 0.45% as she has hypernatraemia
B. Continue treatment. She is on the correct dose of insulin for DKA
C. This is hyperosmolar hyperglycaemic state (HHS); change to sodium chloride 0.45% and continue the iv insulin
D. This is hyperosmolar hyperglycaemic state (HHS); continue the sodium chloride 0.9% and stop the iv insulin until the blood glucose is stable
E. This is hyperosmolar non-ketotic coma (HONK) and she should be on 0.5 units insulin/hour

DIABETES AND ENDOCRINOLOGY | QUESTIONS

11. A 74-year-old patient was admitted with hyperosmolar hyperglycaemic state (HHS). Her plasma glucose was 62 mmol/L, serum sodium 152 mmol/L, and calculated osmolality 389 mosmol/kg. Intravenous sodium chloride 0.9% was started. Six hours later her capillary blood glucose was 28.6 mmol/L and was still dropping with just intravenous fluid replacement.

    Her repeat blood tests at six hours were as follows.

    ```
    Investigations:
       serum sodium          160 mmol/L     (137-144)
       serum potassium       5.0 mmol/L     (3.5-4.9)
       serum urea            22.4 mmol/L    (2.5-7.0)
       serum creatinine      213 µmol/L     (60-110)
       plasma glucose        27.7 mmol/L
       serum osmolality      356 mmol/L     (278-300)
    ```

    What is the next step in management?
    A. Change the fluids to glucose 5% and start a variable-rate insulin infusion
    B. Change to sodium chloride 0.45% and start 0.5 units insulin per hour
    C. Continue sodium chloride 0.9% and start a variable-rate insulin infusion
    D. Continue sodium chloride 0.9% and start insulin at 2 units per hour
    E. Make no changes to the current treatment

12. A 47-year-old woman known to have Turner syndrome presented to the acute medical unit with central chest pain. It came on suddenly four hours previously while playing tennis. She felt dizzy and light-headed. Glyceryl trinitrate (GTN) eased the pain but it hadn't resolved completely.

    She had not been seen by the endocrine team for several years having not attended follow-up appointments. She was on no regular medication. She had come back from a walking holiday in North America six days ago. She smoked 20 cigarettes per day and drank 10 units of alcohol per week.

    On examination, her blood pressure was 165/65 mmHg in the right arm and 140/45 mmHg in the left arm. There was an early diastolic murmur.

    ```
    Investigations:
       serum troponin T      274 ng/L       (<14)
       D-dimer               1.3 mg/L       (<0.5)

       chest X-ray:          small left pleural effusion.

       ECG:                  anterior T-wave inversion.
    ```

    What is the most likely diagnosis?
    A. Aortic dissection
    B. Coarctation of the aorta
    C. Myocardial infarction
    D. Myocarditis
    E. Pulmonary embolus

13. A 37-year-old man presented to the acute medical unit with a severe headache of two days' duration. It came on gradually and was the worst headache he had ever had. Simple analgesia had not helped. He had gained 3 stone in weight in the last year, had stopped exercising because of weakness, and had been started on citalopram recently for depression.

There was no photophobia or neck stiffness. He had vomited but this was unrelated to eating and he felt better lying down. A CT head and lumbar puncture were both normal.

On examination, he was overweight (BMI 34), with plethoric features and bruised skin. Fundoscopy showed grade 3 hypertensive retinopathy. His pulse rate was 87 beats per minute and regular, his blood pressure was 210/140 mmHg right arm, and 205/142 mmHg left arm. Heart sounds were normal and the apex beat was forceful. Peripheral pulses were equal and intact. There were no renal bruits present. His respiratory examination was normal. The abdominal examination showed abdominal skin striae. Neurological examination was normal.

```
Investigations:

  ECG: left ventricular hypertrophy

  chest X-ray: cardiomegaly

  serum sodium                         145 mmol/L       (137-144)
  serum potassium                      3.1 mmol/L       (3.5-4.9)
  serum urea                           4.5 mmol/L       (2.5-7.0)
  serum creatinine                     67 µmol/L        (60-110)
  estimated glomerular filtration      >90 mL/min       (>90)
    rate
  plasma glucose                       13.2 mmol/L

  urine dip: glucose 2 +, no protein, no blood, no
    leucocytes, no nitrites
```

After treating the blood pressure, what is the best investigation to establish the aetiology of the hypertension?

A. Echocardiogram
B. Renal ultrasound
C. Renin-aldosterone ratio
D. Twenty-four hour urinary-free cortisol
E. Twenty-four hour urinary metanephrines

14. **A 78-year-old woman was admitted to the acute medical unit with community-acquired pneumonia. She was otherwise fit and well with no other significant past medical history. Her admission blood tests showed an elevated calcium level. She had no symptoms of hypercalcaemia.**

```
Investigations:
    serum-corrected calcium            2.80 mmol/L         (2.20-2.60)
    serum phosphate                    0.5 mmol/L          (0.8-1.4)
    serum sodium                       134 mmol/L          (137-144)
    serum potassium                    4.5 mmol/L          (3.5-4.9)
    serum urea                         6.5 mmol/L          (2.5-7.0)
    serum creatinine                   87 µmol/L           (60-110)
    serum albumin                      43 g/L              (37-49)
    serum alkaline phosphatase         110 U/L             (45-105)
    serum alanine aminotransferase     23 U/L              (5-35)
    serum total bilirubin              12 µmol/L           (1-22)
    serum C reactive protein           146 mg/L            (<10)
    haemoglobin                        143 g/L             (130-180)
    white cell count                   16.6 × 10$^9$/L     (4.0-11.0)
    neutrophil count                   14.5 × 10$^9$/L     (1.5-7.0)
    platelet count                     453 × 10$^9$/L      (150-400)
```

What is the most likely diagnosis?

A. Lung malignancy with bone metastases
B. Multiple endocrine neoplasia type I
C. Myeloma
D. Primary hyperparathyroidism
E. Tertiary hyperparathyroidism

15. A 55-year-old nurse was admitted to the acute medical unit with an episode of hypoglycaemia. She was found unconscious at home by her husband and the paramedic crew at the scene measured her capillary blood glucose at 1.3 mmol/L and treated her with 1 mg glucagon intramuscularly and an infusion of glucose 10%. Her blood glucose responded to this treatment and the intravenous glucose was stopped on arrival in hospital. Forty-five minutes later her blood glucose dropped to 2.6 mmol/L, so the glucose 10% infusion was restarted and the patient was given a sandwich to eat.

    She did not have a history of diabetes. She was the main carer for her 63-year-old husband who had multiple health problems including a stroke, obesity, and type 2 diabetes (on oral hypoglycaemic agents). There was no history of previous hypoglycaemia, she was on no medication, and was normally fit and well.

    The blood glucose had been stable on the glucose 10% infusion for four hours and the patient was eating normally. The glucose infusion was stopped. Two hours later she had a further episode of hypoglycaemia. The blood glucose dropped to 2.0 mmol/L.

    What is the most likely diagnosis?
    A. Dumping syndrome
    B. Factitious hypoglycaemia due to inappropriate sulphonylurea administration
    C. Insulinoma
    D. Non-islet cell tumour hypoglycaemia
    E. Reactive hypoglycaemia

16. An anaesthetist doing a list in day-case theatres asked for advice. The first patient on the list had type 1 diabetes controlled by a continuous subcutaneous insulin infusion (CSII or insulin pump). The operation was not expected to last longer than an hour, so the patient should be eating and drinking within 2–3 hours of the operation finishing. The blood glucose reading was 7 mmol/L and the surgeon was due in theatre in the next ten minutes to start the case.

    What do you advise?
    A. Keep the pump running at the usual basal rate and monitor the blood glucose hourly
    B. Keep the pump running but increase the basal rate to compensate for the stress of the operation and monitor blood glucose hourly
    C. Keep the pump running but reduce the basal rate to compensate for the patient being anaesthetized and less active and monitor blood glucose hourly
    D. Stop the pump and start a variable-rate insulin infusion (VRII)
    E. Stop the pump for the duration of the procedure and restart once the patient has recovered from the procedure

17. A 26-year-old woman presented to the acute medical unit with palpitations, tremor, and anxiety. She gave a six-month history of weight loss and oligomenorrhoea. She complained of dry, gritty eyes, which were more prominent than usual, and she'd developed a non-tender swelling in her neck. She was usually fit and well, took no over-the-counter supplements, and was on no regular medication. She had not been able to exercise at the gym due to fatigue and was finding the stairs difficult. Her mother had hypothyroidism following radioactive iodine treatment, her twin sister had type 1 diabetes, and a cousin had coeliac disease. She was not using any contraception and wanted to get pregnant.

On examination, she had clammy palms and a fine tremor more obvious on extension of the arms. Her pulse rate was 112 beats per minute and regular and her blood pressure was 125/73 mmHg. Cardiovascular, respiratory, and abdominal examination was normal. She was unable to stand from a chair without using her arms.

She had lid lag and lid retraction with proptosis. There was no ophthalmoplegia or chemosis. There was a palpable smooth moderately sized goitre with no retrosternal extension and a bruit.

```
Investigations:
    ECG: sinus tachycardia
    chest X-Ray: normal
    serum thyroid-stimulating      <0.05 mU/L        (0.4-5.0)
      hormone
    serum free T4                  64.3 pmol/L       (10.0-22.0)
    serum free T3                  13.5 pmol/L       (3.0-7.0)
```

All other blood tests were normal.

What is your first-line treatment?

A. Carbimazole 40 mg od
B. Propranolol 40 mg tds
C. Propylthiouracil 200 mg bd
D. Refer for treatment with radio-iodine (I^{131})
E. Thyroxine 50 mcg od

18. A 42-year-old man presented to the emergency department with confusion and agitation. He had been vomiting profusely for the last 12 hours. He had no significant past medical history and was not on any regular medication. He was confused and was trying to leave the department. He denied heavy alcohol use.

On examination, his pulse rate was 110 beats per minute, blood pressure was 100/55 mmHg, respiratory rate 20 breaths per minute, and oxygen saturation 98% on air. Cardiovascular and respiratory examination were normal, his abdomen was soft on palpation with some epigastric tenderness, and bowel sounds were present.

```
Investigations:
    serum sodium        112 mmol/L      (137-144)
    serum potassium     3.0 mmol/L      (3.5-4.9)
    serum urea          14.3 mmol/L     (2.5-7.0)
    serum creatinine    145 µmol/L      (60-110)
```

What is the correct management of his hyponatraemia?

A. Demeclocycline 300 mg orally tds
B. Fluid restrict to 500 mL in 24 hours
C. Give 0.45% sodium chloride 500 mL intravenously
D. Give 0.9% sodium chloride 500 mL intravenously
E. Give 1.8% sodium chloride 500 mL intravenously

19. A 78-year-old woman was being treated for community-acquired pneumonia. On admission, she was taking furosemide 40 mg once daily; this had been stopped for four days. Her serum sodium was 126 mmol/L (137–144 mmol/L) on admission and was now 124 mmol/L. She was clinically euvolaemic.

Her paired osmolalities were as follows.

```
Investigations:
    serum osmolality    240 mosmol/kg   (278-300)
    urine osmolality    420 mosmol/kg   (350-1000)
```

What is the best management of her hyponatraemia?

A. Fluid restrict to 750 mL in 24 hours
B. Intravenous 0.9% sodium chloride 1000 mL over eight hours
C. Restart furosemide 40 mg daily
D. Start demeclocylcine 300 mg three times a day (tds)
E. Start tolvaptan 15 mg daily

DIABETES AND ENDOCRINOLOGY | QUESTIONS

20. An 84-year-old woman presented to the acute medical unit having fallen at home. She had a past medical history of hypertension, ischaemic heart disease, and osteoarthritis. She was frail and used a wheeled zimmer frame to mobilize. Her regular medication included aspirin, bendroflumethiazide, simvastatin, amlodipine, and paracetamol.

```
Investigations:
   urine dipstick      positive to leucocytes and nitrites
   serum sodium        124 mmol/L    (137-144)
```

What is the best next step to manage her hyponatraemia?
A. Fluid restrict to 1 L in 24 hours
B. Intravenous 0.9% saline
C. Send urine and serum osmolalities
D. Start trimethoprim
E. Stop bendroflumethiazide

21. A 34-year-old man with Addison's disease presented to the acute medical unit with diarrhoea and vomiting. His normal medication was hydrocortisone 10 mg in the morning, 5 mg at midday, and 5 mg in the evening. On examination, his heart rate was 100 beats per minute and his blood pressure was 86/54 mmHg.

What is the correct management of his steroid therapy?
A. Convert him to prednisolone 40 mg daily
B. Double his hydrocortisone dose to 20 mg/10 mg/10 mg and give it intravenously
C. Double his oral hydrocortisone dose to 20 mg/10 mg/10 mg
D. Give intravenous hydrocortisone 100 mg once daily
E. Give intravenous hydrocortisone 100 mg four times a day

22.
A 64-year-old woman was admitted to the acute medical unit with polyuria and polydipsia. She described needing to pass urine at least three times every night, and was constantly thirsty. She was drinking regularly overnight and taking a glass of water to bed. She had a past medical history of hypertension, ischaemic heart disease, and bipolar disorder. She was taking aspirin, lithium, and bisoprolol.

```
Investigations:
    serum sodium            145 mmol/L         (137-144)
    serum potassium         4.5 mmol/L         (3.5-4.9)
    serum urea              11.5 mmol/L        (2.5-7.0)
    serum creatinine        188 µmol/L         (60-110)
    plasma glucose (random) 7.2 mmol/L
    serum osmolality        370 mosmol/kg      (278-300)
    urine osmolality        165 mosmol/kg      (350-1000)
```

What is the most likely diagnosis?

A. Cranial diabetes insipidus
B. Nephrogenic diabetes insipidus
C. Pre-renal acute kidney injury
D. Type 1 diabetes mellitus
E. Type 2 diabetes mellitus

23.
A 48-year-old woman presented to the acute medical unit with palpitations. She described nearly a year of palpitations associated with sweating, headaches, and feeling unwell. Her family reported that she went pale during the episodes. She had no past medical history and was not on any regular medication. On examination, her heart rate was 90 beats per minute and regular, blood pressure was 170/65 mmHg, and respiratory rate was 16 breaths per minute. Cardiorespiratory examination was normal.

```
Investigations:
    ECG:              sinus rhythm
    chest X-ray:      normal
    urine dipstick:   no blood or protein
```

What test is likely to be most useful in reaching a diagnosis?

A. Serum renin-aldosterone ratio
B. Twenty-four-hour ambulatory blood pressure monitor
C. Twenty-four-hour holter monitor
D. Twenty-four-hour urinary 5HIAA
E. Twenty-four-hour urinary metanephrines

chapter 5

DIABETES AND ENDOCRINOLOGY

ANSWERS

1. D. Propranolol 40 mg tds

This woman has subacute (or De Quervain's) thyroiditis. This is an inflammatory disorder of the thyroid that is assumed to be viral in origin. It is often preceded by a non-specific viral illness. The main symptoms are malaise, fever, pain, and tenderness in the neck, which may be a prominent symptom as well as those associated with the presence of excessive amounts of thyroid hormones (e.g. palpitations, tremor, and anxiety). Histology shows leucocytic and granulomatous infiltration of the thyroid gland with follicle disruption. Characteristic giant cells are present.

It is caused by the release of pre-formed thyroid hormone from the thyroid gland and, as such, doesn't require treatment with anti-thyroid medication. Treatment is aimed at reducing inflammation with non-steroidal anti-inflammatory drugs (NSAIDs) or steroids, especially when pain is a problem (e.g. prednisolone 20–40 mg/day for two weeks and titrated down). Beta-blockers would be the first-line treatment to control the sympathetic symptoms of thyrotoxicosis (e.g. tachycardia, tremor, and anxiety symptoms). The thyrotoxicosis can last for three to eight weeks and may be followed by a period of transient hypothyroidism afterwards. About 10% of cases will be hypothyroid long term.

Some women develop post-partum thyroiditis but this typically occurs within the first six months after delivery. It occurs in up to 7% of women. Up to 50% of women have positive anti-thyroid peroxidase (TPO) antibodies.

De Groot L. Thyroid Disease- www.thyroidmanager.org. Accessed November 2015.

Wass J, Owen K. Oxford handbook of endocrinology and diabetes. Oxford University Press, 2014.

Wass J, Stewart P et al. Oxford textbook of endocrinology and diabetes. Oxford University Press, 2011.

2. E. Start a calcium gluconate infusion intravenously

The patient is still symptomatic and hypocalcaemic, despite three boluses of calcium gluconate. Start an infusion of calcium gluconate. Dilute 10 ampoules of 10 mL 10% calcium gluconate in either sodium chloride 0.9% or glucose 5%. This is 22 mmol of calcium. Start at 50 mL/hr and titrate to maintain calcium in the low normal range; 0.30–0.40 mmol/kg of elemental calcium should increase serum calcium by 0.5–0.75 mmol/L. If the hypocalcaemia is likely to persist, oral vitamin D in the form of an activated vitamin D supplement (e.g. 1- alfacalcidol) should be commenced.

The post-operative hypocalcaemia after thyroidectomy may be due to hypoparathyroidism either due to inadvertent removal or interruption of blood supply. Symptoms and signs appear between one and seven days post-op depending on the severity of insult. The other cause of hypocalcaemia after thyroidectomy is due to calcium retention by bone. Thyrotoxicosis leads to demineralization of the bones, and so this can be restored once the hyperthyroid state is resolved.

Parathyroid hormone has role in activating vitamin D (conversion of 25-hydroxyvitamin D3 to 1,25-hydroxy vitamin D3) in the kidneys, so the best response to hypocalcaemia is from giving activated vitamin D that doesn't require hydroxylation in the kidneys.

Hypomagnesaemia needs to be corrected before hypocalcaemia will resolve.

Oral calcium replacement is appropriate in asymptomatic patients or with corrected Ca^{2+} >1.8 mmol/L.

Kronenberg H, Melmed S. Williams textbook of endocrinology. Saunders, 2007.

Wass J, Stewart P et al. Oxford textbook of endocrinology and diabetes. Oxford University Press, 2011.

3. C. Pituitary apoplexy

The pituitary gland sits in the pituitary fossa. This is in the sphenoid bone and is adjacent to the cavernous sinus. Within the cavernous sinus are the internal carotid artery and the following cranial nerves: IIIrd (oculomotor), IVth (trochlear nerve), VIth (abducens), and Vth (trigeminal—ophthalmic and maxillary division). The pituitary gland is connected to the hypothalamus via the pituitary stalk; above the pituitary gland lies the optic chiasm.

An increase in size of a pituitary adenoma causes compression of the optic chiasm leading to visual disturbance—the classic one being a bitemporal hemianopia. When there is haemorrhage into a large pituitary tumour, there is usually destruction of the pituitary gland and compression of the surrounding structures by the enlarged gland. The cranial nerves that pass through the cavernous sinus are then affected and cause cranial nerve palsies; this is not seen with other causes of intracranial haemorrhage.

Pituitary apoplexy may be a result from haemorrhage into a pituitary adenoma, after head trauma, skull base fracture, or in association with diabetes and hypertension, sickle cell anaemia, or acute hypovolaemic shock (e.g. Sheehan's syndrome).

Clinically, it presents with headache, neck stiffness, cranial nerve lesions, cardiovascular collapse, and change in consciousness. If it is a functioning adenoma, then symptoms and signs of hormone excess will also be present. However, there can also be sudden hypopituitarism.

Signs: hypotension, ophthalmoplegia, hypoglycaemia, coma, and signs of subarachnoid haemorrhage can be present when blood has leaked into the subarachnoid space.

Imaging: haemorrhage into the pituitary. An MRI will provide the best imaging. Pituitary profile: a short synacthen test does not provide useful information in the first six weeks after an acute event.

Treatment: liaise with the local neurosurgical centre and endocrinologist as trans-sphenoidal decompression is indicated if there are signs of IIIrd (oculomotor) nerve palsy, or other nerve compression that fails to improve; optimal recovery occurs if surgery is done within the first eight days of presentation. However, treatment with dopamine agonists is appropriate if it is a prolactinoma, as rapid shrinkage and decompression can occur. Conservative management is appropriate for those patients with no focal neurological signs. Acute steroid replacement is given if there is a suspicion of hypoadrenalism.

Pituitary function often doesn't recover, so long-term hormone replacement is needed for the adrenal, thyroid, and gonadal axis. Long-term follow-up imaging shows the development of an empty sella as the pituitary tissue atrophies.

Grossman A. Pituitary Disease and Neuroendocrinology http://endotext.org. Accessed November 2015.

Kronenberg H, Melmed S. Williams textbook of endocrinology. Saunders, 2007.

Sam A, Meeran K. Lecture notes diabetes and endocrinology. Wiley-Blackwell, 2009.

Wass J, Stewart P et al. Oxford textbook of endocrinology and diabetes. Oxford University Press, 2011.

DIABETES AND ENDOCRINOLOGY | ANSWERS

4. A. Refer to GP to follow up the result of the HbA1c

The patient is asymptomatic and has not had a diagnostic blood glucose reading.

Diagnosis and initial treatment of diabetes: the diagnostic criteria for diabetes changed in January 2011. This, for the first time, allowed for the use of the HbA1c in the diagnosis of diabetes rather than relying on the oral glucose tolerance test. The HbA1c cannot be used for diagnosis in the following patients:

- *All* children and young people
- Patients of any age suspected of having type 1 diabetes
- Patients with symptoms of diabetes for less than two months
- Patients at high diabetes risk who are acutely ill (e.g. those requiring hospital admission)
- Patients taking medication that may cause rapid glucose rise (e.g. steroids, antipsychotics)
- Patients with acute pancreatic damage, including pancreatic surgery
- In pregnancy
- Presence of genetic, haematological, and illness-related factors that influence HbA1c and its measurement

Diagnostic criteria: an HbA1c >48 mmol/mol is the cut-off point for diagnosing diabetes; however, if glucose tolerance tests have diagnosed diabetes and the HbA1c is <48 mmol/mol, this does not rule out diabetes.

Previous World Health Organization (WHO) criteria were: diabetes symptoms (i.e. polyuria, polydipsia, and unexplained weight loss) plus:

- a random venous plasma glucose concentration $\geq$11.1 mmol/L; or
- a fasting plasma glucose concentration $\geq$7.0 mmol/L (whole blood $\geq$6.1 mmol/L); or
- two-hour plasma glucose concentration $\geq$11.1 mmol/L two hours after 75 g anhydrous glucose in an oral glucose tolerance test (OGTT).

With no symptoms, diagnosis should not be based on a single glucose determination but requires confirmatory plasma venous determination. At least one additional glucose test result on another day with a value in the diabetic range is essential, either fasting, from a random sample, or from the two-hour post-glucose load. If the fasting or random values are not diagnostic, the two-hour value should be used.

National Institute for Health and Care Excellence (NICE) guidance for the treatment of type 2 diabetes has structured patient education as the core of treatment. At diagnosis, all patients should have the opportunity to take part in an education programme (e.g. DESMOND (Diabetes Education and Self Management for Ongoing and Newly Diagnosed)) that focuses on diet and lifestyle to encourage a healthy, balanced diet with appropriate activity levels (current recommendation is for 30 minutes of physical activity five times per week). If after three months of diet and lifestyle interventions the HbA1c is still >48 mmol/mol then medication, usually metformin, is introduced.

National Institute for Health and Care Excellence. NICE Guideline 28: Type 2 diabetes in adults: management. December 2015.

World Health Organization. Use of Glycated Haemoglobin (HbA1c) in the Diagnosis of Diabetes Mellitus, 2011. http://www.who.int/diabetes/publications/report-hba1c_2011.pdf

5. D. Contact the diabetes team to arrange for the patient to start insulin

This man has type 1 diabetes—slim build and short duration of symptoms point towards this diagnosis. There is no sign of any other endocrinopathies. Starting on oral hypoglycaemic agents would be the wrong thing to do. In newly diagnosed type 2 diabetes, oral hypoglycaemic agents are usually started after a three-month trial of diet and lifestyle. All newly diagnosed patients with type 2 diabetes should be referred for community education (e.g. DESMOND; other programmes exist).

He does not need to be admitted for intravenous insulin at a variable or fixed rate; he is eating and drinking and does not have ketoacidosis. Adult patients are rarely admitted to start insulin. The best course of action is to contact the diabetes team to arrange patient education and the commencement of insulin. If the patient had presented out of hours, many hospitals have guidelines in place for the administration of long-acting insulin od as an outpatient (often done on ambulatory day units) until the patient is seen by the diabetes team. This prevents unnecessary admissions to hospital. Patients newly diagnosed with Type 1 diabetes should be invited to attend a structured education programme approximately six months after diagnosis as per NICE guidance NG17.

National Institute for Health and Care Excellence. NICE Guideline 17: Type 1 diabetes in adults: diagnosis and management. August 2015.

Definition and diagnosis of Diabetes Mellitus and Intermediate Hyperglycaemia. World Health Organization/International Diabetes Federation. 2006. ISBN: 978 92 4 159493 6.

6. C. Intravenous insulin

There is hyperglycaemia and hypertriglyceridaemia present. The amylase is consistent with pancreatitis but this will be secondary to the hypertriglyceridaemia, so it is important to treat this. Insulin decreases triglyceride levels by activating lipoprotein lipase which metabolizes chylomicrons. If the glucose is normal, or insulin doesn't bring down the triglycerides adequately, then plasmapheresis is an appropriate treatment to remove the excess triglycerides. This should be done in a critical care setting and the patient needs to be haemodynamically stable. A lipid-lowering agent would need to be started pre-discharge.

Reiner Z, Catapano A, De Baker G, et al. European Society of Cardiology/European Atherosclerosis Society Guidelines for the Management of Dyslipidaemias. European Heart Journal 2011;32: 1769–1818. doi: 10.1093/eurheartj/ehr158.

7. B. Levothyroxine 50 mcg od

This patient is known to have a diagnosis of hypothyroidism and has not taken her levothyroxine for three months, thus making her significantly under-treated (TSH >95, fT_4 <5.0). She is bradycardic and hypotensive but is fully conscious. She does not need a temporary pacing wire at the time of her assessment; if she was cardiovascularly unstable then this would need to be considered. Carbimazole is used to treat hyperthyroidism. When replacing thyroid hormone it is recommended to start at a low dose and titrate up to avoid causing problems by rapidly increasing metabolic demand. In the elderly, the recommended starting dose of levothyroxine is 25 mcg. Liothyronine via a nasogastric tube is used for patients in a coma or with cardiovascular instability. There is no consensus on the best regimen to use but an accepted regimen is: Levothyroxine 300–500 mcg iv or via a nasogastric tube as a starting dose, followed by 50–100 mcg daily until the patient is able to take oral medication or Liothyronine 5–20 mcg slowly iv (be cautious, as it may precipitate undiagnosed heart disease) followed by 5–20 mcg iv 4–12 hourly until sustained improvement is seen and then convert to Levothyroxine. If hypoadrenalism is suspected, give hydrocortisone 50–100 mg iv qds initially. If possible, a baseline cortisol and ACTH should be measured.

Care on an Intensive Care Unit would be appropriate for the comatosed patient. Also, consider the development of other autoimmune diseases (e.g. primary hypoadrenalism and coeliac disease). If a patient has one autoimmune disease they are more likely to develop another—rarely, they can all present at the same time.

Undiagnosed coeliac disease could potentially cause malabsorption of levothyroxine. Ferrous sulphate combines with levothyroxine to form a ferrous–thyroxine complex and so should be taken at a separate time of the day. Other medications that interfere with the absorption of levothyroxine are calcium carbonate, orlistat, antacids, and cholestyramine, as well as soy products. Levothyroxine should be taken four hours before or after these medications.

Okosieme O, Gilbert J, et al. Management of primary hypothyroidism: statement by the British Thyroid Association Executive Committee. Clinical Endocrinology 2015; 0: 1–10. doi: 10.1111/cen.12824.

8. C. Short synacthen test

In primary hypoadrenalism there is loss of glucocorticoid and mineralocorticoid production from the adrenal cortex. The adrenal medulla is usually intact. The classic electrolyte disturbance in primary hypoadrenalism (Addison's disease) is hyponatraemia (in about 90%) and hyperkalaemia (about 65%). Hyperkalaemia occurs because of the loss of aldosterone production. In secondary hypoadrenalism, hyperkalaemia doesn't occur because aldosterone production is unaffected. Hyponatraemia is partly due to sodium depletion but also vasopressin levels are elevated, resulting in an increase in free water retention. Reversible changes to liver enzymes may also occur.

Hypercalcaemia (6%) may also occur. This is partly due to a reduction in calcium removal by the kidney and an increase in mobilization of calcium from bone stores. Thyroid stimulating hormone (TSH) can be elevated in primary hypoadrenalism due to a loss of feedback on the pituitary gland; however, hypothyroidism may also be present and rarely can present at the same time as a new diagnosis. Other autoimmune syndromes can also be present, so it is prudent to screen at the initial presentation. The pigmentation in primary hypoadrenalism occurs because of ACTH drive from the pituitary gland; ACTH is thought to stimulate the melanocortin-2 receptor and so cause the development of pigmentation. There can be pigmentation in the buccal mucosa, in addition to palmar creases and the skin. In secondary hypoadrenalism ACTH is absent, so there is no increased pigmentation.

Primary hypoadrenalism is diagnosed by a short synacthen test and a failure to increase cortisol levels to above 550 nmol/L is diagnostic. A paired cortisol and ACTH is useful to demonstrate an elevated ACTH in primary hypoadrenalism.

In primary hypoadrenalism, glucocorticoid and mineralocorticoid replacement is required, so patients should be discharged on hydrocortisone and fludrocortisone. Typical replacement doses are fludrocortisone 100 mcg od and hydrocortisone 10 mg on waking, 5 mg at midday and 5 mg at 5.00 p.m. to try to mimic the normal circadian secretion of cortisol. Follow-up with an endocrinologist is required.

Kronenberg H, Melmed S. Williams textbook of endocrinology, Saunders, 2007.

Montoli A et al. Hypercalcaemia in Addison's disease: caliciotropic hormone profile and bone histology. Journal of Internal Medicine December 1992; 232(6): 535–540.

Muls E et al. Etiology of hypercalcaemia in a patient with Addison's disease. Calcified Tissue International 1982; 34(6): 523–526.

9. D. Increase the insulin to 10 units per hour

National guidelines in the United Kingdom recommend the use of a weight based (0.1 units/kg/hr) fixed-rate insulin infusion to treat DKA, to continue basal analogues (i.e. glargine, detemir or degludec), and the use of venous gas for the confirmation of DKA in the majority of patients. The use of a weight based insulin dose has come about because, as a population, we are more overweight and consequently more insulin resistant.

The patient in this scenario should have been started on 10 units/hour when first assessed.

Adequate insulin is required to suppress ketosis; it is important to remember that it is the acidosis that is the primary treatment target and not the blood glucose. If acidosis has not resolved but normoglycaemia is present then glucose 10% should be added to the fluid regimen to maintain the blood glucose within acceptable limits. Bicarbonate is rarely used in the treatment of DKA as the acidosis resolves once an adequate insulin dose is started.

Basal insulins (glargine, detemir, degludec) are continued as it helps to minimize the hyperglycaemia that often follows DKA, ensures that there is some insulin in the system should there be cannula or pump problems, and means that the iv insulin can be stopped more easily.

Venous gas samples read slightly lower than arterial blood gas samples but, in this case, more of an improvement should have been seen given the duration of treatment.

Joint British Diabetes Societies Inpatient Care Group. The management of diabetic ketoacidosis in adults. Second edition. September 2013.

National Institute for Health and Care Excellence. NICE Guideline 17: Type 1 diabetes in adults: diagnosis and management, 2015.

10. D. This is hyperosmolar hyperglycaemic state (HHS); continue the sodium chloride 0.9% and stop the iv insulin until the blood glucose is stable

The diagnosis is hyperosmolar hyperglycaemic state (HHS). This used to be known as hyperosmolar non-ketotic (HONK) coma.

The diagnostic of HHS is made with the combination of dehydration plus osmolality >320 mosmol/kg and a blood glucose >30 mmol/L in the absence of ketoacidosis. Calculated osmolality is 2(Na$^+$) + glucose + urea (this patient's calculated osmolality is 398.9 mosmol/kg).

The Joint British Diabetes Society produce guidelines for the management of HHS. Initial management is with sodium chloride 0.9% (+/– potassium) without insulin. Insulin should only be started at a reduced rate (0.05 units/kg) at presentation if there is significant ketosis (urine >2 +, blood >1 mmol/L) or if the blood glucose is falling by less than 5 mmol/hour despite adequate fluid resuscitation. In the first 24 hours, the aim is to keep blood glucose levels between 10–15 mmol/L. There are significant fluid losses, typically between 110–220 mL/kg (e.g. 7.7–15.4 L in a 70 kg person).

Joint British Diabetes Societies Inpatient Care Group. The Management of Hyperosmolar Hyperglycaemic State (HHS) in Adults with Diabetes. August 2012.

11. E. Make no changes to the current treatment

In HHS, you should expect a fall in blood glucose of at least 5 mmol/hour with fluids alone, as in this case. An initial increase in sodium is expected and is not an indication for sodium chloride 0.45%. For each 5.5 mmol/L reduction in glucose, the sodium may rise by 2.4 mmol/L. This is because in marked hyperglycaemia water moves from the intracellular space into the extracellular space due to the osmotic effect of glucose, leading to dilution of extracellular solutes including sodium (often termed pseudohyponatraemia). As the glucose is corrected, the osmotic effect lessens and the measured serum sodium rises, reflecting the true sodium levels.

Insulin given without adequate fluid resuscitation in HHS shifts fluid, glucose, and electrolytes into the intracellular space and causes circulatory collapse because there is a deficit in the extracellular space.

Hillier et al. Hyponatraemia: evaluating the correction factor for hyperglycaemia. American Journal of Medicine April 1999; 106(4): 399–403.

Zeitler P et al. Pediatric Endocrine Society. Hyperglycemic Hyperosmolar Syndrome in Children: Pathophysiological considerations and guidelines for treatment. Journal of Pediatrics 2011; 158(1): 9–14.

12. A. Aortic dissection

Turner syndrome is gonadal dysgenesis with partial or complete absence of one X chromosome (45 XO) caused by a sporadic nondisjunction of chromosomes.

The classic phenotype is short stature, webbing of the neck (25–40%), micrognathia, low-set ears, high arched palate, cubitus valgus, and shield-like chest. Also associated is lymphoedema, congenital renal abnormalities (horseshoe kidney), hypothyroidism, osteoporosis, short fourth/fifth metacarpals, and cardiac abnormalities.

The cardiac abnormalities occur in 20–50% of patients with Turner syndrome and include coarctation of the aorta (10% and the commonest abnormality). Other cardiac abnormalities are bicuspid aortic valve, mitral valve prolapse, partial anomalous venous drainage, hypoplastic left heart syndrome, and aortic root dilatation.

All patients with Turner syndrome should have an echo every 3–5 years depending on the cardiac abnormalities. Patients with risk factors for dissection and rupture need more frequent follow-up.

Bondy C. Aortic dissection in Turner syndrome. Current Opinion in Cardiology 2008; 23(6): 519–526.

13. D. Twenty-four hour urinary-free cortisol

The most likely underlying diagnosis is Cushing's syndrome. The patient has depression, is overweight with plethoric features, and striae are present on abdominal examination. The biochemical profile is consistent with mineralocorticoid excess and the blood glucose level is diagnostic for diabetes.

There is no blood or protein in the urine and there are no masses palpable in the abdomen, which makes a renal cause less likely. Pulses are equal and there are no murmurs present making a cardiac cause unlikely. Renovascular disease (e.g. renal artery stenosis) can also cause hypertension and hypokalaemia via the renin-angiotensin-aldosterone system (secondary hyperaldosteronism).

The electrolytes would also be consistent with Conn's syndrome but the presence of an elevated glucose, increased BMI, abdominal striae, and depression makes Cushing's syndrome more likely but it is important to rule out the other causes of endocrine hypertension as the patient may just be overweight with undiagnosed diabetes (but unlikely).

A phaeochromocytoma needs to be considered as it can also be associated with diabetes but there is no mention of palpitations, sweating, anxiety, or other features of a pheochromocytoma.

Endocrine follow-up will need to be arranged and if the first test is negative and there is a high index of suspicion then it should be repeated as there is a false negative rate of 5–10% with 24-hour urinary-free cortisol and cyclical Cushing's syndrome is a possibility.

Nieman L, Ilias I., Evaluation and treatment of Cushing's syndrome. The American Journal of Medicine 2005; 118(12): 1340–1346. doi: org/10.1016/j.amjmed.2005.01.059

14. D. Primary hyperparathyroidism

The commonest causes of hypercalcaemia are:

1. Primary and tertiary hyperparathyroidism
2. Malignancy—myeloma, bony metastases, humoral hypercalcaemia (paraneoplastic)

Less common causes are:

1. Hyperthyroidism
2. Addison's disease
3. Vitamin D toxicity
4. Thiazide diuretics
5. Renal failure
6. Immobilization
7. Vitamin A toxicity
8. Familial hypercalcaemic hypocalcuria
9. Sarcoidosis

Symptoms of hypercalcaemia are renal stones, abdominal pain, constipation, depression, arthralgia ('stones, bones, groans, psychic moans'), thirst, polyuria, and polydipsia. Often, the hypercalcaemia associated with primary hyperparathyroidism is asymptomatic.

Primary hyperparathyroidism has an incidence of 1 in 500 in the general population. It is most common in postmenopausal women. In primary hyperparathyroidism there is an inappropriately high parathyroid hormone (PTH) for the level of calcium. The commonest cause is a single parathyroid adenoma (85%); parathyroid hyperplasia occurs in 14% and in <1% the cause is parathyroid carcinoma. Multiple Endocrine Neoplasia (MEN) syndromes are associated with parathyroid hyperplasia rather than a discrete adenoma and occur in younger patients; there may be a family history.

Calcium and phosphate homeostasis is controlled by PTH and vitamin D. The main function of PTH is to maintain calcium within normal ranges. When calcium levels fall there is a rise in PTH, which has direct effects on bone and kidneys and indirect effects on the gastrointestinal tract.

In the kidney, PTH enhances renal calcium absorption and promotes the 1-hydroxylation of 25-hydroxyvitamin D3. 1,25-dihydroxyvitamin D3 increases absorption of calcium from the gastrointestinal tract. PTH and 1,25-dihydroxyvitamin D3 also have effects on bones to increase resorption of calcium from the bones to increase calcium. PTH inhibits renal phosphate reabsorption, which leads to low serum phosphate levels and phosphaturia.

Hyperparathyroidism is not a benign condition and can lead to osteoporosis, renal stones, renal impairment, and heart disease.

Andersson et al. Primary hyperparathyroidism and heart disease—a review. European Heart Journal October 2004; 25(20): 1776–1787.

Kronenberg H, Melmed S. Williams Textbook of Endocrinology. Saunders, 2007.

Wass J, Owen K. Oxford handbook of endocrinology and diabetes. Oxford University Press, 2014.

Wass J, Stewart P et al. Oxford textbook of endocrinology and diabetes. Oxford University Press, 2011.

15. B. Factitious hypoglycaemia due to inappropriate sulphonylurea administration

There is no past history of hypoglycaemia, and the patient has access to medication (at home and at work) that would cause hypoglycaemia. Despite appropriate treatment, the hypoglycaemia persists throughout the day suggesting an ongoing stimulus to insulin secretion (e.g. ingestion of medication).

In patients with an insulinoma there is a history of fasting hypoglycaemia, hypoglycaemia several hours after eating or brought on by exercise. Persisting hypoglycaemia such as in this patient would typically be seen in an insulinoma that had been present for some months before, so there would usually be a history of hypoglycaemia prior to the initial presentation. A paired glucose, insulin, and c-peptide would show hypoglycaemia (blood glucose <2.2 mmol/L) with an inappropriately high c-peptide and insulin level. The gold standard diagnostic test is a 72-hour fast but often patients do no need to fast for that long to become hypoglycaemic. In exogenous insulin administration, c-peptide levels would be low.

Reactive (postprandial) hypoglycaemia occurs three to four hours after food and is due to disordered insulin secretion from the pancreas. A prolonged oral glucose tolerance test will pick up the hypoglycaemia three to four hours after a 75 g oral glucose load. It is thought to be a prediabetic condition and is managed initially by a low glycaemic index (GI) diet.

Dumping syndrome has a similar aetiology to reactive hypoglycaemia. It occurs after gastric surgery (e.g. weight-loss surgery or gastrectomy) due to a rapid transit of food and excessive insulin release 1.5–3 hours after eating. Small meals with a low GI are used to manage the hypoglycaemia.

Non-islet cell tumour hypoglycaemia is a rare phenomenon associated with non-islet cell tumours. It has been associated with a wide variety of tumours. The hypoglycaemia is caused by 'big' insulin-like growth factor-II. On investigation, hypoglycaemia is associated with a low insulin and c-peptide level and the sample needs to be analysed for IGF-1 and IGF II.

Diagnosing hypoglycaemia needs a full drug history (of the patient and family members) and questioning regarding the timing of hypoglycaemia in relation to eating, activity, etc. Establishing the resolution of symptoms with consumption of carbohydrate also helps to confirm hypoglycaemia.

Causes of hypoglycaemia:

Fasting hypoglycaemia:

- Endogenous hyperinsulinaemia
  * Insulinoma
  * Nesidioblastosis (ß -cell hyperplasia)
  * Insulin antibodies
- Non-islet cell tumour
  * Mesenchymal
  * Epithelial
  * Haematopoietic
- Drugs
  * Insulin, sulphonylurea
  * Ethanol
  * Quinine
  * Salicylates
  * Haloperidol
- Hormonal deficiencies
  * Cortisol
  * Growth hormone
  * Glucagon
  * Catecholamine
- Critical organ failure
  * Hepatic disease
  * Cardiac disease
  * Renal disease
  * Sepsis
  * Prolonged starvation

Post-prandial (reactive) hypoglycaemia:

- Congenital deficiencies in enzymes of carbohydrate metabolism
  * Glycogen storage disease
- Alimentary hypoglycaemia

Wass J, Owen K. Oxford handbook of endocrinology and diabetes. Oxford University Press, 2014.

Wass J, Stewart P et al. Oxford textbook of endocrinology and diabetes. Oxford University Press, 2011.

16. A. Keep the pump running at the usual basal rate and monitor the blood glucose hourly

If the patient is having an elective procedure and will not miss more than one meal and the pre-operative blood glucose level is between 4 and 12 mmol/L, then it is safe to proceed with the pump running at the usual basal rate with hourly monitoring of the blood glucose levels. The cannula needs to be placed away from the operation site. Post-operatively, the patient can then manage their blood glucose levels as normal.

If the patient is going to miss more than one meal or the blood glucose is more than 12 mmol/L then the pump should be removed (and put in a safe place) or turned off and a variable-rate insulin infusion (VRII) should be started.

If the patient experiences hypoglycaemia intra-operatively—treat the hypoglycaemia normally and retest in 15 minutes. If there are repeated episodes of hypoglycaemia then the basal rate is too high; the pump should be stopped and a VRII started.

There are little data on the use of continuous subcutaneous insulin infusions (CSII) in surgery, so recommendations are based on expert opinion.

CSII is used to treat patients with type 1 diabetes. It is approved by NICE for those patients that fail to reach HbA1c targets despite intensive management with multiple daily injections with analogue insulin and carbohydrate counting or due to severe disabling hypoglycaemia. The patient wears an insulin pump that contains a reservoir of short-acting analogue insulin (not actrapid), which is attached to the patient via a short length of fine-bore tubing connected to a special cannula placed in the subcutaneous tissues. Modern pumps are about the size of a pager. It is not an artificial pancreas.

Insulin is continually infused at a pre-programmed rate over a 24-hour period with variations throughout the 24-hour period to account for changes in hormone levels and activity (basal rate). Some patients have different basal rates for work and weekends/holidays which reflect the effect of a stressful or physical job on insulin requirements (e.g. lower basal rates for physical jobs, higher rates for stress, lower rates needed for relaxing weekends or the hormonal changes during the menstrual cycle). There is the ability to set a temporary basal rate should the need arise (e.g. exercise, stress). The patient will bolus insulin when eating based on the carbohydrate content of the meal but also to correct for hyperglycaemia.

There is no basal insulin taken, so if the pump is disconnected, accidentally stopped, or if there is kinking of the tubing etc., hyperglycaemia and ketoacidosis can follow more rapidly than in patients on subcutaneous injections of insulin.

The pump should not be stopped or removed unless an alternative means of insulin delivery is available.

If a patient on CSII is admitted to hospital and is still able to use their pump then do not swap to another means of insulin delivery. If there is DKA or the patient is unconscious or unable to manage the pump then either swap to VRII or subcutaneous insulin until CSII can be restarted. Always involve the diabetes team at the earliest opportunity.

Boyle et al. Guidelines for application of continuous subcutaneous insulin infusion (insulin pump) therapy in the peri-operative period. Journal of Diabetes Science and Technology 2012; 6: 184–190.

National Institute for Health and Care Excellence. Technology Appraisal Guidance 151. Continuous subcutaneous insulin infusion for the treatment of diabetes mellitus. July 2008, revised 2011.

17. C. Propylthiouracil 200 mg bd

This patient has blood tests and a history consistent with hyperthyroidism due to Graves' disease, so needs anti-thyroid medication as a first-line treatment. She is also keen to get pregnant and is not currently using any contraception, so propylthiouracil is the first-line treatment as it is safer in pregnancy. Propranolol is useful for treating the sympathetic symptoms of thyrotoxicosis (e.g. palpitations, anxiety, tremor, etc.) but doesn't treat the underlying cause. Thyroxine is used to treat hypothyroidism. Radio-iodine (I^{131}) is not the first-line treatment for hyperthyroidism in the UK. In the USA, I^{131} is often the first-line treatment for hyperthyroidism as the higher iodine content in the water makes anti-thyroid medication less effective. Patients with hyperthyroidism are normally managed as an outpatient.

Patients need to be advised of the side effects of carbimazole and propylthiouracil (rash, agranulocytosis) and not to stop taking the anti-thyroid medication without being advised to by a doctor.

All patients with thyrotoxicosis need to be referred to an endocrinologist for long-term management and follow-up.

Features of hyperthyroidism are:
- Palpitations
- Increased appetite and weight loss (sometimes weight gain)
- Hair loss
- Heat intolerance, clamminess
- Tremor
- Diarrhoea
- Oligomenorrhoea/amenorrhoea
- Pruritis
- Irritability and emotional lability

Signs of hyperthyroidism:
- Tremor, hyperreflexia
- Clammy palms and palmar erythema
- Sinus tachycardia, atrial fibrillation
- Hair loss
- Proximal myopathy
- Lid lag and lid retraction
- Congestive cardiac failure
- Rarely periodic paralysis

Features of Graves' disease:
- Thyroid acropachy
- Pretibial myxoedema
- Goitre
- Ophthalmopathy—dry, gritty eyes; exopthalmos (proptosis); chemosis, ophthalmoplegia; pain or pressure in the eyes; peri-orbital oedema; keratitis; optic nerve dysfunction. This often needs referral to ophthalmology
- Family history of autoimmune disease

De Groot L. http://endotext.org, thyroid disease manager. Accessed January 2013.

Wass J, Owen K. Oxford handbook of endocrinology and diabetes. Oxford University Press, 2014.

Wass J, Stewart P et al. Oxford textbook of endocrinology and diabetes. Oxford University Press, 2011.

18. D. Give 0.9% sodium chloride 500 mL intravenously

When assessing and investigating patients with hyponatraemia, the first assessment should be of fluid status. This patient has been vomiting and is tachycardic; he has acute, symptomatic hypovolaemic hyponatraemia. He needs volume and sodium replacement, so 0.9% sodium chloride should be used, and his sodium reassessed closely, every 1–2 hours initially (use the blood gas analyser for rapid real-time results). Rapid correction is needed until neurological symptoms resolve, usually achieved by a rise in serum sodium of 1–2 mmol/L/hr for 3–4 hours (3–8 mmol/L), to prevent further cerebral oedema and seizures. His sodium should not be corrected quickly into the normal range, but to a safe level (i.e.120 mmol/L). The target correction rate for any form of hyponatraemia is no more than 10–12 mmol in the first 24 hours, so although you should correct his sodium quickly initially, his serum sodium in 24 hours should not be over 122–124 mmol/L.

Symptoms of hyponatraemia depend on the rate of fall of the sodium. Symptoms include anorexia, headache, nausea, vomiting, lethargy, personality change, muscle cramps/weakness, confusion, ataxia, drowsiness, hyporeflexia, seizures, coma, and death. This patient's confusion is likely secondary to his hyponatraemia, which, given the history, is likely to have fallen quickly. The risk of central pontine myelinolysis from rapid over-correction is more likely to occur if the rate of fall has been slow. In this case, the risk of cerebral oedema from acute hyponatraemia is high and the risk of central pontine myelinolysis from rapid sodium correction is low.

If the patient is fitting or comatosed, hypertonic saline is indicated, with very close monitoring of sodium levels. In this case 1.8% sodium chloride could be used but the dose of 500 mL stat is too fast and needs to be given in a more controlled way. Stronger solutions (e.g. 3%) can also be used; the dose needs to be calculated according to the solution used and the sodium deficit of the patient and desired rise.

Ellison D, Berl T. The syndrome of inappropriate antidiuresis. The New England Journal of Medicine 2007; 356: 2064–2072.

Gheorghiade M et al. Vasopressin V2 Receptor Blockade with Tolvaptan versus fluid restriction in the treatment of hyponatraemia. American Journal of Cardiology 2006; 97(7): 1064–1067.

19. A. Fluid restrict to 750 mL in 24 hours

This is the syndrome of inappropriate diuretic hormone (SIADH). In SIADH, the hyponatraemia is dilutional. Urine osmolality is inappropriately high (over 100 mosmol/kg, often 400–500 mosmol/kg) in the face of low-serum osmolality, indicating an inability of the kidneys to dilute the urine. To diagnose SIADH, the patient must be clinically euvolaemic with normal hepatic, renal, cardiac, thyroid, and adrenal function. You cannot diagnose SIADH in a patient on diuretics, and these should be stopped for at least 48 hours prior to osmolality measurements.

SIADH is often caused by drugs, malignancy, or pathology in the respiratory or central nervous system (infection, tumours, trauma, etc.).

As the hyponatraemia in this case is dilutional, the mainstay of treatment is fluid restriction. If this doesn't work, demeclocycline can be used. Demeclocycline is a tetracycline antibiotic that induces nephrogenic diabetes insipidus by reducing the effects of anti-diuretic hormone (ADH) in the collecting tubule.

Tolvaptan is a selective V2 receptor antagonist. It is licensed for the treatment of SIADH, but can cause rapid correction of hyponatraemia and should not be combined with fluid restriction. Close monitoring of serum sodium is mandatory.

Ellison D, Berl, T. The syndrome of inappropriate antidiuresis. The New England Journal of Medicine 2007; 356: 2064–2072.

Gheorghiade M et al. Vasopressin V2 Receptor Blockade with Tolvaptan versus fluid restriction in the treatment of hyponatraemia. American Journal of Cardiology 2006; 97(7): 1064–1067.

20. E. Stop bendroflumethiazide

Bendroflumethiazide is a very common cause of hyponatraemia and is the most likely cause in this patient. Paired osmolalities are not helpful in a patient taking diuretics. She may well have a urinary tract infection, but this is unlikely to be causing her hyponatraemia. Bendroflumethiazide should be stopped and her serum sodium rechecked in a few days.

Ellison D, Berl, T. The syndrome of inappropriate antidiuresis. The New England Journal of Medicine 2007; 356: 2064–2072.

Gheorghiade M et al. Vasopressin V2 Receptor Blockade with Tolvaptan versus fluid restriction in the treatment of hyponatraemia. American Journal of Cardiology 2006; 97(7): 1064–1067.

DIABETES AND ENDOCRINOLOGY | ANSWERS

21. E. Give intravenous hydrocortisone 100 mg four times a day

All patients with hypoadrenalism should be told sick-day rules, which include doubling their normal oral steroids if they have a fever of more than 37.5°C or have an infection, taking 20 mg hydrocortisone if they experience nausea or serious injury, and taking 100 mg intramuscular hydrocortisone (which they should keep at home) if they vomit, then call a doctor.

This patient is in adrenal crisis and needs intravenous hydrocortisone. Giving it intravenously allows a faster onset of action and bypasses gut absorption. It needs to be given six-hourly due to the short half-life. Adequate fluid replacement should also be given.

Wass J, Howlett T et al. Caring for patients with Addisons; information for GPs. ADSHG/ACAP/007/ May 2015. http://www.addisons.org.uk

22. B. Nephrogenic diabetes insipidus

The clinical picture of polyuria, polydipsia, and nocturia, and the biochemical profile is consistent with diabetes insipidus. Diabetes insipidus is diagnosed with a water-deprivation test. A lack of response (failure to concentrate the urine) to desmopressin would suggest nephrogenic diabetes insipidus. Concentrating urine in response to desmopressin is consistent with cranial diabetes insipidus. In most cases of psychogenic polyipsia, the urine concentrates appropriately in response to water deprivation and desmopressin isn't necessary. This patient needs referral to an endocrinologist. Nephrogenic diabetes insipidus in adults is most often caused by lithium toxicity or hypercalcaemia. Up to 20% of patients taking lithium develop impairment of urinary concentration due to dysregulation of the aquaporin system in the collecting duct. This is usually, but not always, reversed on stopping the lithium.

In diabetes insipidus, urine specify gravity is 1.005 or less, urine osmolality is less than 300 mosmol/kg, with plasma osmolality greater than 287 mosmol/kg. Polyuria and a high serum osmolality suggests nephrogenic diabetes insipidus.

Trepiccione F, Christensen B. Lithium-induced nephrogenic diabetes insipidus: new clinical and experimental findings. Journal of Nephrology 2010; 23(16): S43–8 (ISSN: 1121–8428).

23. E. Twenty-four-hour urinary metanephrines

The episodic nature of her symptoms and the complaints of headache, sweating, and palpitations with hypertension suggests she might have a phaeochromocytoma. Phaeochromocytoma is rare, and associated with a hereditary syndrome 30% of the time (e.g. von Hippal-Lindau, multiple endocrine neoplasia type 2, succinate dehydrogenase mutations).

Phaeochromocytoma is diagnosed by detecting elevated levels of metanephrines in the blood or urine, and then localization is needed with CT or MRI. Young patients also need genetic screening and referral to an endocrinologist. Surgical resection of the tumour is the treatment of choice. Careful preoperative management of blood pressure and fluid status is required.

Ilias I, Pacak K. A clinical overview of heochromocytomas/paragangliomas and carcinoid tumors. Nuclear Medicine and Biology August 2008; 35(1): S27–S34. doi: 10.1016/j.nucmedbio.2008.04.007

chapter 6

ELDERLY CARE AND STROKE

QUESTIONS

1. **An 82-year-old man was brought to the emergency department by the police. He was found causing a disturbance in a supermarket. He was known to live alone and had no known family. His GP had recently referred him to the memory clinic and social services, but he had not yet been seen. His temperature was 38.5°C; he had a bruise over his right eye, and looked unkempt. He was resistant to any other examination or intervention and was fighting with staff and trying to leave the emergency department.**

    What medication should be prescribed?
    A. 1 mg haloperidol intramuscularly
    B. 10 mg haloperidol intramuscularly
    C. 1 mg lorazepam intramuscularly
    D. 2 mg lorazepam orally
    E. 2.5 mg olanzapine orally

2. **A 92-year-old woman was brought to the emergency department after being found on the floor at home. She had a history of hypertension and atrial fibrillation (AF) and was taking warfarin. On examination, her Glasgow Coma Score was 13/15 and she had power of 3/5 in her left arm and leg. Her CT head showed a large right subdural haematoma.**

    What is the most appropriate treatment?
    A. Prothrombin complex concentrate 50 units/kg intravenously
    B. Recombinant factor VIIa 90 micrograms/kg intravenously
    C. Vitamin K 5 mg intravenously and fresh frozen plasma 12 mL/kg intravenously
    D. Vitamin K 5 mg intravenously and prothrombin complex concentrate 50 units/kg intravenously
    E. Vitamin K 10 mg orally and prothrombin complex concentrate 50 units/kg intravenously

3. You reviewed a 60-year-old woman who was brought to ambulatory care clinic with chest pain. She was accompanied by her son. The son expressed concern about his mother's memory.

   What is the most common cause of early onset dementia?
   A. Alcohol-related dementia
   B. Alzheimer's disease
   C. Frontotemporal dementia
   D. Kuf's disease
   E. Vascular dementia

4. **Which of the following drugs used to treat dementia is available in a transdermal preparation?**
   A. Donepezil
   B. Galantamine
   C. Memantine
   D. Rivastigmine
   E. Rotigotine

5. **Which of the following investigations are not routinely recommended for the investigation of suspected dementia?**
   A. B12 and folate
   B. CT or MRI head
   C. Serum calcium levels
   D. Syphilis serology
   E. Thyroid function tests

6. An 86-year-old man was assessed in the emergency department after a house fire caused by a pan left on the stove. His neighbours were concerned that he had become increasingly confused, and felt he shouldn't be living on his own anymore. He had a diagnosis of Alzheimer's disease, but had refused help. He had a daughter who lived some distance away. He was continually trying to leave the ward to go home, stopping him made him angry, and the other patients were becoming distressed.

   What is the most appropriate next step in management?
   A. A best-interests meeting should be arranged
   B. A formal capacity assessment should be carried out
   C. He should be discharged home with a care package
   D. His daughter should be contacted
   E. An IMCA should be appointed

ELDERLY CARE AND STROKE | QUESTIONS

7. **What is important when deciding whether a person has capacity to make a decision?**
   A. The ability to communicate the decision by any means possible
   B. The ability to retain the information for a set period of time
   C. The level of formal education
   D. A mini-mental test score of 27 or over
   E. The severity of the dementia

8. **Which is true regarding power of attorney?**
   A. Enduring Power of Attorneys can be used as soon as all parties have signed up to them, even before someone loses their mental capacity
   B. Lasting Power of Attorney replaced Enduring Power of Attorney in 2005
   C. A personal and welfare Lasting Power of Attorney's decision takes priority over an advanced directive
   D. A properties and affairs Lasting Power of Attorney can only take effect when the donor has lost capacity
   E. There are two types of Enduring Power of Attorney: one for properties and affairs, and the other for personal and welfare

9. **A 68-year-old woman attended the emergency department after a 15-minute episode of left arm weakness. She had no significant past medical history. On examination, her heart rate was 100 beat per minute and irregular, and her blood pressure was 150/90 mmHg. Her arm weakness had resolved and she had no speech impairment. Her ECG showed atrial fibrillation.**

   What should her management include?
   A. Clopidogrel 75 mg daily
   B. A diffusion-weighted MRI scan of brain within one week
   C. An echocardiogram within 24 hours
   D. Low molecular weight heparin until fully anticoagulated
   E. Referral for carotid endarterectomy within one week of symptom onset if there is significant carotid stenosis

10. **An 88-year-old man was referred to the acute medical unit by his GP with increasing shortness of breath and a cough with green sputum. On further questioning, he complained of choking on his food for a number of months and double vision for even longer. On examination, he had a left partial ptosis, but otherwise his cranial nerve examination was normal. He was generally weak in all muscle groups; his reflexes were normal.**

    Which is the most important investigation?
    A. Acetylcholinesterase antibodies
    B. Chest X-ray
    C. MR scan of brain
    D. Spirometry
    E. Thyroid function tests

11. **A 55-year-old man presented with a right-sided hemiparesis. He responded to voice and had a National Institute of Health stroke score (NIHSS) of 24. A CT head scan confirmed an infarct of more than 50% in the territory of the middle cerebral artery on the left. He had no past medical history.**

    Which of the following criteria are <u>not</u> important in deciding whether he should be referred for a decompressive hemicraniectomy?

    A. He is less than 60 years of age
    B. He scores 1 on item 1a of the NIHSS
    C. He was previously fit
    D. The infarct volume is more than 50% of the MCA territory on CT
    E. The NIHSS score is more than 15

12. **A 78-year-old man presented to the acute care of the elderly clinic with a six-month history of declining mobility. His wife had noticed he was increasingly forgetful and sometimes unaware of episodes of nocturnal incontinence. He had a past medical history of hypertension, hypercholesterolaemia, and benign prostatic hypertrophy. He took bendroflumethiazide 2.5 mg, simvastatin 40 mg, and doxazosin 2 mg. On examination, he had a broad-based shuffling gait. His mini-mental state examination was 22/30.**

    What is the most likely diagnosis?

    A. Lewy body dementia
    B. Normal pressure hydrocephalus
    C. Prostate cancer with spinal bone metastases
    D. Urinary tract infection
    E. Vascular dementia

13. **A 93-year-old woman presented to the emergency department in January having been found unresponsive in her flat. The paramedics stated the flat was very cold. No other medical information was available and she lived alone. On examination, her heart rate was 45 beats per minute and blood pressure 82/50 mmHg. She was hypotonic in all four limbs and had dilated sluggish pupils. Her ECG showed sinus rhythm with abnormal positive deflections occurring at the junction between the QRS complex and the ST segment.**

    Which treatment will address the underlying cause?

    A. Intravenous antibiotics
    B. Intravenous hydrocortisone
    C. Intravenous liothyronine
    D. Intravenous thrombolysis
    E. Rewarming

14. An 88-year-old man was admitted to the acute medical unit from his nursing home with a two-month history of general fatigue and lethargy. The nursing home staff described a very poor oral intake and declining mobility. He complained of low mood and bilateral leg pain. On examination, he had a widespread purpuric rash and some ecchymoses.

    What is the most appropriate treatment?
    A. Intramuscular hydroxycobalamin
    B. Intravenous phytomenadione
    C. Oral ascorbic acid
    D. Oral vitamin D 800 international units
    E. Oral vitamin D 50,000 international units

15. A 93-year-old woman was admitted to the acute medical unit with a fall and left hip pain. She was unable to mobilize. Her past medical history included chronic kidney disease stage 3, a previous TIA, previous alcohol abuse, and she was a smoker. Her left hip X-ray showed a loss of cortical bone with a partial fracture of the femoral neck.

    ```
    Investigations:
        serum-corrected calcium         2.10 mmol/L     (2.20-2.60)
        serum phosphate                 0.6 mmol/L      (0.8-1.4)
        serum alkaline phosphatase      175 U/L         (45-105)
        plasma parathyroid hormone      6.1 pmol/L      (0.9-5.4)
    ```

    What is the most likely underlying cause?
    A. Osteoporosis
    B. Paget's disease
    C. Primary hyperparathyroidism
    D. Renal osteodystrophy
    E. Vitamin D deficiency

16. A 46-year-old man was admitted to the emergency department at 05:30 with right-sided weakness and dysphasia. His wife woke at 04:30 to a bang as he got out of bed and fell to the floor. She noticed he could not get up and had incoherent speech so phoned an ambulance. She last saw him well at 22:30 the previous night. He had no past medical history and was not on any regular medication. He was a gardener and had smoked 20 cigarettes per day, since the age of 20. He drank two cans of lager four times per week.

On examination, he responded to voice. His heart rate was 76 beats per minute, blood pressure was 160/92 mmHg, respiratory rate was 12 breaths per minute, and oxygen saturation 99% on room air. He had a right-sided facial weakness and a right homonymous hemianopia. He had receptive and expressive dysphasia with only occasional intelligible words. Power was 2/5 in the right arm and right leg, reflexes were diminished, and he had an upgoing plantar response on the right. There was sensory neglect on the right side. The left side was normal. On bedside swallowing assessment, he choked on sips of water. His NIHSS was 20.

He had an urgent unenhanced CT head scan, which was normal.

Blood results were as follows.

```
Investigations:
  haemoglobin                        140 g/L              (130-180)
  white cell count                   9.0 × 10⁹/L          (4.0-11.0)
  platelet count                     220 × 10⁹/L          (150-400)
  international normalized ratio     1.0                  (<1.4)
  activated partial                  36 s                 (30-40)
    thromboplastin time
  random serum glucose               5.2 mmol/L
```

What is the next best step in management?

A. Alteplase 0.9 mg/kg intravenously
B. Aspirin 300 mg orally
C. Aspirin 300 mg rectally
D. Sodium chloride 0.9% 250 mL intravenously
E. Tenecteplase 50 mg intravenously

17. An emergency department doctor has asked for your advice. She would like to discharge an 85-year-old man who sustained a significant elbow laceration after a brief syncopal episode. He did not remember the episode. He was sat in a chair, had no warning symptoms, lost consciousness and recovered quickly afterwards. He could not recall any previous episodes.

    On examination, his heart rate was 60 beats per minute, blood pressure was 130/70 mmHg, and oxygen saturation 95% on air.

    ```
    Investigations:
      troponin T 35 ng/L (<14)
      ECG: sinus rhythm, right bundle branch block, left axis deviation
      chest X-ray: nil focal
    ```

    What is the most appropriate management?
    A. Admission for cardiac monitoring
    B. Arrange a CT pulmonary angiogram
    C. Discharge with GP follow-up
    D. Discharge with outpatient 24-hr tape and echocardiogram
    E. Immediate cardiology review

18. An 87-year-old man was admitted with a six-month history of recurrent falls and poor gait pattern.

    What is the most appropriate method of assessing his risk of falls?
    A. Assessment of muscle weakness using the MRC scale
    B. Get-up-and-go test
    C. Grip strength test
    D. Modified Barthel index
    E. Romberg's test

19. A previously fit and well 82-year-old woman was witnessed to be unconscious at the wheel of her car before it swerved and hit a lamp post. She had no prodrome and recovered rapidly having only sustained minor injuries. She was not taking any regular medication. She lived in a rural location and was keen to drive again as she cared for her husband who had dementia.

    What is the most appropriate driving advice?
    A. Can drive unless investigations are abnormal
    B. Licence revoked
    C. No driving for one year if a cause is found and treated
    D. No driving for four weeks
    E. No driving for six months if no cause is found

20. **A 76-year-old woman attended the emergency department with sudden onset of vertigo. She had a minor head injury one week prior to these symptoms commencing. The episodes were short-lived and occurred more at night. She had a past medical history of atrial fibrillation (AF) and hypertension. Her medications included aspirin 75 mg and atenolol 50 mg. On examination, she had latent onset of geotropic rotatory nystagmus on lateral gaze.**

    What is the most likely diagnosis?
    A. Horizontal semi-circular canal benign paroxysmal positional vertigo
    B. Labyrinthitis
    C. Ménière's disease
    D. Posterior circulation cerebral infarction
    E. Posterior semi-circular canal benign paroxysmal positional vertigo

21. **An 82-year-old woman presented to the emergency department following three falls over the last week. She had a past medical history of idiopathic Parkinson's disease.**

    Which is <u>least</u> likely to reduce her risk of falls?
    A. Dual-chamber cardiac pacing if she has cardioinhibitory carotid sinus hypersensitivity
    B. Exercise programme incorporating balance, gait, and strength training
    C. Home environment assessment and intervention
    D. Medication review
    E. Multifocal lenses

22. **An 86-year-old woman was admitted following an accidental fall and sustained a fractured right neck of femur. She had a past medical history of deep vein thrombosis six weeks prior to admission, stage 3 chronic kidney disease, type 2 diabetes mellitus, cognitive impairment, and hypertension. The patient underwent repair of her fractured neck of femur.**

    ```
    Investigations:
      serum urea                              12.6 mmol/L    (2.5–7.0)
      serum creatinine                        195 µmol/L     (60–110)
      estimated glomerular filtration rate    29 mL/min      (>90)
      haemoglobin                             92 g/L         (115–165)
      mean cell volume                        72 fL          (80–96)
      calcium, phosphate, and vitamin D levels were normal
    ```

    What is the most appropriate management of her osteoporosis?
    A. Intravenous zoledronic acid
    B. Oral alendronate
    C. Strontium ranelate
    D. Subcutaneous denosumab
    E. Subcutaneous teriparatide

23. A 78-year-old woman living in a residential home was admitted to the acute medical unit following four falls over a six-week period. She had a past medical history of type 2 diabetes mellitus, depression and anxiety, postural hypotension, and oesophagitis. An ECG showed a prolonged QTc.

    Which drug is most likely to be increasing her risk of falls?

    A. Amitriptyline
    B. Calcium and vitamin D
    C. Fludrocortisone
    D. Gliclazide
    E. Omeprazole

24. An 88-year-old man was admitted to the acute medical unit by his GP from a nursing home with lower back pain. He had type 2 diabetes mellitus and was bed bound following a total anterior circulation stroke six months ago. He tolerated a puréed diet and had urinary incontinence. On examination, he had a grade 4 sacral pressure sore. His temperature was 38.9°C.

    Which is the most important immediate intervention?

    A. Avoid catheterization
    B. Complete an incident form
    C. High-specification foam mattress
    D. Nutritional assessment using MUST score
    E. Referral to surgical team

25. A 25-year-old woman was admitted to the acute medical unit after a syncopal episode. She had been previously diagnosed with anxiety and chronic fatigue syndrome. On further questioning, she described recurrent episodes of light-headedness, nausea, and palpitations, which were often triggered by changes in posture.

    On examination, her heart rate was 80 beats per minute and lying blood pressure was 125/60 mmHg. Standing her heart rate was 120 beats per minute and blood pressure was 120/60 mmHg.

    ECG showed normal sinus rhythm.

    What is the most likely diagnosis?

    A. Anxiety-related
    B. Aortic stenosis
    C. Hyperthyroidism
    D. Paroxysmal atrial fibrillation (AF)
    E. Postural tachycardia syndrome (PoTS)

ELDERLY CARE AND STROKE | QUESTIONS

26. A 65-year-old woman was admitted to the acute medical unit on multiple occasions after collapses while out visiting her friends. She had no recollection of the events but quickly recovered after each episode. Her friends reported that the episodes usually occurred while seated at a table and talking in a group.

She was referred for a tilt-table test. On the day she attended for her test, the doctor performing it decided to perform carotid sinus massage first.

Which of the following would help in confirming carotid sinus hypersensitivity?

A. Drop in systolic blood pressure of 20 mmHg
B. Greater than three second pause on the ECG
C. Loss of consciousness with no change in blood pressure or heart rate on ECG
D. Transient arm and face weakness on the opposite side to where the carotid massage is being performed
E. Two to three second pause on the ECG

27. A 70-year-old man was admitted to an orthopaedic ward after a fall and fractured left neck of femur. The orthopaedic foundation 2 doctor noted he had a postural drop in blood pressure of 10 mmHg and felt dizzy on standing. The patient had a history of diabetes mellitus and was taking metformin 500 mg twice daily.

Once he had recovered from his operation, he was referred to a syncope clinic for further assessment.

Which of the following most supports the diagnosis of orthostatic hypertension?

A. An asymptomatic fall in systolic blood pressure of ≥20 mmHg on active standing for three minutes
B. An asymptomatic fall in systolic blood pressure to less than 100 mmHg on active standing for three minutes
C. The induction of loss of consciousness in the absence of hypotension or bradycardia on tilt-testing
D. A symptomatic episode of bradycardia and hypotension at three minutes on tilt-testing
E. A symptomatic progressive fall in blood pressure on tilt-testing ≥20 mmHg

28.

An 86-year-old man was admitted to the acute medical unit with community-acquired pneumonia. He had a past medical history of hypertension and was taking bendroflumethiazide 2.5 mg once daily.

His chest X-ray showed a right middle lobe pneumonia.

His initial blood results are as follows.

```
Investigations:
  haemoglobin                      130 g/L              (130-180)
  white cell count                 22 × 10⁹/L           (4.0-11.0)
  neutrophil count                 18 × 10⁹/L           (1.5-7.0)
  serum sodium                     130 mmol/L           (137-144)
  serum potassium                  3.7 mmol/L           (3.5-4.9)
  serum urea                       6.8 mmol/L           (2.5-7.0)
  serum creatinine                 115 µmol/L           (60-110)
  serum C-reactive protein         44 mg/L              (<10)
  serum total protein              70 g/L               (61-76)
  serum albumin                    30 g/L (37-49)
  serum total bilirubin            21 µmol/L            (1-22)
  serum alanine aminotransferase   40 U/L (5-35)
  serum alkaline phosphatase       190 U/L              (45-105)
```

He was treated with intravenous antibiotics and discharged home with community support on oral antibiotics after 48 hours.

Six weeks later, the patient was seen in the acute medicine follow-up clinic.

He was feeling well. His chest X-ray showed resolution of his pneumonia.

His repeat blood tests were as follows.

```
Investigations:
  haemoglobin                      131 g/L              (130-180)
  white cell count                 5.3 × 10⁹/L          (4.0-11.0)
  neutrophil count                 3.2 × 10⁹/L          (1.5-7.0)
  serum sodium                     135 mmol/L           (137-144)
  serum potassium                  3.4 mmol/L           (3.5-4.9)
  serum urea                       6.5 mmol/L           (2.5-7.0)
  serum creatinine                 112 µmol/L           (60-110)
  serum C-reactive protein         2 mg/L               (<10)
  serum total protein              70 g/L               (61-76)
  serum albumin                    34 g/L               (37-49)
  serum total bilirubin            20 µmol/L            (1-22)
  serum alanine aminotransferase   35 U/L               (5-35)
  serum alkaline phosphatase       196 U/L (45-105)
```

What is the best management for his persistently elevated alkaline phosphatase?

A. Myeloma screen
B. Nothing unless he develops any symptoms
C. Recheck serum alkaline phosphatase in six months
D. Referral to a gastroenterologist
E. Urinary Bence Jones protein

29. A 79-year-old man was admitted to the acute medical unit after an acute coronary syndrome. He had a past medical history of ischaemic heart disease, heart failure, type 2 diabetes, chronic kidney disease, and osteoarthritis. He lived independently and was virtually housebound due to poor mobility and breathlessness. His wife had died six months ago. During his initial assessment, the junior doctor was concerned by the patient's withdrawn demeanour and, on further questioning, he admitted to poor sleep, reduced appetite, and feelings of worthlessness.

    Which tool would <u>not</u> be useful in assessing his depressive symptoms?
    A. Barthel index
    B. BASDEC
    C. Beck inventory
    D. GDS
    E. HADS

30. **A 72-year-old woman was admitted to the acute medical unit, as she was no longer able to mobilize at home due to left hip pain. This had developed over a four-month period but had worsened over the week prior to admission.**

    As part of your assessment you arranged a pelvic X-ray.

    Investigations:

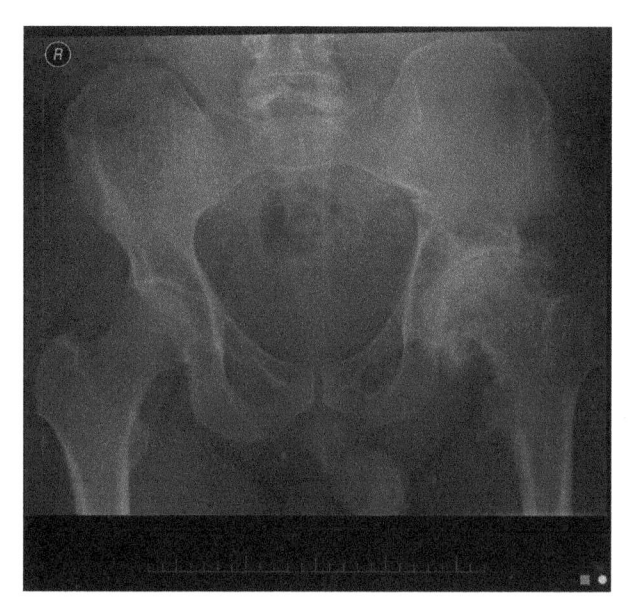

    Figure 6.1 Pelvic X-ray.

    What is the most likely cause for her reduced mobility?
    A. Fractured neck of femur
    B. Incarcerated femoral hernia
    C. Myeloma
    D. Osteoarthritis
    E. Paget's disease

chapter 6

ELDERLY CARE AND STROKE

ANSWERS

1. A. 1 mg haloperidol intramuscularly

This man is likely to be suffering from delirium, probably on the background of dementia. He needs urgent investigation and treatment but is currently a risk to himself. National Institute for Health and Care Excellence (NICE) guidance only recommends pharmacological treatment with small doses of haloperidol or olanzapine if a patient presents a danger to himself or others, and verbal and non-verbal de-escalation techniques are ineffective or inappropriate. It is unlikely that this patient will take any oral medication. Antipsychotics should be used with caution or not at all in patients with Parkinson's disease or Lewy body dementia.

National Institute for Health and Care Excellence. Clinical Guideline 103. Delirium: prevention, diagnosis and management. July 2010.

2. D. Vitamin K 5 mg intravenously and prothrombin complex concentrate 50 units/kg intravenously

The CT head scan shows a large acute subdural on the right. This is a life-threatening bleed and the immediate priority is to reverse the warfarin. Intravenous vitamin K is given at the same time as the prothrombin complex concentrate (PCC) to switch on endogenous synthesis of vitamin K-dependent clotting factors. PCC is preferred to fresh frozen plasma (FFP) in this setting; it can be administered rapidly in less volume and is more efficacious. FFP should only be used if PCC is not available; however, all hospitals should stock a four-factor PCC. Recombinant factor VIIa is not recommended for emergency anticoagulation reversal.

Markris M, Von Keen J et al. Guideline on the management of bleeding in patients on antithrombotic agents. British Journal of Haematology November 2012; 160(1): 35–46.

3. B. Alzheimer's disease

Early onset dementia is defined as dementia presenting before the age of 65 years. It can be difficult to diagnose because non-Alzheimer's aetiologies and unusual dementias are more common. Despite this, Alzheimer's disease remains the most prevalent cause of dementia between the ages of 45–64 (35 per 100,000), followed by vascular dementia (17.9 per 100,000), frontotemporal dementia (15.4 per 100,000), and then alcohol-related dementia (13.6 per 100,000). Kuf's disease is the major adult form of neuronal ceroid lipofuscinosis, caused by mutations in CLN6. It can present with dementia and seizures.

Rogers B, Lippa C. A clinical approach to early onset inheritable dementia. American Journal of Alzheimer's Disease and Other Dementias 2012; 27(3): 154–161.

Harvey R, Skelton-Robinson M, Rossor M. The prevalence and causes of dementia in people under the age of 65 years. Journal of Neurology, Neurosurgery & Psychiatry 2003; 74(9): 1206–1209.

ELDERLY CARE AND STROKE | **ANSWERS** | 171

4. D. Rivastigmine

Donepezil, galantamine, and rivastigmine are acetylcholinesterase inhibitors and can be used for the treatment of mild to moderate Alzheimer's disease. Rivastigmine is available in a transdermal patch. Memantine is a glutamate receptor antagonist and can be used for moderate Alzheimer's disease in patients who are unable to take acetylcholinersterase inhibitors, and for patients with severe disease. Rotigotine is a dopamine receptor agonist available as a patch and used for the treatment of Parkinson's disease; it's not a treatment for dementia.

National Institute for Health and Care Excellence. Technology Appraisal 217. Donepezil, galantamine, rivastigmine, and memantine for the treatment of Alzheimer's disease. March 2011.

5. D. Syphilis serology

A dementia screen should be performed at presentation. This should include routine haematology, biochemistry (electrolytes, glucose, calcium, and renal and liver function), thyroid function tests, and B12 and folate levels. An MSU should be sent if delirium is suspected. A chest X-ray or ECG would be appropriate if presenting acutely on the admissions unit. Syphilis serology and HIV testing should only be done if clinically suspected. CSF examination is only appropriate if CJD or other forms of rapidly progressing dementias are being considered. An EEG may be useful in a suspected delirium, CJD, or seizures associated with dementia. Structural imaging using MRI or CT should be used to rule out other causes or cerebral pathology and help identify subtypes. A single-photon emission computed tomography (SPECT) is useful to identify Alzheimer's disease from vascular dementia and frontotemporal dementia in the setting of a memory clinic.

National Institute for Health and Care Excellence. Clinical Guideline 42. Dementia: supporting people with dementia and their carers in health and social care. November 2006 (revised April 2014).

6. B. A formal capacity assessment should be carried out

All of the options may well be appropriate; however, the most important first step would be to make an assessment of capacity. The Mental Capacity Act 2005 aims to empower and protect people of 16 years of age and over, who lack capacity to make certain decisions for themselves because of illness, learning disabilities, or mental health problems. The five main principles of the Act are: there is a presumption of capacity; the right for individuals to be supported to make their own decisions; it should not be assumed that someone lacks capacity simply because their decisions might seem unwise or eccentric; if someone lacks capacity, anything done on their behalf must be done in their best interests; and, if someone lacks capacity, before making a decision on their behalf, all alternatives must be considered and the option chosen should be the least restrictive of their basic rights and freedoms.

Great Britain. Mental Capacity Act 2005. http://legislation.gov.uk

7. A. The ability to communicate the decision by any means possible

According to the law, a person is defined as being unable to make decisions for themselves if they are not able to undertake at least one of the following: understand information given to them; retain that information long enough to be able to make a decision; weigh up the information available to make a decision; and communicate their decision by any possible means, including talking, using sign language, or even through simple muscle movements such as blinking an eye or squeezing a hand.

Great Britain. Mental Capacity Act 2005. http://legislation.gov.uk

8. A. Enduring Power of Attorneys can be used as soon as all parties have signed up to them, even before someone loses their mental capacity

The Mental Capacity Act 2005 created a new type of power of attorney called Lasting Power of Attorney (LPA). LPAs replaced Enduring Power of Attorneys (EPAs) in 2007, when the Mental

Capacity Act came into force. EPAs remain valid provided that both the donor of the power and the attorney signed the document prior to 1 October 2007. There are two types of LPA: a property and affairs LPA and a personal welfare LPA. A personal welfare LPA only takes effect when the donor lacks capacity to make decisions. However, a property and affairs LPA can take effect as soon as it is registered, even while the donor still has capacity, unless the donor specifies otherwise. EPAs can be used as soon as all parties have signed up to them, even before someone loses their mental capacity (assuming the EPA has not been drafted to the contrary). Only when the person granting the EPA loses their mental capacity does the EPA have to be registered with the Office of the Public Guardian. Any existing EPA only applies to finance and property matters, so even if someone already has one, they can make an additional LPA for personal welfare decisions.

Great Britain. Mental Capacity Act 2005. http://legislation.gov.uk

9. E. Referral for carotid endarterectomy within one week of symptom onset if there is significant carotid stenosis

The ABCD^2 score is validated and used to classify transient ischaemic attack into low, moderate, or high risk for developing a stroke. This woman scores 4, which is high risk and requires urgent referral to a specialist within 24 hours for assessment and investigation according to NICE guidance. She should initially be treated with 300 mg aspirin, prior to anticoagulation with warfarin or a novel oral anticoagulant (NOAC). People who have symptomatic carotid stenosis (70–99% according to the European Carotid Surgery Trialists' collaborative group criteria) should be assessed for carotid endarterectomy within one week and undergo surgery within two weeks.

ABCD^2 score:

- Age: <60 = 0, ≥60 = 1
- BP: <140/90 mmHg = 0, systolic ≥140 mmHg +/or diastolic ≥90 mmHg = 1
- Clinical features: unilateral weakness = 2, speech disturbance = 1, other = 0
- Duration: <10 minutes = 0, 10–59 minutes = 1, ≥60 minutes = 2
- Diabetes = 1

Modified from *The Lancet*, 366, Rothwell P et al., 'A simple score (ABCD) to identify individuals at high early risk of stroke after transient ischaemic attack', pp. 29–36, Copyright (2005), with permission from Elsevier.

- Risk of stroke:

Risk (score)	2 days	7 days	90 days
Low risk (<4)	1%	1.2%	3.1%
Moderate risk (4 or 5)	4.1%	5.9%	9.8%
High risk >5	8.1%	11.7%	17.8%

Modified from *The Lancet*, 369, Jonhston SC et al., 'Validation and refinement of scores to predict very early stroke risk after transient ischemic attack', pp. 283–292, Copyright (2007), with permission from Elsevier.

Johnston S, Rothwell P, Nguyen-Huynh M et al. Validation and refinement of scores to predict very early stroke risk after transient ischaemic attack. Lancet 2007; 369/9558: 283–292.

National Institute for Health and Care Excellence. Clinical Guideline 68. Stroke and transient ischaemic attack in over 16s: diagnosis and initial management. July 2008.

Rothwell P, Giles M, Flossmann E et al. A simple score (ABCD) to identify individuals at high early risk of stroke after transient ischaemic attack. Lancet 2005; 366/9479: 29–36.

Walter K. Stroke after transient ischaemic attack: dealing in futures. Lancet 2007; 369: 251–252.

ELDERLY CARE AND STROKE | ANSWERS

10. C. Spirometry

This man has myasthenia gravis. It has a bimodal distribution, with peaks in the second and third decade for young women, and another peak in the eighth decade in men. Acetylcholinesterase antibodies have 80–96% sensitivity and are an important diagnostic test, but will not help in the initial emergency management of this case. It is important that as soon as a myasthenia crisis is suspected in a patient that spirometry is monitored; a forced vital capacity less than 15–20 mL/kg of ideal body weight (around 1 L) should raise concern about impending respiratory failure.

National Institute of Neurological Disorders and Stroke. Myasthenia Gravis fact sheet. 2010. NIH Publication No. 10–768.

11. C. He was previously fit

Malignant middle cerebral artery syndrome usually presents within 2–5 days of stroke onset and has a mortality rate of 80%. It occurs in younger patients without brain atrophy. The guidelines for referral for decompressive hemicraniectomy according to NICE are:

- referred within 24 hours of onset of symptoms and treated within a maximum of 48 hours
- aged 60 years or under
- clinical deficits suggestive of infarction in the territory of the middle cerebral artery, with a score on the NIHSS of more than 15
- a decrease in the level of consciousness to give a score of 1 or more on item 1a of the NIHSS (which equates to verbally rousable or worse)
- signs on CT of an infarct of at least 50% of the middle cerebral artery territory, with or without additional infarction in the territory of the anterior or posterior cerebral artery on the same side, or infarct volume greater than 145 cm^3 on diffusion-weighted MRI

Although you would always consider the patients pre-morbid condition, this is not a criteria for treatment in the NICE guidelines.

National Institute for Health and Care Excellence. Clinical Guideline 68. Stroke and transient ischaemic attack in over 16s: diagnosis and initial management. July 2008.

12. B. Normal pressure hydrocephalus

This patient's wife described the typical triad of normal pressure hydrocephalus (NPH): gait apraxia, urinary incontinence, and dementia. Although he does have vascular risk factors, there is no other history or neurological findings suggestive of vascular dementia, such as a sudden deterioration or hyperreflexia. Patients with Lewy body dementia classically describe visual hallucinations and disturbances in alertness, as well as some Parkinsonism. The clinical history is too long for a urinary tract infection. Prostate cancer and bone metastases would not explain the cognitive changes.

National Institute for Health and Care Excellence. Interventional procedure guideline 263. Lumbar infusion test for the investigation of normal pressure hydrocephalus. June 2008.

13. E. Rewarming

This patient shows clinical signs that could be consistent with hypothermia. The ECG description of a J wave confirms this. Hence, rewarming is the most appropriate next step. This presentation could represent an addisonian crisis or hypothyroid coma but there is no suggestion of these as an underlying cause. You would always give intravenous steroids with intravenous liothyronine. Some of the ECG changes in hypothermia may mimic acute coronary syndrome. Sepsis may be an underlying cause and sepsis-induced hypothermia can cause the same ECG changes as environmental hypothermia, but in this case the history is suggestive of environmental hypothermia.

Polderman K. Mechanisms of action, physiological effects, and complications of hypothermia. Critical Care Medicine July 2009; 37(7 Suppl): S186–202.

14. C. Oral ascorbic acid

Vitamin C deficiency occurs in the elderly population due to poor oral intake and poor diet. Patients present with abnormal bleeding, perifollicular haemorrhages, bleeding gums, corkscrew hairs, purpura, and ecchymoses. Other symptoms include poor wound healing and muscle/joint/bone pain. Diagnosis is made by demonstrating an increased bleeding time and low-plasma vitamin C. Treatment is with oral vitamin C (ascorbic acid).

Donald I, Bruce S, Newton J. Healthy Eating for Older People—British Geriatric Society Best Practice Guide. 2011. http://www.bgs.org.uk

15. E. Vitamin D deficiency

Vitamin D deficiency is common in the elderly population especially those who are institutionalized or housebound and have very limited sunlight exposure. 25-hydroxyvitamin D levels of less than 50 nmol/L indicate insufficiency; levels less than 30 nmol/L indicate deficiency. Patients need replacement first (protocols vary, but commonly recommend 300,000 IU if deficient e.g. 50 000 IU capsules once weekly for six weeks.) then maintenance of 800–1,000 IU per day. Most combined calcium and vitamin D preparations contain 400 units of vitamin D per tablet so a dose of two tablets per day is adequate for maintenance but not for replacement. Biochemically, patients may have a low-serum calcium, high-alkaline phosphatase, and high-parathyroid hormone due to secondary hyperparathyroidism. Vitamin D deficiency contributes to osteoporosis by decreasing intestinal uptake of calcium. Biochemistry is normal in primary osteoporosis, although alkaline phosphatase may be elevated if there is a fracture.

National Osteoporosis Society. 2013. Vitamin D and Bone Health: A Practical Clinical Guideline for Patient Management.

16. C. Aspirin 300 mg rectally

This patient has had an ischaemic stroke. He fulfils most of the criteria for stoke thrombolysis, except the timing of onset of symptoms is unknown. He was last seen well seven hours prior to assessment and appeared to wake up with symptoms, so his stroke could have happened at any time between 22:30 and 04:30; therefore, he is ineligible for thrombolysis and should be treated with aspirin, which should be rectal or via a nasogastric tube as his swallow is unsafe.

Thrombolysis in stroke

Alteplase (recombinant tissue plasminogen activator) is currently the only licensed thrombolytic agent for stroke. It is licensed for acute ischaemic stroke within 4.5 hours of symptom onset after exclusion of intracranial haemorrhage in patients aged 18–80 (although most centres will thrombolyse off licence in the over 80s) and in patients with an NIHSS of 4–25.

Exclusion criteria:

From the history

Absolute contraindications:

- Active internal bleeding
- Major surgery or serious trauma within last 14 days
- Clinical diagnosis of subarachnoid haemorrhage even if CT normal
- Treatment-dose heparin (low molecular weight or unfractionated) within 24 hours

Relative contraindications:

- Recent CVA, head injury, or cranial surgery (within three months)
- Seizure at stroke onset
- Any history of intracranial haemorrhage, brain tumour, intracranial AVM, or aneurysm
- Recent (<48 hours) lumbar puncture or (<1 week) arterial/venous puncture at non-compressible site

- Pregnancy (very little evidence, each case needs to be assessed individually)
- Current warfarin treatment if INR is more than 1.7 (not a contraindication if INR is less than or equal to 1.7)

On assessment

- Coma (Glasgow Coma Score <8)
- Severe stroke (NIHSS >25)
- NIHSS <4 except isolated disabling symptoms (e.g. severe dysphasia, homonymous hemianopia)
- Rapidly improving symptoms or signs
- Capillary blood glucose <2.8 or >22.0 mmol/L (if hypoglycaemic treat with 50% glucose and reassess)
- Systolic blood pressure >185 mmHg and/or diastolic >110 mmHg after treatment with labetolol or nitrates

If lab results available (but do not wait for results if not available)

- Platelets <100
- INR >1.7
- APPT >1.2
- Plasma glucose <2.8 or >22.0 mmol/L

On CT brain

- Intracranial haemorrhage
- Other pathologies

Evidence:

Current evidence supports thrombolysis up to 4.5 hours after the onset of symptoms, but the earlier the treatment, the better the outcome (see Table 6.1).

Table 6.1 Timing of thrombolysis and odds of a good outcome.

Timing of thrombolysis	Increased odds of a good outcome
within 90 minutes	2.6
91–180 minutes	1.6
181–270 minutes	1.3
271–360 minutes	no improvement

Adapted from *The Lancet*, 375, 9727, Lees KR et al., 'Time to treatment with intravenous alteplase and outcome in stroke: an updated pooled analysis of ECASS, ATLANTIS, NINDS, and EPITHET trials', pp. 1695–1703., Copyright (2010) with permission from Elsevier.

Number needed to treat for a good outcome with thrombolysis within 4.5 hours is 8.

For every 100 patients who are thrombolysed, 32 will benefit, 3 will get worse, and 65 will be unchanged.

Ongoing trials in stroke thrombolysis are looking at 'wake-up' stroke (as in this patient), and hypothermia after stroke.

Other evidence for the treatment of acute stroke

- Admit to a specialist stroke unit
- Aspirin 300 mg/day for two weeks in ischaemic stroke, then clopidogrel or full anticoagulation if appropriate
- Oxygen only if hypoxic (no benefit of supplemental oxygen if normal oxygen saturation)

- Temperature control and lowering of fever
- Blood sugar control (4–11 mmol/L)
- Ensure hydration and nutrition
- Early mobilization
- Continue statins if patients are already taking them
- Carotid imaging if anterior circulation stroke and carotid endarterectomy appropriate
- Blood pressure control—initially only if hypertension emergency
- Surgical referral for decompressive hemicraniectomy if MCA infarction if NICE criteria are met

Royal College of Physicians (RCP) National Clinical Guidelines for Stroke (Fourth Edition) 2012.

Lees KR, Bluhmki E, von Kummer R et al. Time to treatment with intravenous alteplase and outcome in stroke: an updated pooled analysis of ECASS, ATLANTIS, NINDS, and EPITHET trials. Lancet 2010; 375(9727): 1695–1703.

National Institute for Health and Care Excellence. Clinical Guideline 68. Stroke and transient ischaemic attack in over 16s: diagnosis and initial management. July 2008.

Thrombolysis Masterclass www.strokeadvancingmodules.org

17. A. Admission for cardiac monitoring

This man has a good story for a cardiac syncope. Factors in this history that would lead you to this diagnosis would be syncope occurring on sitting down, absence of prodromal symptoms, and the immediate recovery. In the presence of bifasicular block, an abnormal ECG, the European Society of Cardiology Guidelines (2009) suggests admission for cardiac monitoring to look for an arrhythmic cause. The inpatient diagnostic yield of such monitoring is low but justified by the potentially life-threatening event. Other features suggestive of cardiac syncope would be exertional syncope, palpitations, chest pain, cardiac risk factors or history of structural cardiac disease, and a family history of sudden cardiac death.

Box 6.1 Clinical features and co-morbidities

From the ESC Guidelines 2009, indications for hospitalization:

Severe structural or coronary artery disease (heart failure, low left ventricular ejection fraction or previous myocardial infarction)

Clinical or ECG features suggesting arrhythmic syncope
- Syncope during exercise or while supine
- Palpitations at the time of syncope
- Family history of sudden cardiac death
- Non-sustained ventricular tachycardia
- Bifascicular block (right bundle branch block and either left anterior or left posterior fascicular block)
- Bradycardia with heart rate below 50 beats per minute or sinoatrial block in the absence of negative chronotropic drugs (e.g. beta-blockers) or physical training
- QRS complex longer than 120 milliseconds
- Prolonged or short QT interval
- Pre-excited QRS complex

ELDERLY CARE AND STROKE | ANSWERS

> **Box 6.1** *(continued)*
> - Right bundle branch block pattern with ST elevation in leads V1-V3 (Brugada pattern)
> - Features suggestive of arrhythmogenic right ventricular cardiomyopathy
>
> Important co-morbidities
> - Severe anaemia
> - Electrolyte disturbance
>
> Reproduced from *European Heart Journal*, 30, Angel M et al., 'Guidelines for the diagnosis and management of syncope (version 2009)', pp. 2631–2671. Copyright (2009) with permission from Oxford University Press.

Guidelines for the diagnosis and management of syncope (version 2009): The Task Force for the Diagnosis and Management of Syncope of the European Society of Cardiology (ESC). European Heart Journal 2009; 30: 2631–2671.

18. B. Get-up-and-go test

All older persons who report a single fall should be observed as they get up from a sitting position, stand without using their arms for support, walk several paces, turn, return to the chair, and sit back in the chair without using their arms for support. Individuals who have difficulty or demonstrate unsteadiness performing this test require further assessment.

Mathias S, Nayak USL, Isaacs B. Get-up and Go Test, 'Balance in elderly patient'. Archives of Physical Medicine and Rehabilitation 1986; 67: 387–389.

The Timed 'Up and Go': a test of basic functional mobility for frail elderly persons. Journal of the American Geriatrics Society 1991; 39: 142–148.

19. E. No driving for six months if no cause is found

This woman's syncope would be classified by the Driver and Vehicle Licensing Agency (DVLA) as 'solitary loss of consciousness likely to be cardiovascular in origin'. The DVLA identifies the following as high risk: abnormal ECG; clinical evidence of structural heart disease; syncope causing injury, occurring at the wheel or while sitting or lying; and more than one episode in the previous six months.

Restrictions apply as stated:

Group 1 vehicle (car, motorcycle)—licence refused/revoked for six months if no cause identified. Can drive four weeks after the event if the cause has been identified and treated.

Group 2 vehicle (lorries, buses)—licence refused/revoked for 12 months if no cause identified. Can drive three months after the event if the cause has been identified and treated.

At-a-glance guide to the current medical standards of fitness to drive: Drivers Medical Group, Driver & Vehicle Licensing Agency, Swansea, November 2014 Edition (including August 2015 amendments).

20. E. Posterior semi-circular canal benign paroxysmal positional vertigo

Classic benign paroxysmal positional vertigo (BPPV) is usually triggered by sudden head movement, typically turning over in bed at night. Symptoms are brief and self-limiting, lasting seconds to a minute. Ménière's disease has a classic triad of sustained vertigo, fluctuating hearing loss, and tinnitus of longer duration. Labyrinthitis can be preceded by viral illness and last days to weeks with a more gradual onset. Central causes of nystagmus classically have different patterns of nystagmus: baseline nystagmus, down-beating, or periodic alternating nystagmus. There may be other neurological symptoms suggestive of a posterior circulation event.

BPPV can be preceded by a head injury; the theory is that debris is dislodged into the semi-circular canals. Posterior semi-circular canal BPPV is more common and identified using the Dix-Hallpike manoeuvre when rotatory geotropic nystagmus (horizontal nystagmus towards the upward ear) is provoked with vertigo symptoms. Lateral semi-circular canal BPPV (also known as horizontal) is diagnosed using the supine roll test. Identifying the type of BPPV has indications for treatment. Posterior canal BPPV responds to the Epley manoeuvre, while horizontal canal responds to the roll manoeuvre (Lempert manoeuvre or barbecue roll manoeuvre or its variations).

Li J, Meyers A, Epley J et al. Benign paroxysmal positional vertigo. Medscape 2013. http://emedicine.medscape.com/article/884261-overview (accessed November 2015)

21. E. Multifocal lenses

The 2010 American Geriatric Society/British Geriatric Society guidelines and NICE guidance recommend older persons who present for medical attention because of a fall, report recurrent falls (≥2) in the past year, or report difficulties in walking or balance (with or without activity curtailment) should have a multifactorial falls risk assessment. This should include a full medical assessment and, in addition, examination of the feet and footwear; functional assessment; assessment of the individual's perceived functional ability and fear related to falling; and environmental assessment, including home safety. Older patients should be advised not to wear multifocal lenses when walking, especially on the stairs.

There are multiple evidence-based interventions but these must be tailored to the individual's risk factors, as follows.

- strength and balance training
- home hazard assessment and intervention
- vision assessment and referral
- medication review and modification/withdrawal
- cardiac pacing if cardioinhibitory carotid sinus hypersensitivity

American Geriatrics Society, British Geriatrics Society. AGS/BGS Clinical Practice Guideline: Prevention of Falls in Older Persons, 2010. http://www.americangeriatrics.org/health_care_professionals/clinical_practice/clinical_guidelines_recommendations/2010/ (accessed November 2015)

National Institute for Health and Care Excellence. Clinical Guideline 161. Falls in older people: assessing risk and prevention. June 2013.

22. D. Subcutaneous denosumab

Denosumab is a human monoclonal antibody which inhibits osteoclast formation, function, and survival, therefore decreasing bone resorption. In 2010, NICE approved denosumab for secondary prevention in the treatment of postmenopausal osteoporosis in patients who are unable to comply with/intolerant of or have a contraindication to alendronate and strontium. There is no dose adjustment required in renal failure. Vitamin D deficiency and hypocalcaemia should be corrected before commencing denosumab. It is a six-monthly subcutaneous injection.

Bisphosphonates should be avoided if creatinine clearance is less than 35 mL/min. They are contraindicated in oesophageal strictures or achalasia and cautioned if there is active upper gastrointestinal bleeding.

Strontium stimulates bone formation and reduces bone resorption. It is now contraindicated in patients cerebrovascular disease; current or previous venous thromboembolic event; ischaemic heart disease; peripheral arterial disease; temporary or prolonged immobilisation; or uncontrolled hypertension.

The World Health Organisation has developed a tool to evaluate fracture risk in patients called the Fracture Risk Assessment Tool (FRAX). The tool includes clinical risk factors with or without bone mineral density to give a ten-year fracture risk probability to help guide treatment with the use of National Osteoporosis Guideline Group (NOGG) guidelines.

National Institute for Health and Care Excellence. Technology Appraisal Guidance 204. Denosumab for the prevention of osteoporotic fractures in postmenopausal women. October 2010.

FRAX: www.shef.ac.uk/FRAX

NOGG: http://www.shef.ac.uk/NOGG/index.html (accessed November 2015)

23. A. Amitriptyline

Amitriptyline is the most likely cause in this case. Tricyclic antidepressants have long been recognized as a contributory factor to falls in older people. Sedation, nocturia, cardiac conduction disturbances, and orthostatic hypotension are some of the postulated mechanisms. Elderly patients are particularly susceptible to the side effects of tricyclic antidepressants. Although omeprazole has been found in some trials to be associated with increased hip fracture, there is no documented increased risk of falls. Gliclazide is less likely to cause hypoglycaemic events in the elderly than the longer-acting oral hypoglycaemics such as glibenclamide. Vitamin D supplementation is one of the only interventions in falls prevention with an evidence base. Fludrocortisone will increase blood pressure and improve symptoms of postural hypotension. The STOPP/START screening tool is helpful in prescribing for older patients.

Gallagher P, Ryan C, Byrne S et al. STOPP (Screening Tool of Older Persons' Prescriptions) and START (Screening Tool to Alert Doctors to Right Treatment): consensus validation. International Journal of Clinical Pharmacology and Therapeutics 2008; 46: 72–83.

24. C. High-specification foam mattress

A high-specification foam mattress is recommended as a for patients with pressure sore. Nutritional assessment using a recognized tool is recommended as nutritional support may be needed to aid healing in this case. Referral to the surgical team may be appropriate given the high grade of pressure sore and signs of systemic sepsis. Osteomyelitis needs to be excluded. In this situation, maintaining a dry, non-contaminated environment will be important to aid healing.

National Institute for Health and Care Excellence. Clinical Guideline 179. Pressure ulcers: prevention and management. April 2014.

EPUAP-NPUAP Guidelines. Prevention and Treatment of Pressure Ulcers: Clinical Practice Guideline. Updated 2014. http://www.npuap.org/resources/educational-and-clinical-resources/prevention-and-treatment-of-pressure-ulcers-clinical-practice-guideline/ (accessed November 2015)

25. E. Postural tachycardia syndrome (PoTS)

Postural tachycardia syndrome (PoTS) is a condition of dysautonomia. The hallmark feature is a rise in pulse rate on standing of more than 30 beats per minute without a corresponding drop in blood pressure. 80% of sufferers are female (especially young women). The presenting symptoms can be varied and non-specific but reflect the wide ranges of autonomic functions (e.g. syncope and presyncope, shaking, anxiety, nausea, palpitations). The condition is often misdiagnosed as chronic fatigue syndrome or anxiety. The diagnosis can be confirmed with a tilt-table test. There are many medical treatments available, including beta-blockers and selective serotonin reuptake inhibitors, but these should only be initiated by a syncope specialist.

http://www.potsuk.org/ (accessed November 2015)

26. B. Greater than three second pause on the ECG

Carotid sinus hypersensitivity results in vagal activation and/or sympathetic inhibition, which causes bradycardia and/or vasodilatation which then causes syncope. The prevalence increases with age and is rare in under 40-year-olds. Carotid sinus hypersensitivity can be diagnosed using carotid sinus massage. The European Society of Cardiology (ESC) Guidelines 2009 recommend massage for ten seconds on each side consecutively in the supine and then erect position with continuous heart rate monitoring and periodic blood pressure measurements. This is contraindicated if there is a history of a TIA or stroke in the previous three months or a carotid bruit (unless carotid studies have excluded a significant stenosis). Carotid sinus massage is positive if syncope is reproduced in the presence of asystole longer than three seconds (cardioinhibitory response) or there is a fall in systolic blood pressure of greater than 50 mm Hg (vasopressor response). An asymptomatic bradycardic or hypotensive episode is less sensitive and specific as false positives are common; in this setting, it would be important to exclude other causes of syncope.

Treatments include reassurance and education. Patients are advised to avoid situations where the neck may be manipulated. Medications that cause a fall in blood pressure should be stopped or reduced where possible. Dual-chamber pacemakers maybe helpful if the carotid sinus hypersensitivity is cardioinhibitory.

Guidelines for the diagnosis and management of syncope (version 2009): The Task Force for the Diagnosis and Management of Syncope of the European Society of Cardiology (ESC). European Heart Journal 2009; 30: 2631–2671.

27. E. A symptomatic progressive fall in blood pressure on tilt-testing of ≥20 mmHg

Normally, standing causes compensatory reflexes so that there is only a small fall in blood pressure (5–10 mmHg) and an increase in pulse rate (10–20 beats per minute). If intravascular volume is depleted or autonomic reflexes impaired, a significant reduction in blood pressure occurs and causes orthostatic hypotension (OH). This is common in the elderly for a number of reasons: a reduction in baroreceptor sensitivity; the use of antihypertensives; and diseases that cause autonomic failure (Parkinson's disease, Lewy body dementia, multisystem atrophy, diabetes, paraneoplastic syndromes) and volume depletion.

The initial investigation for OH is 'active standing'; the patient arises from supine to erect and the BP is measured for three minutes. It is diagnostic if there is a significant drop in systolic blood pressure (≥20 mmHg, or systolic BP falls to less than 90 mmHg) and the patient is symptomatic. When 'active standing' is not diagnostic, or the symptoms could be neurocardiogenic (reflex) syncope or OH, then it would be appropriate to progress to a tilt-table test in order to reproduce the symptoms. It is important to rule out structural heart disease beforehand. The tilt table is set in a quiet room with minimal distractions. The patient is initially monitored for five minutes supine. The purpose-built couch then tilts the head up to 60–70° smoothly and quickly within ten seconds. The patient is encouraged to report symptoms. There is beat-to-beat ECG and BP monitoring from a device attached to a finger. This is the passive phase and lasts for 20–45 minutes or until symptoms are reproduced. If neurocardiogenic syncope is suspected and the passive test has been negative, then 300–400 mcg of GTN may be given. Orthostatic hypotension is diagnosed if there is a slow, progressive, and significant (≥20 mmHg) decrease in systolic blood pressure on passive tilting with or without symptoms. If symptoms are reproduced either in the passive or active phase (after GTN) and there is reflex hypotension/bradycardia, then this is diagnostic of neurocardiogenic (reflex) syncope.

Guidelines for the diagnosis and management of syncope (version 2009): The Task Force for the Diagnosis and Management of Syncope of the European Society of Cardiology (ESC). European Heart Journal 2009; 30: 2631–2671.

ELDERLY CARE AND STROKE | ANSWERS

28. B. Nothing unless he develops any symptoms

Results of common laboratory tests need to be interpreted with care in older adults. Multiple confounding factors make interpreting results in older patients more difficult. There are physiological changes associated with ageing; there is a higher prevalence of chronic conditions, changes in nutrition and fluid consumption, and multiple medications to consider. With some tests, older adults have higher than normal values (e.g. ESR, alkaline phosphatase) and others a lower (e.g. haemoglobin, white cell count, albumin, and potassium), and some remain unchanged. So, laboratory values falling outside the normal ranges may indicate benign or pathological conditions and values within the expected normal reference range may indicate new or progressive pathologic conditions (e.g. creatinine). Therefore, it is important to consider the patient as a whole, their weight, co-morbidities, medication, and then focus on goals of treatment. Goals of treatment for older patients need to be individualized; for some frail patients it is inappropriate to concentrate on disease prevention and risk reduction, and more on symptom control.

In this case, the alkaline phosphatase is slightly raised, it remains unchanged over the six weeks, and the patient is asymptomatic, so no further tests need to be requested unless he develops symptoms.

Physiological basis of aging and geriatrics. Fourth edition. Edited by Paola S Timiras. New York, Informa Healthcare, 2007. ISBN: 978-0-8493-7305-3.

29. A. Barthel index

The Barthel index is an ordinal scale designed to measure performance in ten activities of daily living, including aspects of continence, self-care, and mobility.

Depression affects 10–15% of adults over the age of 65 living in the UK, with an even higher proportion in hospitalized patients. Risk factors for depression in the older adult include social isolation, bereavement, institutionalization, poor physical health, and cognitive impairment. Depression must be considered as a coexisting diagnosis and a possible cause of cognitive impairment in this age group. Screening for alcohol abuse and co-morbid conditions/medication side effects should be considered. Any evidence of suicidal ideation should prompt further inpatient assessment. Care must be taken when considering antidepressants due to increased sensitivity to side effects and increased drug interactions.

There are various screening and scoring tools available. The geriatric depression scale (GDS) was developed as a screening and assessment tool specifically for depression in older adults. It consists of 30 questions, but there is a shorter version: GDS-15. It can also be used in patients with mild to moderate cognitive impairment. The hospital anxiety and depression scale (HADS) is a self-rating scale measuring symptoms of depression and anxiety during the previous week. The HADS is validated for all ages. The brief assessment schedule depression cards (BASDEC) consists of 19 cards in large print to which the patient must answer 'yes' or 'no'. This can be more user-friendly for frail, medically unwell elderly patients. The Cornell scale for depression in dementia has been specifically developed to assess signs and symptoms of major depression in patients with dementia using a semi-structured interview.

Wilson K, Mottram P, Sivanranthan A et al. Antidepressants versus placebo for the depressed elderly (Cochrane Review). The Cochrane Library, Issue 4, 2001.

30. D. Osteoarthritis

The X-ray shows joint space narrowing, subchondral sclerosis, and cyst formation, consistent with the history suggesting osteoarthritis in the left hip. Osteoarthritis is a common cause of disability and reduced mobility in older adults. There is joint pain and deformity due to degeneration of articular cartilage and new bone formation at joint margins. Non-pharmacological treatment includes weight loss, exercise, and orthotics. Analgesia and intra-articular steroid injection can be considered.

Subluxation can also be a consequence of severe osteoarthritis. Referral to orthopaedic surgeons for joint replacement is an option in severe cases. A detailed history, appropriate imaging, and other investigations should be undertaken with this degree of severity, or if there are atypical features.

Multiple myeloma can cause hypercalcaemia, renal impairment, and anaemia along with characteristic lytic lesions on the X-ray. Paget's disease can be associated with a raised alkaline phosphatase and distortion and overgrowth of the involved bone. The chronic background in this case makes septic arthritis unlikely and the absence of trauma excludes fractured neck of femur unless there is an underlying bone lesion.

Gout and pseudogout should be considered in acute single joint disease and uric acid can be useful. Rheumatoid arthritis has a more bilateral symmetrical onset with early morning stiffness and swelling around the MCP joints. Stiffness in the shoulder and hip girdles should prompt an ESR to look for polymyalgia rheumatica.

BSR and BHPR Guidelines for the management of polymyalgia rheumatica. May 2011.

chapter 7

RENAL MEDICINE AND UROLOGICAL PROBLEMS

QUESTIONS

1. **A 54-year-old man attended the emergency department with a five-day history of fevers and night sweats. There were no other symptoms. He had received a pre-emptive live donor renal transplant from his wife four months earlier upon reaching end-stage renal failure due to IgA nephropathy. The patient's medications included: tacrolimus 4 mg two times daily (bd), mycophenolate mofetil 500 mg three times a day (tds), prednisolone 7.5 mg once a day (od), and nifedipine M/R 10 mg bd.**

```
Investigations:
  haemoglobin                   112 g/L           (130-180)
  white cell count              5.4 × 10⁹/L       (4.0-11.0)
  neutrophil count              3.2 × 10⁹/L       (1.5-7.0)
  lymphocyte count              0.16 × 10⁹/L      (1.5-4.0)
  platelet count                202 × 10⁹/L       (150-400)
  serum sodium                  137 mmol/L        (137-144)
  serum potassium               4.4 mmol/L        (3.5-4.9)
  serum urea                    6.6 mmol/L        (2.5-7.0)
  serum creatinine              122 µmol/L        (60-110)
  serum bilirubin               23 µmol/L         (1-22)
  serum alkaline phosphatase    120 U/L           (45-105)
  serum alanine                 131 U/L           (5-35)
    aminotranferase
  serum albumin                 32 g/L            (37-49)
  serum C-reactive protein      74 mg/L           (<10)

  urinalysis: blood + protein +
```

What is the most likely diagnosis?

A. CMV disease
B. Pneumocystis jiroveci pneumonia
C. Post-transplant lymphoproliferative disorder
D. Recurrent IgA nephropathy
E. Urinary tract infection

2. A 25-year-old man attended the emergency department with a headache. There were no focal neurological signs. His symptoms resolved after a period of observation. No further investigation was planned and he was due to be discharged home. A foundation year 1 doctor (in the UK) was completing his discharge summary and noted that his urinalysis showed blood + + on admission and again prior to discharge. Urine microscopy was normal and there was no growth on culture.

Examination revealed a blood pressure of 118/74 mmHg.

```
Investigations:
    serum sodium        140 mmol/L      (137-144)
    serum potassium     3.9 mmol/L      (3.5-4.9)
    serum urea          4.1 mmol/L      (2.5-7.0)
    serum creatinine    67 µmol/L       (60-110)
```

The foundation year 1 doctor (in the UK) asked you what to advise the patient's GP to do next?

A. Order a renal ultrasound
B. Repeat dipstick urine and perform urine protein:creatinine ratio
C. Repeat MSU and start trimethoprim 200 mg bd
D. Urine cytology and refer to urology
E. Urine protein:creatinine ratio and refer to nephrology

3. A 66-year-old man was admitted three days ago with urinary sepsis. He was febrile at 39.7°C and hypotensive on admission with a blood pressure of 74/45 mmHg. Blood and urine cultures had both grown gram-negative rods. Renal ultrasonography showed normal-sized unobstructed kidneys.

He had partially responded to intravenous fluids, a single dose of gentamicin, and three days of oral ciprofloxacin. He had become breathless.

On examination, his temperature was 37.1°C and pulse 83 beats per minute. His blood pressure was 125/78 mmHg and respiratory rate was 20 breaths per minute. On auscultation of his chest, he had crackles to the mid-zones bilaterally. His fluid balance charts showed he had 10.5 L of fluid input and 1 L of urine output over a three-day period. Urine output for the last 12 hours was less than 100 mL. He had been prescribed insulin:dextrose infusions repeatedly due to persistent hyperkalaemia 6.5 mmol/L (3.5–4.9).

```
Investigations:
    Admission      serum creatinine     88 µmol/L      (60-110)
    Day 1          serum creatinine     147 µmol/L     (60-110)
    Day 2          serum creatinine     332 µmol/L     (60-110)
    Day 3          serum creatinine     590 µmol/L     (60-110)
```

The critical care team had reviewed him but felt he had single-organ failure and could be managed on the ward. The nearest acute dialysis unit was 30 miles away.

What should be your next action?

A. Furosemide infusion 240mg/24h
B. Further fluid challenge
C. Renal-dose dopamine on coronary care unit
D. Re-refer to critical care
E. Transfer to renal unit for dialysis

4. **A 55-year-old woman presented to the acute medical unit with a one-week history of worsening lower limb oedema. She was generally fit and well and her only medication was ibuprofen as required for intermittent back pain.**

   Investigations:
serum sodium	140 mmol/L	(137–144)
serum potassium	4.3 mmol/L	(3.5–4.9)
serum bicarbonate	22 mmol/L	(20–28)
serum urea	7.8 mmol/L	(2.5–7.0)
serum creatinine	95 µmol/L	(60–110)
serum bilirubin	12 µmol/L	(1–22)
serum alkaline phosphatase	90 U/L	(45–105)
serum alanine aminotranferase	34 U/L	(5–35)
serum albumin	14 g/L	(37–49)

   urinalysis: protein + + + +
   ECG: normal sinus rhythm
   CXR: normal lung fields and heart size

   Which test is most likely to provide a diagnosis?
   A. HbA1C and fasting glucose
   B. Anti-PLA2R antibody assay
   C. Renal biopsy
   D. Renal ultrasound
   E. Serum-free light chains, serum and urine electrophoresis

5. **A 30-year-old bodybuilder was visiting his mother on the acute medical unit when he developed acute severe right loin pain and visible haematuria. A renal stone was suspected. The busy urology registrar asked for confirmation of the diagnosis before reviewing the patient.**

   What is the best choice of imaging to confirm renal calculi?
   A. Magnetic resonance urography
   B. Non-contrast helical CT urogram
   C. Plain abdominal radiography
   D. Plain intravenous urogram
   E. Renal ultrasound

RENAL MEDICINE AND UROLOGICAL PROBLEMS | QUESTIONS

6. A 72-year-old man presented with a six-week history of fever, shortness of breath, night sweats, sinusitis, anorexia, muscle pains, and a weak left wrist. During initial investigations his GP had found persistent non-visible haematuria and treated him with trimethoprim. Urine culture had been negative on three occasions.

   On examination, his temperature was 37.8°C, his pulse was 105 beats per minute, and blood pressure 138/75 mmHg. His oxygen saturation was 90% on air. No cardiac murmurs were audible and there were no peripheral signs of infective endocarditis.

   ```
   Investigations:
     haemoglobin              87 g/L              (130-180)
     white cell count         13.5 × 10⁹/L        (4.0-11.0)
     neutrophil count         11.9 × 10⁹/L        (1.5-7.0)
     lymphocyte count         1.5 × 10⁹/L         (1.5-4.0)
     platelet count           380 × 10⁹/L         (150-400)
     serum creatinine         335 µmol/L          (60-110)
     serum C-reactive protein 135 mg/L            (<10)

     urine microscopy: blood + +, no white cells; granular casts present

     CXR showed bilateral pulmonary infiltrates in an alveolar
       filling pattern
   ```

   Which non-invasive test is the best to support the likely diagnosis?
   A. ANCA titre
   B. Anti-GBM titre
   C. Induced sputum for acid-fast bacilli
   D. Nerve conduction studies
   E. Transthoracic echocardiography

7. A 68-year-old man was on the vascular ward two days following a left below-knee amputation. He had an episode of bloody diarrhoea two hours ago, and was complaining of severe abdominal pain. He appeared peripherally shut down. On examination, his pulse rate was 90 beats per minute and his blood pressure was 122/55 mmHg.

   He had taken his regular medications including ramipril, furosemide, metformin, simvastatin, and aspirin that morning. An arterial blood gas showed a lactate of 6.7 mmol/L (0.5–1.6); preoperatively, his serum creatinine was 147 µmol/L (60–110).

   The surgical registrar wanted to confirm the extent of his ischaemic bowel before planning surgery.

   What is the most appropriate manoeuvre to reduce his risk of contrast-induced acute kidney injury (CI-AKI)?
   A. Intravenous N-acetylcystine
   B. Perform non-contrast CT scan abdomen
   C. Pre-hydration with intravenous 0.9% sodium chloride
   D. Stop ramipril and metformin and defer scan for 48 hours
   E. Use high-osmolality iodinated contrast medium

8. A 43-year-old man presented to the acute medical unit due to abnormal blood results. His GP had taken blood earlier that day as he had been feeling lethargic for three months and nauseated for the last four days.

   Blood pressure on arrival was 182/90 mmHg.

   ```
   Investigations:
      haemoglobin                 81 g/L              (130–180)
      MCV                         82.1 fL             (80–96)
      white cell count            6.4 × 10⁹/L         (4.0–11.0)
      platelet count              390 × 10⁹/L         (150–400)
      serum sodium                136 mmol/L          (137–144)
      serum potassium             5.6 mmol/L          (3.5–4.9)
      serum urea                  42.4 mmol/L         (2.5–7.0)
      serum creatinine            785 µmol/L          (60–110)
      serum corrected calcium     1.89 mmol/L         (2.20–2.60)
      serum C-reactive protein    3 mg/L              (<10)
      no previous blood results were available

      urinalysis: protein + +

      ECG: LVH but otherwise normal
   ```

   What is the most useful next investigation?
   A. ANCA titre
   B. CT urogram
   C. Parathyroid hormone
   D. Renal biopsy
   E. Renal ultrasonography

9. A 69-year-old man returned to the ward after a diagnostic coronary angiogram. Diffuse coronary disease was found but no lesions were deemed suitable for angioplasty. The recommendation on the angiogram report was to continue his current maximal medical treatment, which included aspirin, atorvastatin, and bisoprolol. There was also a comment that a 'drive by' renal angiogram was performed at the end of the procedure showing what appeared to be bilateral 50% stenoses at the renal artery ostia. His blood pressure of 128/80 mmHg was similar to his blood pressure pre-procedure.

   His estimated glomerular filtration rate (MDRD) pre-procedure was 58 mL/min (>60), with no deterioration in function over the last 18 months.

   Renal ultrasound showed bilateral 10 cm-long unobstructed kidneys.

   What is your next step in his management?
   A. Formal renal arteriogram
   B. MR renal angiography
   C. Proceed as per angiogram report
   D. Refer to nephrology
   E. Refer to vascular surgery

10. **A 36-year-old man was admitted to the acute medical unit with shortness of breath and cough and was diagnosed with pneumonia after a chest X-ray showed left lower-lobe consolidation. His admission blood tests showed the following.**

    ```
    Investigations:
       serum urea          23.4 mmol/L      (2.5-7.0)
       serum creatinine    364 µmol/L       (60-110)
    ```

    A catheter was inserted to monitor fluid balance. His urine output was 5 ml per hour over the last six hours. Blood tests done six months previously showed a urea 4.4 mmol/L and creatinine 118 µmol/L.

    Using the RIFLE criteria, which stage of acute kidney injury does he have?

    A. End-stage
    B. Failure
    C. Injury
    D. Loss
    E. Risk

11. A 28-year-old woman was referred to the acute medical unit reporting decreased urine output. She received a cadaveric renal transplant eight months earlier after developing progressive renal failure due to chronic pyelonephritis and reflux nephropathy.

On admission, she was apyrexial and alert with a fine peripheral tremor, intermittent nystagmus, and a blood pressure of 188/92 mmHg. Mild peripheral oedema was present. Her transplanted kidney was palpable and non-tender. Ultrasound scan identified a normal appearance of the urinary bladder and transplant kidney with normal arterial Doppler profiles.

Six weeks prior to admission, her blood results showed the following.

```
Investigations:
   haemoglobin           122 g/L           (130-180)
   white cell count      4.8 × 10⁹/L       (4.0-11.0)
   serum sodium          134 mmol/L        (137-144)
   serum potassium       4.1 mmol/L        (3.5-4.9)
   serum creatinine      128 µmol/L        (60-110)

   urine dip: blood + protein +
```

On admission, her results were as follows.

```
Investigations:
   haemoglobin           122 g/L           (130-180)
   white cell count      4.0 × 10⁹/L       (4.0-11.0)
   serum sodium          131 mmol/L        (137-144)
   serum potassium       5.9 mmol/L        (3.5-4.9)
   serum creatinine      288 µmol/L        (60-110)

   urine dip: blood + protein +
```

What is the most appropriate next step?

A. Administer 1000 mL 0.9% sodium chloride over two hours
B. Commence broad-spectrum antibiotics
C. Intravenous labetalol
D. Request antinuclear antibody, anti-neutrophil cytoplasmic antibody, and anti-glomerular basement membrane antibody analysis
E. Request a tacrolimus level

12. **A 78-year-old woman was referred to the acute medical unit with progressive malaise and swelling around her ankles and knees. She was diagnosed with rheumatoid arthritis 34 years earlier. Symptoms had been moderately well controlled with weekly methotrexate and intermittent courses of oral and intra-articular corticosteroids, and naproxen.**

On examination, she had pitting oedema up to the lower thigh. Blood pressure was 102/45 mmHg. Moderate crepitations were heard at both lung bases. She had a 2/6 pan-systolic murmur, best heard at the right sternal edge. There were numerous ecchymoses but no evidence of synovitis, cellulitis, or cutaneous vasculitis.

```
Investigations:
  haemoglobin                        108 g/L           (115-165)
  platelet count                     360 × 10⁹/L       (150-400)
  serum creatinine                   288 µmol/L        (60-110)
  estimated glomerular filtration    33 mL/min         (>60)
    rate
  serum albumin                      19 g/L            (37-49)
  serum electrophoresis: polyclonal excess IgG; no serum
    paraprotein identified
  antinuclear antibodies: weakly positive
  serum C3/C4 levels: normal

  urine dip: no blood, protein + + + +, leucocyte esterase +,
    nitrites negative
```

What is the most likely cause for her swelling?

A. Amyloidosis
B. Cryoglobulinaemia
C. Infective endocarditis
D. Lupus nephritis
E. Methotrexate-induced liver failure

13. A 56-year-old man born in the UK, was referred to hospital after he developed progressive breathlessness over one week. He had no significant medical history and was not prescribed any medications. He had not travelled abroad for the last ten years. He was a smoker.

On arrival, he was tachypnoeic at rest, pale, and unwell. His temperature was 37.5°C, pulse 115 beats per minute, and blood pressure 171/92 mmHg. His oxygen saturation was 90% on 4 L/min oxygen via nasal cannula.

```
Investigations:
   serum creatinine              1085 µmol/L      (60-110)
   haemoglobin                   68 g/L           (130-180)
   serum C-reactive protein      252 mg/L         (<10)
   serum electrophoresis: no serum paraprotein identified
   antinuclear antibodies: negative
   serum C3/C4 levels: normal

   urine dipstick: no sample available

   chest X-ray: bilateral airspace shadowing
```

Which is the most likely diagnosis?

A. Anti-glomerular basement membrane disease
B. Granulomatosis with polyangiitis (Wegener's)
C. Microscopic polyangiitis
D. Mycoplasma pneumonia
E. Squamous cell carcinoma of the lung

14. **A 68-year-old woman with diabetes and chronic kidney disease stage 4 attended the walk-in centre with dysuria and urinary frequency. She had no known allergies. She was apyrexial with a blood pressure of 142/84 mmHg.**

    ```
    Investigations:
      Urine dipstick revealed:
      Blood                    + +
      Protein                  + + +
      Leucocyte esterase       + +
      Nitrites                 positive
    ```

    Blood and urine samples were sent for analysis, as follows.

    ```
    Investigations:
      serum creatinine                   302 µmol/L      (60-110)
      estimated glomerular filtration    18 mL/min       (>60)
        rate
      serum potassium                    5.9 mmol/L      (3.5-4.9)

      urine culture: coliforms
      sensitivities: trimethoprim, cefalexin, meropenem,
        nitrofurantoin
    ```

    What is the most appropriate treatment?
    A. Cefalexin
    B. Meropenem
    C. Nitrofurantoin
    D. No antimicrobial therapy
    E. Trimethoprim

15. A 56-year-old man was referred with left loin pain, fever, and dysuria. His GP treated him for an uncomplicated proven E. Coli urinary tract infection just over a year ago. He had no other past medical history.

On examination, his temperature was 38.2°C, pulse rate 90 beats per minute, and blood pressure 128/78 mmHg. Urine dipstick analysis confirmed the presence of leucocyte esterase and nitrites.

The following laboratory results were received.

```
Investigations:
    serum creatinine            95 µmol/L       (60-110)
    serum C-reactive protein    121 mg/L        (>10)

    urine culture: >10⁵ colony forming units of E. Coli
    sensitivities: trimethoprim, cefalexin, co-amoxiclav,
      nitrofurantoin
```

After 48 hours of intravenous co-amoxiclav, he was apyrexial and his symptoms had resolved.

Which further investigations are not indicated at this stage?

A. Abdominal radiograph
B. Fasting serum glucose
C. Post-micturition bladder volume scan
D. Prostate specific antigen
E. Ultrasound kidneys

16. A 25-year-old woman presented to the acute medical unit with progressive leg swelling and marked fatigue 14 weeks into her first pregnancy. Her medication included folic acid 400 μg per day and a multivitamin preparation. Her symptoms had developed over two to three weeks. She had no significant medical history. On systemic enquiry, she reported slight dyspnoea on exertion with a dry cough, and infrequent rapid palpitations. She had no gastroenterological or neurological symptoms.

    On examination, she appeared fatigued and pale. Her temperature was 36.7°C, pulse 96 beats per minute, and blood pressure 175/98 mmHg. A gravid uterus was palpable. Chest auscultation was unremarkable. A 2/6 pan systolic murmur was audible throughout the praecordium.

    Urine dipstick analysis revealed blood + +, protein + + + +, leucocyte esterase +, nitrites negative.

    ```
    Investigations:
       serum creatinine     108 μmol/L        (60-110)
       serum albumin        18 g/L            (37-49)
       white cell count     4.0 × 10⁹/L       (4.0-11.0)
       haemoglobin          89 g/dL           (115-165)
       platelets            91 × 10¹²/L       (150-400)

       chest X-ray: clear lung fields, normal cardiac outline
    ```

    What is the most likely cause of her symptoms?
    A. Inferior vena cava thrombosis
    B. Pre-eclampsia
    C. Systemic lupus erythematosus
    D. Tuberculosis
    E. Urinary tract infection

17. You see a 65-year-old man in the emergency department. He presented after a four-day history of nausea and vomiting. He had a past medical history of hypertension and bipolar disorder, both of which had been well controlled for many years. He had continued taking his regular medication ramipril and lithium.

    Initial blood pressure was 65/34 mmHg but this improved to 123/70 mmHg following 7 L of intravenous normal saline. The nurses were increasingly concerned about his respiratory rate, which was 40 breaths per minute.

    Which of the following is not an indication for urgent dialysis?
    A. Diuretic-resistant pulmonary oedema with oligoanuria
    B. Serum creatinine of 1245 μmol/L
    C. Serum lithium of 4.3 mmol/L
    D. Serum potassium 7.1 mmol/L after attempted medical treatment
    E. Uraemic pericarditis

18. **A 67-year-old man was admitted to the acute medical unit from the emergency department with a two-day history of right upper quadrant pain, fever, and dyspnoea.**

His temperature was 38.8°C, pulse 110 beats per minute, blood pressure was 85/60 mmHg and respiratory rate 32 breaths per minute. Treatment was immediately commenced with intravenous piperacillin and tazobactam, along with intravenous fluid resuscitation. Non-contrast computerized tomography identified a gallbladder empyema for which the patient underwent percutaneous drainage. Blood cultures and samples from the drain were positive for enterococcus species and sensitive to amoxicillin.

Antibiotics and intravenous fluid therapy were continued over the next 48 hours while he remained nil-by-mouth. Drain output was 250 mL in the first 24 hours and 80 mL in the second 48 hours. His progress was documented; see Table 7.1.

Table 7.1 Patient observations and blood results on admission and then at 6, 24, and 48 hours after admission.

	On admission	6 hours after admission	24 hours after admission	48 hours after admission
Pulse (beats per minute)	110	95	88	85
Blood pressure (mmHg)	85/60	110/70	115/72	118/75
Respiratory rate (breaths per minute)	32	22	16	22
Urine output (mL/hour)		25	75	200
Sodium (mmol/L)	135	137	137	140
Potassium (mmol/L)	5.0	4.1	4.2	4.5
Creatinine (µmol/L)	252	201	158	121
Bicarbonate (mmol/L)	15	16		20
Lactate (mmol/L)	7.2	4.1		1.0
pH	7.19	7.30		7.27
Base excess	−15	−8		−10
pCO_2 (kPa)	4.0	4.2		5.1
Anion gap (mmol/L)	28	19		10

What is the most likely cause of the persistent acidaemia?
A. Bicarbonate loss from biliary drainage
B. Excess chloride administration
C. Ketoacidosis
D. Ongoing septicaemia
E. Respiratory insufficiency

19. A 53-year-old man was admitted after a three-day history of nausea and vomiting. Past medical history included formation of an ileostomy nine months ago following large bowel excision for synchronous bowel and caecal tumours. He also had hypertension. His was taking loperamide 2 mg as required and bendroflumethiazide 2.5 mg once daily.

On arrival, he was dyspnoeic and obtunded. You assessed him urgently as he had become less responsive and you were unable to palpate a femoral pulse. In line with your hospital's policy, you commenced cardiopulmonary resuscitation and summoned the cardiac arrest team. Following 1 L intravenous Hartmann's he had return of spontaneous circulation with a blood pressure of 70/30 mmHg.

```
Investigations:
  Arterial blood gas:
  pH              7.02          (7.35-7.45)
  pO2             15.4 kPa      (11.3-12.6)
  pCO2            6.3 kPa       (4.7-6.0)
  bicarbonate     8 mmol/L      (21-29)
  lactate         6.9 mmol/L    (0.5-1.6)
  potassium       5.0 mmol/L    (3.5-4.9)
```

Your foundation year 1 doctor (in the UK) asks you which fluid to give next?
A. 1.4% sodium bicarbonate
B. 8.4% sodium bicarbonate
C. Hartmann's solution
D. Hydroxyethyl starch
E. No further fluid, transfer for dialysis

20. You were preparing to hand over to the night team at 8.30 p.m. The core medical training (in the UK) year 1 doctor asked you to review a 92-year-old man she had just seen on the acute medical unit. His GP referred him as he had frank pus draining from a suprapubic catheter. This was inserted six months ago for bladder outflow obstruction secondary to benign prostatic hypertrophy. This followed a failure to pass a urethral catheter. He had been judged unsuitable for transurethral resection of prostate.

Your core medical training (in the UK) year 1 doctor diagnosed him as having a catheter-associated urinary tract infection, gave him 240 mg intravenous gentamicin, and removed the catheter. She was now unable to insert a replacement catheter along the original tract or palpate a bladder, and wanted advice on how to proceed.

What is the most appropriate next step in management?
A. Attempt suprapubic catheter insertion via fresh puncture
B. Attempt urethral catheter with further gentamicin cover
C. Contact on-call radiologist for urgent bladder ultrasound
D. Contact on-call urologist tomorrow morning
E. Contact on-call urologist tonight

chapter 7

RENAL MEDICINE AND UROLOGICAL PROBLEMS

ANSWERS

1. A. CMV disease

The combination of fever, night sweats, and hepatitis in the context of recent solid organ transplantation is highly suggestive of CMV disease. This should be confirmed by quantitative PCR rather than through CMV IgG/IgM serology, as the latter can be misleading in the immunosuppressed. Treatment is with intravenous ganciclovir, although oral valganciclovir may be appropriate in less severe cases, or once disease responds to IV treatment.

Post-transplant lymphoproliferative disorder might also present with night sweats, fevers, and moderately raised inflammatory markers, but would be unusual this soon after transplantation.

Atypical respiratory infection is seen following solid organ transplantation. There are no clinical features to suggest the diagnosis in this case, although a chest X-ray as part of the initial assessment would be indicated. Similarly, there are no clinical features to suggest urinary tract infection. Blood and protein in the urine may simply be a manifestation of pre-existing IgA disease. Urine microscopy and culture should, however, still be performed in an immunosuppressed patient with a positive urine dipstick and fever.

Baker R, Jardine A, Andrews P. Post-operative care of the kidney transplant recipient. UK Renal Association, 5th edition, final version (5 February 2011).

2. B. Repeat dipstick urine and perform urine protein:creatinine ratio

Asymptomatic non-visible haematuria (a-NVH) in a man aged less than 40 is unlikely to have a urological cause. Abnormal renal function (eGFR <60), hypertension (BP >140/90 mmHg), or proteinuria (urine protein:creatinine ratio >50 mg/mmol) would all be triggers for further nephrology assessment. Either visible haematuria or non-visible haematuria with urinary symptoms should be investigated by a urologist regardless of age. Transient causes of haematuria—namely, urinary tract infection—should always be excluded before further investigation or onward referral is contemplated.

Joint Consensus Statement on the Initial Assessment of Haematuria BAUS/RA Guidelines. http://www.renal.org/docs/default-source/what-we-do/RA-BAUS_Haematuria_Consensus_Guidelines.pdf

3. D. Re-refer to critical care

This man has stage 3 acute kidney injury according to the AKIN diagnostic criteria. He remains oligoanuric despite enthusiastic fluid resuscitation and appropriate treatment of his septic focus.

Despite theoretical benefits, neither furosemide nor low-dose dopamine have been shown to be effective in this situation. He is clinically fluid overloaded and a further fluid challenge would most likely be harmful. Due to the combination of pulmonary oedema and resistant hyperkalaemia, he is not fit for transfer to a regional renal centre for dialysis. He should, therefore, be re-referred to critical care team for renal replacement therapy and transferred to a renal unit once stable.

Transfer criteria and AKI management resources (London AKI Network guidelines). http://www.londonaki.net/clinical/guidelines-pathways.html

4. C. Renal biopsy

This woman is likely to have nephrotic syndrome, defined by hypoalbuminaemia, proteinuria >3 g/day (or urine PCR >300), and oedema.

The differential diagnosis includes membranous nephropathy, focal segmental glomerulosclerosis, minimal change disease, IgA nephropathy, amyloidosis, membranoproliferative glomerulonephritis, lupus nephritis, and diabetic nephropathy. M-type phospholipase A2 receptor autoantibodies (PLA2R—found in 70–80% of patients with idiopathic membranous nephropathy), autoimmune profile, complement levels, and a myeloma screen might point towards a specific renal diagnosis but would not obviate the need for biopsy. Renal ultrasound would be indicated to demonstrate normal renal anatomy prior to a biopsy, but would be unlikely to provide a diagnosis alone. Although diabetic nephropathy is the most common cause of nephrotic range proteinuria, the absence of a previous history of either diabetes or of microvascular complications makes it less likely in this case.

Woodward N, Harber M. 'Kidney Biopsy', Practical nephrology, edited by Harber M. London: Springer-Verlag, 2014.

5. B. Non-contrast helical CT urogram

Non-contrast helical CT urogram has the best diagnostic accuracy (sensitivity 95%) and is now considered the gold-standard investigation for renal colic. An intravenous urogram has a sensitivity of 70–90% and may fail to detect radiolucent stones. Plain radiography has a sensitivity of 45–60% and ultrasonography a sensitivity of 37–64%. MR urography is a useful tool, often limited by time taken to scan and competing imaging priorities in the radiology department.

National Institute for Health and Care Excellence Clinical Knowledge Summaries: Renal or ureteric colic – acute. Secondary Care Investigations and Treatment. Updated April 2015. http://cks.nice.org.uk/renal-or-ureteric-colic-acute#!scenario

6. A. ANCA titre

The symptoms and initial investigations suggest a small vessel vasculitis with renal, respiratory, and neuronal involvement such as granulomatosis with polyangiitis (GPA)—formerly known as Wegener's granulomatosis. This diagnosis would be supported by a positive cANCA on immunofluorescence and PR3 antigen on ELISA. The differential diagnosis includes microscopic polyangiitis, which would also be likely to demonstrate ANCA positivity (pANCA/MPO positive). The diagnosis would usually be confirmed with renal biopsy.

Anti-GBM disease is a cause of pulmonary–renal syndrome but does not typically present with neurological signs or symptoms.

Endocarditis can be associated with ANCA positivity and a similar picture of blood results; echocardiography is helpful if diagnostic uncertainty is raised by a subsequent positive blood culture, atypical ANCA or renal biopsy findings, or development of a new murmur.

Nerve conduction studies might confirm a mononeuritis in the context of new wrist drop, but would not in itself provide a diagnosis.

Della Rossa A, Cioffi E, Elefante E et al. Systemic vasculitis: an annual critical digest of the most recent literature. Clinical and Experimental Rheumatology May–June 2014; 32(Suppl 82(3)): 98–105.

7. C. Pre-hydration with intravenous 0.9% sodium chloride

Using a minimum dose of low-osmolality iodinated contrast medium may be helpful in reducing the risk of contrast induced acute kidney injury (CI-AKI). Non-contrast CT may not yield a diagnosis in this setting. The clinical scenario here precludes delaying imaging; omitting nephrotoxic medication and metformin should be considered for semi-urgent and elective contrast-enhanced imaging.

Recent meta-analysis and RCT data does not support the routine use of N-acetylcystine. Both 0.9% sodium chloride (1 mL/kg/h for 12 hours pre- and post-procedure) and isotonic sodium bicarbonate have been shown to be effective at reducing the risk of CI-AKI.

Prevention of Contrast Induced Acute Kidney Injury (CI-AKI) In Adult Patients: http://www.renal.org/docs/default-source/guidelines-resources/joint-guidelinesPrevention_of_Contrast_Induced_Acute_Kidney_Injury_CI-AKI_In_Adult_Patients.pdf

8. E. Renal ultrasonography

The most pressing question here is whether this man has an acute reversible pathology (including renal tract obstruction) or established chronic renal disease. There are some features here to suggest chronic disease, such as the normocytic anaemia, hypocalcemia, and ECG findings supporting longstanding hypertension.

Ultrasound (US) is preferred to CT for initial assessment of renal size, symmetry, and the diagnosis of hydronephrosis. US findings such as small smooth kidneys or polycystic kidney disease would usually indicate an end-stage chronic process in this setting and the diagnostic yield from further investigation may be small.

Renal biopsy may be indicated if the US shows relatively normal-sized kidneys or immunological testing proves positive, but is not the first-line test.

ANCA testing might be helpful but the relatively clear urine and suppressed inflammatory markers count against an acute vasculitis.

Parathyroid hormone assay would be indicated as part of assessment of renal bone disease in the context of probable chronic kidney disease with hypocalcaemia, but is unlikely to contribute directly to the renal diagnosis

The Renal Association: The UK eCKD Guide. www.renal.org/ckd (accessed November 2015).

9. C. Proceed as per angiogram report

Two recent large randomized controlled trials have failed to demonstrate a benefit in renal or cardiovascular outcomes from renal artery stenting compared with maximal medical therapy in renal artery stenosis. In this man's case, with well-controlled blood pressure and stable renal function, there is no indication for further investigation. He should be treated aggressively for cardiovascular risk as suggested by the interventional cardiologist.

There is still some uncertainty as to whether patients with very severe renal artery stenosis (>80%) might benefit from intervention.

Young patients with hypertension and a finding of fibromuscular dysplasia on renal angiography do not behave in the same way as those with atheroscletotic renal disease, and may still benefit from renal artery angioplasty.

Cooper C, Murphy T, Cutlip D et al. Stenting and medical therapy for atherosclerotic renal-artery stenosis. NEJM 2013.

The ASTRAL Investigators. Revascularization versus medical therapy for renal-artery stenosis. New England Journal of Medicine 2009; 361: 1953–1962.

10. B. Failure

The RIFLE criteria were developed by the Acute Dialysis Quality Initiative to standardize the definition of acute kidney injury. They identify three stages of acute kidney injury (Risk, Injury, Failure) and two outcome classes (Loss and End-stage).

The criteria are as follows.

- **Risk:** creatinine increased × 1.5 baseline OR GFR decrease >25% OR urine production of <0.5 mL/kg/hr for 6 hours
- **Injury:** creatinine increased × 2 baseline OR GFR decrease >50% OR urine production <0.5 mL/kg/hr for 12 hours
- **Failure:** creatinine × 3 baseline or creatinine >354 μmol/L (with a rise of >44) (>4 mg/dL) OR GFR decrease >75% OR urine output below 0.3 mL/kg/hr for 24 hours or anuria for 12 hours
- **Loss:** persistent AKI or complete loss of kidney function for more than four weeks
- **End-stage renal disease:** complete loss of kidney function for more than three months

Acute renal failure - definition, outcome measures, animal models, fluid therapy and information technology needs: the Second International Consensus Conference of the Acute Dialysis Quality Initiative (ADQI) Group', pp 204–212. Copyright © 2004 Bellomo et al.; licensee BioMed Central Ltd. This figure is from an Open Access article: verbatim copying and redistribution of this article are permitted in all media for any purpose, provided this notice is preserved along with the article's original URL (http://www.ccforum.com/content/8/4/R204)

The Acute Kidney Injury Network then modified these criteria to include a creatinine rise of >26.4 μmol/L in stage 1 (Risk), reflecting the clinical significance of small rises in creatinine.

The Kidney Disease Improving Global Outcomes group combined these criteria into stage 1, 2, or 3 AKI, reflecting stages Risk, Injury, and Failure with the addition of the creatinine criteria as outlined in the earlier list.

Bellomo R, Ronco C, Kellum J et al. Acute renal failure—definition, outcome measures, animal models, fluid therapy and information technology needs: the Second International Consensus Conference of the Acute Dialysis Quality Initiative (ADQI) Group. Critical Care August 2004; 8(4): R204–212. Epub: 24 May 2004.

Kidney Disease: Improving Global Outcomes. Clinical practice guideline on acute kidney injury. 2011. http://www.kdigo.org

Mehta R, Kellum J, Shah S et al. Acute Kidney Injury Network: report of an initiative to improve outcomes in acute kidney injury. Critical Care 2007; 11(2): R31.

11. E. Request a tacrolimus level

Acute renal transplant dysfunction can be due to 'standard' causes of acute kidney injury or transplant-specific causes:

- Vascular problems—renal artery stenosis, renal vein occlusion
- Outflow problems—ureteric stenosis, pre-transplant urological disease
- Infection—urinary tract infection, sepsis from systemic infections, BK virus nephropathy
- Rejection—T cell mediated, antibody mediated
- Medication effects—calcineurin inhibitor (ciclosporin, tacrolimus) toxicity
- *De novo* or recurrent intrinsic renal disease—glomerulonephritis, haemolytic uraemic syndrome

In this case, there is no supportive evidence of systemic or urinary tract bacterial infection, or vascular problem. *De novo* glomerulonephritis would be very unlikely and the slight urine dipstick abnormalities have not changed. It is, therefore, most likely that the patient either has an episode of rejection or calcineurin inhibitor toxicity. The mild neurological symptoms, hypertension, and hyperkalaemia would be consistent with calcineurin inhibitor toxicity and a tacrolimus (or ciclosporin) level would be crucial. Given the importance of confirming a diagnosis in this situation, it would be prudent to prepare the patient for a renal transplant biopsy at the earliest opportunity.

Sweny P. 'Renal transplantation', Oxford textbook of medicine. Edited by Warrell D, Cox T, Firth J. 5th edition. Oxford: OUP, 2010.

12. A. Amyloidosis

She has nephrotic syndrome based on the presence of oedema, depressed serum albumin, and heavy proteinuria. The proteinuria should be quantified by protein:creatinine ratio or 24-hour urine collection to confirm 'nephrotic range' (protein:creatinine ratio >300 mg/mmol or 24-hour protein >3 g/d). Cryoglobulinaemia and lupus nephritis are unlikely as serum complement levels are not depressed. Her low blood pressure (as a result of cardiac or adrenal involvement) and bruising are consistent with amyloidosis. A renal biopsy can confirm the diagnosis, revealing glomerular and perivascular deposition of amorphous pink material on haematoxylin and eosin (H&E) stain that shows apple-green birefringence when stained with Congo Red. AA amyloidosis secondary to her chronic inflammatory process is more likely than AL or hereditary causes.

Dember L. Amyloidosis-associated kidney disease. JASN December 2006; 17(12): 3458–3471.

13. A. Anti-glomerular basement membrane disease

The patient has a pulmonary–renal syndrome. Pulmonary–renal syndromes may be autoimmune or infective.

Autoimmune:

- ANCA—positive small vessel vasculitis
  - Granulomatosis with polyangiitis (Wegener's)
  - Microscopic polyangiitis
  - Eosinophilic granulomatosis with polyangiitis (EGPA) (formerly Churg Strauss)
- Other vasculitides
  - Associated with systemic lupus erythematosus
  - Cryoglobulinaemia
- Anti-glomerular basement membrane (GBM) disease

Infective:

- Mycoplasma, legionella, leptospirosis
- Cytomegalovirus, Hanta virus
- Tuberculosis
- As part of septic shock multi-organ failure

Cancer-related renal disease is usually related to chemotherapy toxicity or, rarely, paraneoplastic glomerulonephritis, particularly membranous nephropathy. Paraneoplastic rapidly progressive glomerulonephritis is extremely uncommon.

In this scenario, the short history, severe uraemia, and anuria ('no sample available') suggest an acute history that would be most consistent with anti-glomerular basement membrane (GBM) disease.

West S, Arulkumaran N, Ind P et al. Pulmonary–renal syndrome: a life-threatening but treatable condition. Postgraduate Medical Journal 2013; 89: 274–283.

14. A. Cefalexin

She has symptomatic bacteruria, hence treatment is warranted. She is not septic and intravenous therapy is not essential, hence meropenem would be an inappropriate first treatment. Nitrofurantoin should not be prescribed for patients with estimated GFR <60 mL/min/1.73 m^2 as it may be ineffective and the side effect profile, particularly neuropathy, is increased. Trimethoprim should be used with caution in patients with CKD stage 4. Trimethoprim competes with creatinine secretion and, hence, causes a rise in creatinine. This is of limited physiological significance; however, trimethoprim can also precipitate hyperkalaemia and be less effective in treating bacteruria with advanced renal dysfunction.

Thomson C, Armitage A. 'Urinary tract infection', Oxford textbook of medicine. Edited by Warrell D, Cox T, Firth J. 5th edition. Oxford: OUP, 2010.

RENAL MEDICINE AND UROLOGICAL PROBLEMS | ANSWERS

15. D. Prostate-specific antigen

Although this man has had an uncomplicated clinical course, this is a recurrent urinary tract infection and warrants further investigation.

Urinary tract infections (UTIs) in males are usually secondary to a structural or functional abnormality. Although UTIs in males are less common than in females, infections are more likely to be complicated leading to pyelonephritis, epididymo-orchitis, or sepsis. Complicated UTIs in males, therefore, warrants further investigation to reduce the risk of future episodes and identify an underlying cause.

Structural abnormalities include calculi within the renal tract, bladder tumours, diverticulae and phimosis; however, the commonest structural abnormalities are benign prostatic hypertrophy and prostate cancer. Most men with UTIs have prostate involvement leading to significant and prolonged elevation of prostate-specific antigen (PSA). It is, therefore, sensible to perform a rectal examination and arrange PSA testing some weeks after the initial episode, as acute readings are not interpretable.

Functional abnormalities include incomplete bladder emptying due to neurogenic bladder (or chronic obstruction), glycosuria, and conditions or treatment leading to immunocompromise.

The diagnostic yield of investigation for a *single* episode of uncomplicated urinary tract infection, without upper tract involvement, in men, is low. Further investigation is not recommended in this setting.

SIGN guidance for treatment and investigation of UTI. http://www.sign.ac.uk/pdf/sign88.pdf (accessed November 2015)

16. C. Systemic lupus erythematosus

This woman has heavy proteinuria, low serum albumin, oedema, and, hence, has nephrotic syndrome.

The commonest cause of nephrotic syndrome in pregnancy is pre-eclampsia. However, pre-eclampsia is defined as *de novo* hypertension and proteinuria after 20 weeks gestation, hence this is excluded as a diagnosis.

Sepsis from urinary tract infection may cause a number of the findings described but her blood pressure, temperature, the duration of events, and the modest urine dipstick signs of infection go against this. Tuberculosis is not supported by the normal chest X-ray and temperature, and would not lead to oedema.

The presence of invisible haematuria and proteinuria on urine dipstick analysis should be assumed to represent a glomerulonephritis until proven otherwise. Serum creatinine levels drop by 50% by the second trimester as a result of increased renal blood flow, hence a reading of 108 μmol/L in this case strongly suggests renal dysfunction—do not be reassured by a 'normal' creatinine concentration during pregnancy. Her systemic symptoms and mild pancytopenia would be consistent with systemic lupus erythematosus (SLE). Screening for other immunological conditions leading to glomerulonephritis, including ANCA-positive vasculitis and anti-glomerular basement membrane disease, would be reasonable. A diagnosis can be confirmed on renal biopsy which can be performed in the standard prone position up to about 24 weeks gestation. Between 24 and 32 weeks gestation, a sitting position may be used. After 32 weeks, it is recommended to delay a biopsy until post-partum and this may necessitate early delivery.

Rahman A, Isenberg DA. 'Systemic lupus erythematosus and related disorders', Oxford textbook of medicine. Edited by Warrell D, Cox T, Firth J. 5th edition. Oxford: OUP, 2010.

17. B. Serum creatinine of 1245 μmol/L

Indications for acute dialysis are:
  a. Refractory hyperkalaemia
  b. Refractory fluid overload
  c. Refractory metabolic acidosis

d. Uraemic pericarditis or encephalopathy

e. Some poisonings

Agent-specific information regarding treatment of poisoning and drug toxicity can be obtained from Toxbase. Compounds with a low volume of distribution and minimal protein binding are suitable for extracorporeal removal by dialysis.

Marked elevations in creatinine and urea are not indications for dialysis in themselves.

Farrington K, Greenwood R. 'Haemodialysis', Oxford textbook of medicine. Edited by Warrell D, Cox T, Firth J. 5th edition. Oxford: OUP, 2010.

National Poisons Information Service Toxbase

18. B. Excess chloride administration

This patient was admitted with sepsis, acute kidney injury, and a high anion gap metabolic acidaemia. Forty-eight hours later, after appropriate treatment, he has a persistent acidaemia with a now normal anion gap.

Causes of a high anion gap metabolic acidaemia can be simplified into:

1. lactic acidosis
2. ketoacidosis
3. uraemia
4. toxins (such as methanol, ethylene glycol, salicylate)

Causes of a normal anion gap metabolic acidaemia can be simplified into:

1. excess urinary bicarbonate loss (renal tubular acidosis)
2. excess gastrointestinal fluid loss (from small or large bowel)
3. exogenous chloride excess

Sodium chloride administration contributes to a normal anion gap metabolic acidaemia, since the difference in chloride concentration between intravenous fluid and serum (154 mmol/L versus approximately 110 mmol/L) is greater than the difference in sodium concentration (154 mmol/L versus approximately 140 mmol/L).

National Institute for Health and Care Excellence. Clinical Guideline 174. Intravenous fluid therapy in adults in hospital. December 2013.

19. C. Hartmann's solution

The role of intravenous sodium bicarbonate as treatment for metabolic acidosis remains controversial with a dearth of high-quality evidence.

In this setting, guidance from the European Resuscitation Council is to avoid use of intravenous sodium bicarbonate as it can lead to worsening intracellular acidosis, have a negative inotropic effect on myocardium, and reduce peripheral oxygen delivery. Crystalloid (either normal saline or Hartmann's solution) is recommended to restore euvolaemia.

Intravenous sodium bicarbonate is helpful in some situations, including acidosis associated with severe hyperkalaemia or tricyclic antidepressant overdose.

It is commonly used in other scenarios—for example, acidosis associated with renal failure or with gastrointestinal bicarbonate loss—but evidence for its use in these settings is less robust.

The acidosis of chronic kidney disease is commonly treated with oral sodium bicarbonate and this has been show to delay progression to dialysis.

The patient is not stable enough for ward-based dialysis at the current time.

Monsieurs K, Nolan J, Bossaert L et al. on behalf of the ERC Guidelines writing group. European Resuscitation Council Guidelines for Resuscitation 2015 Section 1. Resuscitation 2015; 95: 1–80.

20. E. Contact on-call urologist tonight

There are British Association of Urological Surgeons (BAUS) guidelines for the management of suprapubic catheters and their complications. These suggest best practice is immediate access to a urology unit in the event of a failed catheter change.

In this scenario, a repeated urethral catheterization attempt is likely to be unhelpful given the background. Blind suprapubic catheter insertion is safe when performed by an experienced operator into a palpable bladder; neither applies here. The pathway to arrange a suprapubic catheter insertion will vary from hospital to hospital and the service may be delivered by the radiology department, but should be part of a multidisciplinary approach led by the urology department.

Harrison, S. C.W., Lawrence, W. T., Morley, R., Pearce, I. and Taylor, J. (2011), British Association of Urological Surgeons' suprapubic catheter practice guidelines. BJU International, 107: 77–85. doi:10.1111/j.1464-410X.2010.09762.x

chapter 8

NEUROLOGY AND OPHTHALMOLOGY

QUESTIONS

1. A 25-year-old woman with partial seizures was admitted to the ITU from the neurology ward after a 45-minute generalized tonic–clonic seizure. The seizure had not resolved with benzodiazepines or phenytoin. It was decided to perform a rapid sequence induction in order to intubate, ventilate, and sedate the patient with a propofol infusion.

   On examination, she was apyrexial with a heart rate of 120 beats per minute and a blood pressure (BP) of 105/80 mmHg. Her respiratory rate was set on the ventilator at 16 breaths per minute and oxygen saturation was 99% with FiO$_2$ of 30%.

   The patient had continuous EEG monitoring attached to her scalp.

   What EEG pattern would indicate that the patient was sedated adequately?
   - A. Background suppression
   - B. Burst suppression
   - C. Diffuse slow rhythm
   - D. Generalized epileptiform discharges
   - E. Unilateral decrease in amplitude

2. An 86-year-old man presented to the acute medical take after being found in his nursing home unresponsive and jerking. The ambulance crew described what looked like seizure activity. This lasted around seven minutes and had terminated spontaneously by the time he reached hospital. He had a history of hypertension, hypercholesterolaemia, ischaemic heart disease, and a previous ischaemic stroke, which had left him with a residual left-sided hemiplegia. He required help with personal care and transfers in the nursing home but was able to get around in a wheelchair and enjoyed watching television and visits from his family.

   The emergency department doctor stated he was initially drowsy but when you assessed him his Glasgow Coma Score (GCS) was 15. He had spastic paralysis of the left arm and leg; the rest of the examination was normal. Full blood count, urea and electrolytes, liver function tests, CRP, ECG, CXR, and urinalysis were all unremarkable. He had a CT of brain which showed an area of old infarction consistent with his previous stroke, extensive small vessel disease, and generalized cerebral atrophy.

   What is the best management strategy?
   A. Discharge with no further investigation or treatment
   B. EEG
   C. LP to rule out encephalitis
   D. MRI brain
   E. Start lamotrigine

3. A 23-year-old chef came to the acute medicine follow-up clinic. He presented with a single generalized tonic–clonic seizure. As an outpatient, he was investigated with an MRI scan of the brain and EEG, which were normal.

   How long does the Driver and Vehicle Licensing Agency (DVLA) state he cannot drive a car?
   A. 3 months
   B. 6 months
   C. 9 months
   D. 12 months
   E. 18 months

4. A 32-year-old student was admitted to the acute medical unit with a one-week history of headache and fever. He had no other symptoms. He was on no regular medications and had no known drug allergies.

   On examination, he was pyrexial with a temperature of 39°C. His heart rate was 110 beats per minute and BP was 115/80 mmHg. His respiratory rate was 22 breaths per minute and oxygen saturation 97% on air. GCS was 15/15. Fundoscopy showed no papilloedema. He had mild weakness of his right lower limb.

   Which investigation(s) should be carried out next to confirm the diagnosis?

   A. Blood culture then lumbar puncture
   B. CT of brain then lumbar puncture
   C. MRI brain
   D. MRI lumbosacral spine then lumbar puncture
   E. Nerve conduction studies

5. A 56-year-old woman presented with a severe headache and vomiting. She had experienced headaches in the past but this was the worst she had ever had. She had no other past medical history and was not on any regular medications.

On examination, she had a temperature of 37.5°C, heart rate 96 beats per minute, BP 158/98 mmHg, respiratory rate 18 breaths per minute, and oxygen saturation 98% on air. Cardiorespiratory and abdominal examinations were normal. GCS was 15/15. She was photophobic and had some neck stiffness. The rest of the nervous system examination was normal. There were no rashes.

A CT of head is shown in Figure 8.1.

Investigations:

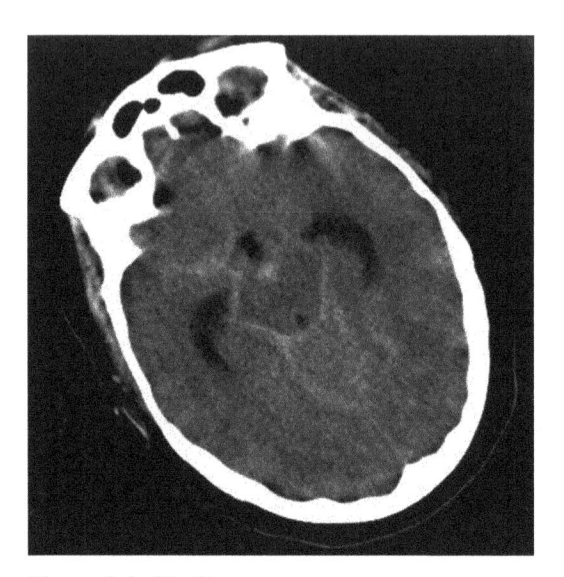

Figure 8.1 CT of head.

What is the next step in management?
A. Intravenous ceftriaxone
B. Intravenous labetalol
C. Intravenous mannitol
D. Lumbar puncture in 12 hours
E. Neurosurgical referral

6. A 75-year-old man presented with headache and confusion. His abbreviated mental test score was 0/10 and no collateral history was available. The paramedics found ramipril, simvastatin, and aspirin at his home. On examination, his GCS was 13/15 (E3, M6, V4). There was no focal neurology.

Investigations:

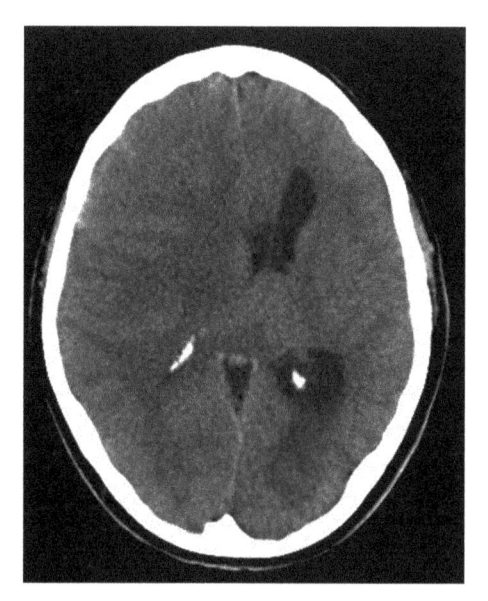

Figure 8.2 CT of head.

What does the CT of head show?
A. Extradural haemorrhage
B. Intracerebral haemorrhage
C. Subarachnoid haemorrhage
D. Subdural haemorrhage
E. Unilateral hydrocephalus

7. A 47-year-old woman was admitted after being found unconscious by her husband. She had a history of oesophageal cancer with known metastases to the lungs and liver. Over the last two weeks she had become increasingly unsteady and had fallen twice. She had an advanced care plan indicating she did not want resuscitation in the event of cardiorespiratory arrest.

   On admission, she had a **GCS** of 4 (E1, M2, V1). Her right pupil was fixed and dilated.

   An urgent **CT** of brain showed multiple brain metastases with associated haemorrhage.

   What is the correct management strategy?
   A. Discussion with the family and end-of-life care
   B. Intravenous dexamethasone and phenytoin
   C. Intravenous recombinant factor VIIa
   D. Intubation and sedation on ICU
   E. Urgent neurosurgical decompression

8. A 23-year-old trainee chef from London presented to the emergency department with diplopia, dysarthria, and dysphagia. On further questioning, it was noted his wife and son were also unwell. They were complaining of nausea, vomiting, and weakness. His son had a dry mouth and said he felt his head was heavy.

   On examination, the patient was apyrexial. His heart rate was 80 beats per minute and **BP** was 140/90 mmHg. His respiratory rate was 18 breaths per minute and oxygen saturation 97% on air. **GCS** was 15/15. Both pupils were dilated and poorly reactive. He had normal sensation on his face, poor palatal movement, bilateral ptosis, and mild right VIIth and left VIth cranial nerve palsies. His peripheral nervous system examination was normal.

   What is the most likely diagnosis?
   A. Anthrax
   B. Botulism
   C. Campylobacter
   D. Diphtheria
   E. Epstein Barr virus

9. A 31-year-old woman was being investigated for bilateral ptosis and slurred speech, which she noted was always worse towards the end of the day. Acetylcholine receptor antibodies were positive. CT chest showed a thymoma.

   What will nerve conduction studies show?

   A. A decrement in the amplitude of the compound muscle action potential to repetitive nerve stimulation at 3 Hz
   B. A decrement in the amplitude of the sensory nerve action potential to repetitive nerve stimulation at 3 Hz
   C. An increase in the amplitude of the compound muscle action potential to a repetitive stimulation at 3 Hz
   D. An increase in the amplitude of the compound muscle action potential to repetitive stimulation at 30 Hz
   E. An increase in the amplitude of the sensory nerve action potential to repetitive nerve stimulation at 3 Hz

10. A 45-year-old dance instructor presented to the emergency department feeling generally unwell. She was concerned that she had not been able to work recently due to weakness. In the last two days, she had become short of breath. On examination, she was apyrexial with a heart rate of 60 beats per minute and a BP of 130/80 mmHg. Her respiratory rate was 20 breaths per minute and oxygen saturation 98% on air. Her chest was clear. Cranial nerve examination was normal. Power in her upper limbs was 3/5 and 2/5 in her lower limbs for all movements. She was areflexic.

    What is the most appropriate monitoring test for predicting the need for ventilation?

    A. Forced expiratory volume in one second
    B. Forced vital capacity
    C. Oxygen saturation
    D. Peak expiratory flow rate
    E. Respiratory rate

11. A 45-year-old dance instructor presented via her GP with a diagnosis of possible transient ischaemic attack. She described blurred vision lasting minutes on three occasions and tingling in her right hand and left hand. This was made worse by her dancing exercise. The patient had also noticed that her balance had been affected on a few occasions and she was concerned about her job.

    Examination revealed normal neurology.

    What is the most likely diagnosis?

    A. Cerebral aneurysm
    B. Cerebrovascular accident
    C. Lead poisoning
    D. Multiple sclerosis
    E. Transient ischaemic attack

12. A 19-year-old man presented to the emergency department after a generalized tonic–clonic seizure. He had never had a seizure before. There was no history of drug or alcohol use and no past medical history. On examination, he had recovered and his GCS was 15/15 with normal cardiac, respiratory, gastrointestinal, and neurological examinations. He was apyrexial. Full blood count, renal and liver function, calcium, and magnesium were all within the normal ranges. He was due to start college the following week.

    What is the best course of action?

    A. Admit for 24 hours' observation
    B. CT head prior to discharge
    C. Driving advice and discharge
    D. Outpatient MRI brain, EEG, and follow-up
    E. Start sodium valproate and discharge

13. A 36-year-old man was admitted with bilateral leg weakness. He presented to hospital as he was unable to stand without assistance for the last three days. He gave a history of self-limiting diarrhoea one week ago. He was on no regular medication and had no past medical history of note. On examination, he had power 3/5 in hip flexion bilaterally and 2/5 in the rest of his lower limb movements. Examination of his upper limbs was normal. He had no cranial nerve abnormalities. Reflexes were absent in his lower limbs and present in his upper limbs.

    A lumbar puncture was performed.

    Which is the most likely finding in the cerebrospinal fluid?

    A. Albumin 0.078 g/L (0.066–0.442)
    B. Glucose 2.1 mmol/L (3.3–4.4)
    C. Lymphocyte count 5/µL (<3)
    D. Total protein 0.85 g/L (0.15–0.45)
    E. White cell count 9/µL (<5)

14. A 63-year-old woman was referred with acute confusion. She had been suffering with a fever, headache, and joint pains for a few days and had been taking paracetamol regularly. This morning, her husband found her in the kitchen where she appeared to be trying to make a cup of tea, but couldn't remember how to work the kettle. She could not tell her husband where she was or what she was doing and became aggressive towards him, which was unlike her. She had a past medical history of hypertension and was taking amlodipine.

    On examination, her temperature was 38.0°C, heart rate 84 beats per minute, BP 154/84 mmHg, respiratory rate 14 breaths per minute, and oxygen saturation 97% on room air. Her GCS was 14/15 (E4, M6, V4). She was confused with an abbreviated mental test of 7/10. On neurological examination, she complained of mild neck pain but there was no focal neurology. Cardiac, respiratory, and gastroenterological examinations were normal.

    CT of brain was normal.

    Lumbar puncture showed the following.

    ```
    Investigations:
      opening pressure    180 mmH2O        (50-180)
      protein             0.54 g/L         (0.15-0.45)
      glucose             3.6 mm/L         (3.3-4.4)
      red cell count      3 cells/µL       (0)
      white cell count    140 cells/µL     (<5) 95% lymphocytes
      gram stain          no organisms
    ```

    What treatment should be urgently initiated?

    A. Intravenous aciclovir 10 mg/kg
    B. Intravenous amoxicillin 2 g
    C. Intravenous ceftriaxone 4 g
    D. Intravenous dexamethsone 10 mg
    E. Intravenous paracetamol 1 g

15. A 29-year-old woman with stable generalized epilepsy was maintained on sodium valproate 500 mg twice a day.

    She wished to start a family—what should you advise her?

    A. Discuss risks with her epilepsy specialist before pregnancy
    B. Reduce dose of sodium valproate to 300 mg twice a day to reduce risks to the foetus
    C. Risks to the foetus are virtually eliminated with folic acid 5 mg per day
    D. Stop all anti-epileptics to eliminate risks to the foetus
    E. Switch to lamotrigine to reduce risks to the foetus

16. A 33-year-old woman had a spontaneous vaginal delivery after 39 weeks of pregnancy. She had suffered with hypertension in pregnancy, which was managed with oral labetalol. Twelve hours after delivery she had a tonic–clonic seizure. BP was 162/118 mmHg.

    What is the best drug management?

    A. Intravenous dexamethasone
    B. Intravenous diazepam
    C. Intravenous hydralazine
    D. Intravenous magnesium sulphate
    E. Intravenous phenytoin

17. An 80-year-old man was admitted to the intensive care unit following a collapse due to a subarachnoid haemorrhage. He was intubated and ventilated but without sedation his GCS was 3/15. You suspect brainstem death.

    Which criterion is consistent with brainstem death?

    A. No cough reflex to bronchial stimulation or gag reflex to pharyngeal stimulation
    B. No eye movement following the slow injection of at least 20 mL of ice-cold water into each ear
    C. No motor response to a sternal rub
    D. No observed respiratory effort in response to disconnection from the ventilator for five minutes and elevation of pCO$_2$ to 5.5 kPa
    E. No pupillary response to changes in ambient light

18. A 64-year-old man presented with left-sided facial weakness. This had started one hour previously. He had a past medical history of hypertension and was taking amlodipine 5 mg once daily. On examination, he was apyrexial, his heart rate was 80 beats per minute, and his BP 160/84 mmHg. He had a left-sided facial droop and was unable to blow out his cheeks or smile. When asked to close his eyes there was visible vertical rotation of the left globe and he was unable to close the left eye fully. His speech was normal and there were no neurological findings in his arms or legs.

    What is the most appropriate next step in management?

    A. Aciclovir 400 mg iv
    B. Alteplase 0.9 mg/kg iv
    C. Aspirin 300 mg orally
    D. CT scan of head
    E. Prednisolone 60 mg orally

19. A 34-year-old woman was referred by her GP with a painful left eye. She described pain that was worse on eye movement. She also complained of blurred vision from the left eye and 'washed out' colour vision. Her symptoms had been coming on over a few days. She had recently been investigated in neurology outpatients for numbness and tingling in her right leg and had undergone an MRI and lumbar puncture. She was waiting for a further appointment to discuss the results. She was not on any treatment and had no other past medical history. On examination, she had pain on all movements of the left eye and her visual acuity was 6/6 on the right and 6/12 on the left. She had a central visual field defect on the left and her pupillary response to light was sluggish.

    What is the best course of action?
    A. Glatiramer
    B. Interferon beta
    C. Plasmapheresis
    D. Pulsed methlyprednisolone
    E. Urgent ophthalmology review

20. An 83-year-old man was referred with a six-month history of leg pain and weakness. It was worse when he was walking and was relieved by sitting down. He also had numbness radiating down both legs. A few months previously he had undergone vascular surgery to improve arterial supply to his legs with a good result; however, this had made no difference to his symptoms. On examination, he had 4/5 power of hip flexion bilaterally. Pain in his thighs was elicited by extension of the lumbar spine and relieved by flexion. Reflexes and sensation were normal. Lower limb pulses were intact. Upper-limb examination was normal.

    Which investigation is likely to reveal the diagnosis?
    A. Angiogram lower limbs
    B. Doppler ultrasound lower limbs
    C. MRI lumbar spine
    D. Plain X-ray lumbar spine
    E. Thyroid stimulating hormone

21. A 65-year-old man was referred to the acute medical unit by his GP with unsteadiness, falls, and confusion. He had a history of hypertension, hypercholesterolaemia, and epilepsy and was taking ramipril, simvastatin, and phenytoin. He had recently started trimethoprim for a urinary tract infection. He smoked 20 cigarettes per day and lived alone. His symptoms of unsteadiness had been coming on over the last few days. On examination, he had slurred speech, nystagmus on horizontal gaze, past-pointing bilaterally, ataxia in all limbs and a broad-based unsteady gait. His abbreviated mental test was 8/10.

    What is the most important investigation?
    A. Blood alcohol level
    B. CT of head
    C. Mid-stream urine sample
    D. MRI brain
    E. Phenytoin level

22. A 45-year-old man presented with bilateral leg weakness. He was normally fit and well, but over the last few days he had become increasingly weak and tired and was now finding it difficult to take even a few steps as his legs gave way and he felt breathless. He had suffered a mild upper respiratory tract infection one week ago, but otherwise had no past medical history. On examination, he was apyrexial, heart rate 80 beats per minute, BP 120/70 mmHg, respiratory rate 12 breaths per minute, and oxygen saturation 98% on air. He had 3/5 power bilaterally in his legs and 4/5 power in his arms. His reflexes were absent in his legs and sluggish in his arms. Sensation was intact. Lumbar puncture revealed CSF protein 1.10 g/L (0.15–0.45). Bedside forced vital capacity was 2 L (40% predicted).

    What should be initiated?
    A. Intravenous immunoglobulin
    B. Intravenous steroids
    C. Mechanical ventilation
    D. Non-invasive ventilation
    E. Plasmapheresis

23. An 83-year-old man was brought to the emergency department by ambulance after being found collapsed at his home. He had a history of ischaemic heart disease, cerebrovascular disease, and atrial fibrillation. He was taking warfarin, ramipril, simvastatin, and bisoprolol. On examination, his heart rate was 90 beats per minute and irregular, BP was 182/94 mmHg, and GCS was 11/15 (E3, M5, V3). He was not compliant with a neurological examination but had a flaccid paralysis of the left arm and leg with neglect of the left side.

```
Investigations:
  International normalized ratio 2.5 (<1.4).
  CT of head showed a deep intracerebral haemorrhage (ICH) in the
    region of the right basal ganglia.
```

What is the next step in management?
  A. Fresh frozen plasma and prothrombin complex concentrate
  B. Neurosurgical intervention
  C. Palliative care only
  D. Vitamin K and fresh frozen plasma
  E. Vitamin K and prothrombin complex concentrate

24. A 76-year-old woman with Parkinson's disease was admitted with confusion and shortness of breath. Her Parkinson's disease was normally controlled with co-beneldopa 125 mg at 8.00 a.m., 11.00 a.m., 2.00 p.m., and 5.00 p.m., and 125 mg controlled release at 8.00 p.m. She lived with her husband and had twice-daily carers to help with personal care. She was usually mobile with a zimmer frame.

On examination, she was pyrexial with signs of right lower lobe pneumonia, which was confirmed on X-ray. Her bedside swallow assessment revealed an unsafe swallow.

How should you manage her Parkinson's disease medication?
  A. Continue Parkinson's disease medication orally with close supervision
  B. Convert her L-dopa dose to a rotigotine transdermal patch
  C. Place a naso-gastric tube and continue the same Parkinson's disease medication
  D. Place a naso-gastric tube and convert the Parkinson's disease medications to soluble forms
  E. Stop all Parkinson's disease medication until formal swallow assessment

25. A 56-year-old man was newly diagnosed with Parkinson's disease. He had been started on rasagiline.

What is the mechanism of action of rasagiline?
  A. Catechol-O-methyl transferase inhibitor
  B. Dopa decarboxylase inhibitor
  C. Dopamine agonist
  D. Dopamine precursor
  E. Monoamine oxidase B inhibitor

26. **A 46-year-old woman was reviewed by the neurology team after presenting with symptoms of idiopathic Parkinson's disease.**

    Which of the following options would not be a viable option for initial therapy?
    A. Co-beneldopa
    B. Co-careldopa
    C. Entacapone
    D. Pramipexole
    E. Rasagiline

27. **A 34-year-old man presented to the emergency department with a severe headache behind his left eye. It had built up over the last 15 minutes and was excruciatingly painful. It was associated with lacrimation of the left eye. He had had a similar episode two days previously and had been investigated with a CT head and lumbar puncture, which were normal. He was pacing around the emergency department and said he could not sit still because of the pain.**

    What is the best initial management?
    A. CT scan of head
    B. High-flow oxygen
    C. Morphine
    D. Paracetamol
    E. Verapamil

28. **A 22-year-old pharmacology student was on the acute medical unit after being admitted for a possible seizure. The emergency alarm was activated because she had collapsed and started shaking. On examination, her eyes were closed and there was shaking of all four limbs, which subsided after four minutes. Her GCS was 8/15 (E1, M5, V2). There was resistance on attempted eye opening. All her limbs were floppy and, although she could not follow commands, there was some purposeful movement in pushing away painful stimuli.**

    What is the best management strategy?
    A. Arrange CT head
    B. Call ICU for airway support
    C. Give intravenous benzodiazepines
    D. Monitor closely for signs of recovery
    E. Tell the patient you are administering benozodiazepines but actually give saline

NEUROLOGY AND OPHTHALMOLOGY | QUESTIONS

29. A 64-year-old man had just been diagnosed with Huntington's disease. His 32-year-old daughter wanted to know the chances of her and her 4-year-old son having inherited the disease.

    What should you tell her?
    A. Her chance of inheriting the Huntington's gene is 25%
    B. Her chance of inheriting the Huntington's gene is 50%
    C. Her son's chance of inheriting the Huntington's gene is 25%
    D. Her son's chance of inheriting the Huntington's gene is 50%
    E. If she does have Huntington's, she can expect her symptom to start at the same time her father's did

30. A 54-year-old man was brought to hospital by the police who found him wandering the streets. He was confused and didn't know where he was. On examination, his vital signs were within normal limits, and he had normal respiratory, cardiovascular, and gastrointestinal examinations. Neurological examination revealed nystagmus to lateral gaze bilaterally and an ataxic gait. He did not have any focal weakness. His abbreviated mental test score was 6/10. A collateral history was obtained from his neighbour over the telephone who stated that he was seen daily in the pub where he would have 4–5 pints of beer every lunch time then would buy a bottle of whisky on his way home. He was not normally confused and was last seen well two days ago.

    Blood tests including full blood count, urea and electrolytes, liver function tests, and CRP were normal. Random plasma glucose was 5.6 mmol/L.

    CT scan of head showed generalized atrophy—no masses, ischaemia, or haemorrhage.

    What treatment should he receive?
    A. Intravenous glucose 10% 250 mL
    B. Intravenous vitamin B + C compound (Pabrinex®) one pair three times daily
    C. Intravenous vitamin B + C compound (Pabrinex®) two pairs three times daily
    D. Oral aspirin 300 mg once daily
    E. Oral thiamine 100 mg twice daily

31. A 72-year-old woman presented with falls and dizziness. She described the dizziness as a spinning sensation associated with nausea. This had been happening off and on over the last two weeks. It seemed to be brought on if she moved quickly or if she turned her head to the right and by turning over in bed. Neurological examination was normal.

    Which would be most helpful in establishing the diagnosis?
    A. Dix–Hallpike test
    B. Epley manoeuvre
    C. Head thrust test
    D. Romberg test
    E. Tilt-table test

NEUROLOGY AND OPHTHALMOLOGY | QUESTIONS

32. **A 66-year-old woman was referred with dizziness, nausea, and vomiting. This had come on suddenly the previous day. She described the room spinning, which was there constantly but worse with any sudden movement. She had suffered flu-like symptoms in the previous week, which were now resolving. On examination, she had horizontal nystagmus with the fast beat towards the right. Speech was normal. There was no past-pointing and finger-nose testing was normal. Gait was normal. Power was 5/5 throughout all limbs. Her hearing was normal.**

    What is the most likely diagnosis?
    A. Benign paroxysmal positional vertigo
    B. Ménière's disease
    C. Transient ischaemic attack
    D. Vertebrobasilar insufficiency
    E. Vestibular neuronitis

33. **A 45-year-old man presented to the acute medical unit with a headache and fever. He had had a flu-like illness for three days, then a headache which was gradually getting worse over the course of the day. On examination, his temperature was 37.5°C, heart rate was 70 beats per minute, BP 110/60 mmHg, respiratory rate 12 breaths per minute, and oxygen saturation 100% on air. Respiratory, cardiovascular, and gastrointestinal examination was normal. He had no focal neurology but had mild neck stiffness and photophobia. Kernig's test was negative.**

    ```
    Investigations:
      CT scan of head was normal.
      Lumbar puncture results were as follows:
      opening pressure          150 mmH2O      (50-180)
      CSF protein               0.45 g/L       (0.15-0.45)
      CSF glucose               4.0 mmol/L     (3.3-4.4)
      serum glucose             5.0 mmol/L
      CSF red cell count        0/µL           (0)
      CSF white cell count      75/µL          (≤5) 97% lymphocytes
      gram stain: no organisms
    ```

    What is the most likely organism causing his symptoms?
    A. Enterovirus
    B. Herpes simplex virus
    C. Herpes zoster virus
    D. Pneumococcus
    E. Tuberculosis

34. A 33-year-old woman was brought into the emergency department via ambulance having a generalized seizure. She had been given 10 mg rectal diazepam in the ambulance and two 4 mg boluses of lorazepam in the emergency department. She had been fitting for 40 minutes. She had an estimated weight of 60 kg.

    What is the next management step?
    A. 4 mg lorazepam intravenously over 1 minute
    B. 600 mg phenytoin intravenously over 20 minutes
    C. 1,000 mg phenytoin intravenously over 2 minutes
    D. 1,000 mg phenytoin intravenously over 20 minutes
    E. 300 mg thiopental sodium intravenously over 1 minute

35. A 69-year-old woman was referred to the acute medical unit by her GP with vertigo and unsteadiness, which started acutely that morning. She had a past medical history of hypertension and smoked 30 cigarettes per day. On examination, her speech was slurred. She had right-sided ptosis and miosis, and decreased sensation over the right side of her face. She had nystagmus and past-pointing on the right. Power was 5/5 throughout all limbs. She had decreased sensation to pain over her left arm, leg, and trunk.

    What is the most likely cause for her symptoms?
    A. Internal carotid artery dissection
    B. Ischaemic stroke
    C. Multiple sclerosis
    D. Pancoast tumour
    E. Syringomyelia

36. A 77-year-old man presented via his GP to the acute medical unit with shortness of breath, cough, and green sputum. On further questioning, he described difficulty swallowing over the last month and choking on his food, which was getting worse. He also described slurred speech and general weakness and fatigue. He complained of increasing difficulty doing up buttons and frequently dropping things. He felt he'd become clumsy and had tripped and stumbled several times. On examination, his speech was nasal. He had weakness and wasting of the muscles of the hand. He had weakness of the legs with increased tone, hyperreflexia and bilateral extensor plantars. There were fasiculations in the muscles of his legs and his tongue. Sensation was normal throughout.

    What is the likely diagnosis?
    A. Cervical myelopathy
    B. Chronic inflammatory demyelinating polyneuropathy
    C. Motor neurone disease
    D. Multiple sclerosis
    E. Syringobulbia

37. **A 72-year-old man was referred to the acute medical unit by his GP with a suspected stroke.** He had left arm weakness, which had come on the previous day while working at his desk. He had a history of hypertension and type 2 diabetes and was taking ramipril, aspirin, and metformin. On examination, he was unable to fully extend his fourth and fifth fingers of the left hand. He had reduced sensation over the fifth finger, adjacent half of the fourth finger and dorsal, and palmar aspects of the medial side of his hand. His grip was weak and he had weakness of abduction of the little finger. Power and sensation in the rest of his forearm was normal. He had a normal cranial nerve examination and normal examination of his other limbs.

    What investigation will confirm the diagnosis?
    A. CT scan of head
    B. MR scan of brain
    C. MR scan of cervical spine
    D. Nerve-conduction studies
    E. X-ray forearm

38. **A 74-year-old man presented with a partial anterior circulation stroke.** His weakness had virtually resolved but he was left with a right homonymous hemianopia.

    What advice should you give him regarding driving?
    A. Driving can continue if he can read a number plate at 20 m
    B. Driving can continue until formal visual field assessment
    C. Driving must cease
    D. Group 1 licence holders can still drive
    E. Group 2 licence holders need formal visual field assessment

39. **A 54-year-old man presented with loss of vision in his right eye.** He had a history of hypertension. The loss of vision had occurred suddenly six hours ago. There was no pain. On examination, his acuity was limited to hand movements only on the right eye. He had a relative afferent pupillary defect on the right. On fundoscopy of his right eye, he had extensive retinal haemorrhages, an oedematous optic disc, and engorged vessels.

    What is the diagnosis?
    A. Amaurosis fugax
    B. Central retinal artery occlusion
    C. Central retinal vein occlusion
    D. Retinal detachment
    E. Vitreal haemorrhage

40. Researchers assessed the effectiveness of parenteral corticosteroids for the relief of acute severe migraine headache in adults. A meta-analysis of randomized controlled trials was undertaken. In total, seven randomized controlled trials were identified that compared single-dose parenteral dexamethasone with placebo. Standard abortive therapy was used in conjunction with both parenteral dexamethasone and placebo in all trials.

The primary outcome was recurrence of acute severe migraine headache within 72 hours of treatment. The results of the meta-analysis were presented in a forest plot (see Figure 8.3). The total overall estimate for dexamethasone compared with placebo in the primary outcome was relative risk (RR) = 0.74 (95% confidence interval: 0.60 to 0.90).*

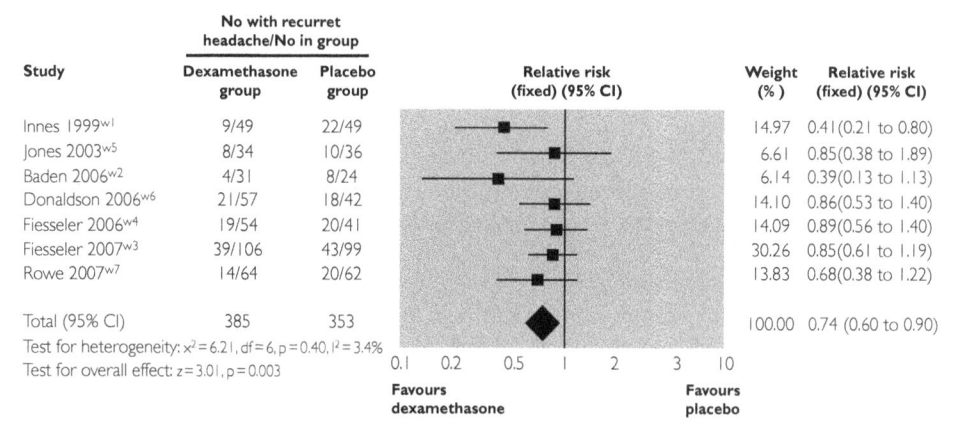

Study	Dexamethasone group	Placebo group	Weight (%)	Relative risk (fixed) (95% CI)
Innes 1999[w1]	9/49	22/49	14.97	0.41 (0.21 to 0.80)
Jones 2003[w5]	8/34	10/36	6.61	0.85 (0.38 to 1.89)
Baden 2006[w2]	4/31	8/24	6.14	0.39 (0.13 to 1.13)
Donaldson 2006[w6]	21/57	18/42	14.10	0.86 (0.53 to 1.40)
Fiesseler 2006[w4]	19/54	20/41	14.09	0.89 (0.56 to 1.40)
Fiesseler 2007[w3]	39/106	43/99	30.26	0.85 (0.61 to 1.19)
Rowe 2007[w7]	14/64	20/62	13.83	0.68 (0.38 to 1.22)
Total (95% CI)	385	353	100.00	0.74 (0.60 to 0.90)

Test for heterogeneity: $x^2 = 6.21$, df = 6, p = 0.40, $I^2 = 3.4\%$
Test for overall effect: $z = 3.01$, p = 0.003

Figure 8.3 Forest plot of the effectiveness of dexamethasone in preventing the recurrence of acute severe migraine headache in adults compared with placebo.

Reproduced from *The BMJ*, I Colman et al., 'Parenteral dexamethasone for acute severe migraine headache: meta-analysis of randomised controlled trials for preventing recurrence', 336, Copyright 2008, with permission from BMJ Publishing Group Ltd.

What is the best interpretation of the total overall estimate for the outcome of recurrence of acute severe migraine headache within 72 hours of treatment with dexamethasone compared with placebo?

A. A reduced risk of 26% of recurrence of acute severe migraine headache within 72 hours of treatment for adults receiving placebo compared with dexamethasone
B. A significantly increased risk of recurrence of acute severe migraine headache within 72 hours of treatment with dexamethasone compared with placebo
C. No significant difference between dexamethasone and placebo in the risk of recurrence of acute severe migraine headache within 72 hours of treatment
D. Risk of recurrence of acute severe migraine headache within 72 hours of treatment was reduced by 74% if receiving dexamethasone compared with placebo
E. Treatment with dexamethasone led to a significantly reduced risk of 26% of recurrence of acute severe migraine headache within 72 hours compared with placebo

* Data included in this question is from I Colman et al., 'Parenteral dexamethasone for acute severe migraine headache: meta-analysis of randomised controlled trials for preventing recurrence', *BMJ*, 2008; 336:1359

chapter 8

NEUROLOGY AND OPHTHALMOLOGY

ANSWERS

1. B. Burst suppression

The principle uses of EEG are to:
1. aid in the diagnosis and identifying the aetiology of epilepsy
2. guide treatment of status epilepticus
3. investigate the cause of disorders of consciousness

The diagnosis of epilepsy remains essentially a clinical diagnosis. The interictal scalp EEG cannot rule out epilepsy and rarely definitively proves the diagnosis. It may identify signs of either an underlying susceptibility to generalized forms of epilepsy or focal abnormalities suggesting the location of an epileptogenic area. Typical spike and wave epileptiform discharges may be seen on the interictal EEG but typically it may be normal or identify non-specific abnormalities so should not be relied on in isolation.

Burst suppression on an EEG consists of short bursts of sharp and slow wave activity alternating with periods of inactivity. In this context it is a sign that the treatment for status epilepticus has induced a sufficiently deep coma to suppress seizures and protect the brain. The pattern may also be seen spontaneously in severe coma. Background suppression would indicate a deeper level of coma or excess sedation. Generalized epileptiform discharges would be a sign of established status epilepticus.

A diffuse slow rhythm on EEG is a non-specific finding suggestive of a disturbance of cerebral activity. It may be seen in conditions such as encephalitis, post-ictal state, cerebrovascular disease, and hypoxic brain injury.

A unilateral reduction in amplitude may indicate something impeding the recording of the EEG from the scalp such as an overlying subdural haematoma.

National Institute for Health and Care Excellence. Clinical Guideline 137. Epilepsies: diagnosis and management. June 2012.

2. E. Start lamotrigine

This patient has presented with a history of a single generalized seizure with a period of post-ictal drowsiness but has now returned to their pre-morbid state.

In the acute setting, single generalized seizures in the elderly will most commonly be secondary to another medical condition such as a metabolic disturbance or acute intracranial pathology such as acute stroke, encephalitis, or a space-occupying lesion. However, once initial investigations have ruled out metabolic disturbance and there is no evidence of ongoing encephalopathy, the commonest cause of epilepsy in the elderly is cerebrovascular disease.

A CT head in this situation is sufficient to rule out a space-occupying lesion such as a tumour or abscess. The role of MRI in investigation of epilepsy is to detect rarer conditions such as hippocampal sclerosis, developmental abnormalities, or causes of encephalopathy not apparent on CT and LP and, therefore, would not be indicated in this age group and clinical setting.

The post-ictal period after a seizure typically lasts a few hours. If the drowsiness/confusion had not resolved then further investigation with an LP would have been the appropriate next step to rule out encephalitis.

After a single generalized seizure in younger patients, anti-epileptic treatment would not usually be initiated. However, as the cause of the seizure in this patient is cerebrovascular disease, the risk of seizure recurrence is very high and, therefore, treatment is indicated.

Seizures after stroke can occur early after stroke within a few days or develop months after the stroke. The seizures are focal in onset and could present as simple partial, complex partial, or, as in this case, secondary generalized.

The choice of anti-epileptic is not influenced directly by age or seizure aetiology but is determined by whether the seizures are focal onset or generalized as well as the side effect profile of the various antiepileptic drugs. The SANAD trial recommends the use of lamotrigine as the first-line agent for focal onset epilepsy. Its main disadvantage is its long dose escalation. Where seizures are more frequent then an alternative drug that would reach a therapeutic dose more rapidly could be indicated. Some drugs are often poorly tolerated in the elderly, such as sodium valproate, which can cause encephalopathy and, more rarely, Parkinsonism.

Marson A et al. The SANAD study of effectiveness of carbamazepine, gabapentin, lamotrigine, oxcarbazepine, or topiramate for treatment of partial epilepsy: an unblinded randomised controlled trial. Lancet 2007; 369(9566): 1000–1015.

3. B. Six months

After a single unprovoked seizure, the DVLA require patients to refrain from driving a car for six months as long as the risk of seizure recurrence is felt to be low (i.e. <20% annual risk). The most significant factors in predicting recurrence are the presence of relevant structural abnormality of the brain on imaging and definite epileptiform activity on EEG. This patient is therefore low risk.

If this patient had had a Group 2 licence then he would have had to be seizure-free for five years, have an estimated annual recurrence risk of <2%, and have been free from any anti-epileptic medication for five years.

If these conditions are not met or there has been a history of more than one seizure within the past five years then the DVLA guidelines for epilepsy apply. Essentially, for a Group 1 licence the patient must be seizure-free for one year, and for a Group 2 licence the patient must have been seizure and anti-epileptic-free for ten years.

It is important to note that these rules apply to all types of seizure, including auras, whether they impair consciousness or not.

There are exceptions to these rules with regard to seizures provoked by other medical conditions or procedures, seizures related to medication adjustment, and those that occur only during or arising from sleep. Some situations are considered only on a case-by-case basis.

There are separate regulations with regard to solitary and recurrent episodes of altered consciousness of uncertain origin, where the driving regulations vary depending on the presence or absence of any seizure markers in the history. The factors to be considered are:

- Absence of reliable prodromal symptoms
- Unconsciousness for more than five minutes
- Amnesia for longer than five minutes
- Sustaining injury
- Tongue biting

- Incontinence
- Remaining conscious but with confused behaviour
- Headache post attack

In all cases, patients should be advised to inform both the DVLA and their motor insurance provider. The DVLA makes the final decision.

Driver and Vehicle Licensing Agency. For medical practitioners: At a glance guide to the current medical standards of fitness to drive. Issued by Drivers Medical Group DVLA, Swansea. November 2014 Edition (including August 2015 amendments). www.gov.uk/government/publications/at-a-glance

4. B. CT of brain then lumbar puncture

This patient has findings consistent with a central nervous system infection. The differential would include meningitis or cerebral abscess. Unimpaired consciousness and lack of papilloedema are poor predictors of normal intracranial pressure.

All patients with suspected intracerebral infection who have an impaired conscious level, confusion, or any focal neurological symptoms or signs should have a CT to rule out a space-occupying lesion before proceeding to a lumbar puncture.

While this patient's history is consistent with meningitis, in which case a lumbar puncture may be safe, the history is also compatible with a cerebral abscess, which could explain the focal neurological signs. A lumbar puncture without excluding this possibility risks brain herniation and death.

Hasbun R, Abrahams J, Jekel J et al. Computed tomography of the head before lumbar puncture in adults with suspected meningitis. New England Journal of Medicine 2001; 345(24):1727–1733.

National Institute for Health and Care Excellence. Clinical Guideline 102. Meningitis (bacterial) and meningococcal septicaemia in under 16s: recognition, diagnosis and management. June 2010.

5. E. Neurosurgical referral

The scan shows high signal within the subarachnoid space in the region of the middle cerebral artery. Eighty-five percent of subarachnoid haemorrhages (SAH) are caused by rupture of an intracerebral aneurysm. Intracerebral aneurysms are typically found on the major vessels of both the anterior (90–95%) and posterior circulation. They are often found at areas of arterial bifurcation within the major vessels making up the circle of Willis.

In approximately 95% of patients with SAH, the diagnosis can be made due to subarachnoid blood being visible on a non-contrast CT head if the scan is done within 24 hours but falls steadily thereafter.

However, a normal CT head does not exclude a diagnosis of SAH. All patients with a history compatible with SAH should go on to have an LP if the CT head is normal. To maximize the sensitivity of the LP it should be done no sooner than 12 hours after onset of the headache and no longer than 2 weeks after the onset.

In the case of a patient presenting with a typical history of SAH more than two weeks after the onset of the headache, discussion with neuroradiology is needed with a view to investigate further with non-invasive imaging or catheter angiogram depending on the index of suspicion of SAH and the age of the patient.

Initial medical management includes appropriate management of impaired consciousness with intubation and transfer to ITU if needed, close fluid balance, management and prevention of hypoxia, metabolic disturbance, hyperglycaemia, and BP instability. Patients should be commenced on nimodipine and transferred as soon as possible to a neurosurgical centre that deals with high volumes of patients as these measures improve outcome.

National Institute for Health and Care Excellence. Interventional Procedure Guidance 106. Coil embolisation of ruptured intracranial aneurysm. January 2005.

NEUROLOGY AND OPHTHALMOLOGY | ANSWERS

6. D. Subdural haemorrhage

Because subdural blood is between the dura mata and arachnoid layers of the meninges, it spreads across the surface of the brain and has a concave shape (CT scan of brain showing acute high-signal subdural blood—see Figure 8.4). Acute subdural blood is hyperdense on CT, whereas chronic subdural are hypodense (see figure 8.2 in question 6). In the subacute phase after 2–3 weeks, the subdural can be isodense with the brain and, therefore, often missed. It is essential to check that sulcal markings extend all the way to the skull. Also, look for ventricular asymmetry and midline shift. The most difficult situation is when there are bilateral small isodense subdural haemorrhages, as both of these features may be absent. In this situation, as well as the sulcal markings, also look for whether the ventricles appear smaller than you would expect for a patient of this age.

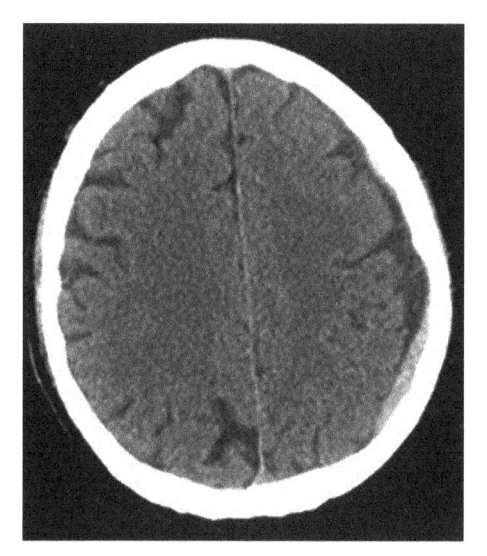

Figure 8.4 Urgent CT of brain.

All subdural haemorrhages causing focal neurological deficit or impaired consciousness should be discussed urgently with a neurosurgeon. However, many patients with subdural haemorrhages can be managed conservatively—in particular, chronic subdural haemorrhages causing no significant mass effect or neurological deficit. It is important to remember that patients with subdural haemorrhage have often also had a significant traumatic brain injury.

Extradural haemorrhage is typically secondary to trauma and often associated with a skull fracture. As the blood accumulates, it strips the dura-mata away from the skull and takes up a more convex shape (CT scan of brain showing an extradural haemorrhage with blood taking up a convex shape—see Figure 8.5). Subarachnoid blood appears within the CSF space on CT head and is, therefore, seen in the basal cisterns and within the sulci most clearly.

Lindsay K, Bone I, Fuller G. Neurology and neurosurgery illustrated, 5th edition. Section IV: Localised neurological disease and its management. Churchill Livingstone, Elsevier. 2010.

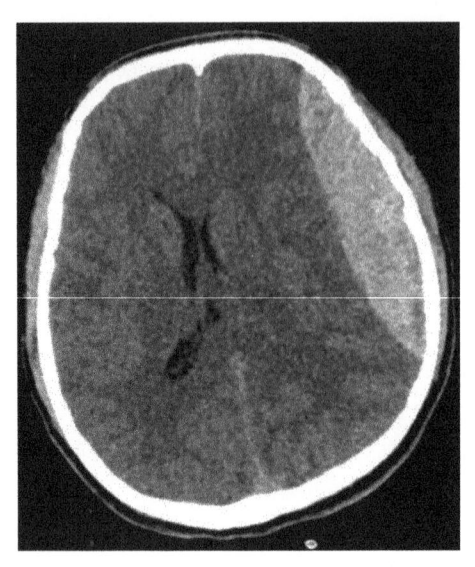

Figure 8.5 CT scan of brain showing an extradural haemorrhage with blood taking up a convex shape.

7. A. Discussion with the family and end-of-life care

This presentation indicates a very poor prognosis and is essentially a peri-arrest situation. Further treatment at this point is unlikely to be compatible with her known wishes or in her best interests.

Although her unconscious state could be secondary to a post-ictal state, the unilateral dilated pupil suggests that the predominant pathology is brain swelling and raised intracranial pressure. Steroid treatment may reduce swelling temporarily and delay deterioration but is unlikely to lead to any improvement at this late stage.

Some superficial solitary cerebral metastases may be amenable to surgery if there is potential for treating the underlying cancer with curative intent or if the primary is unknown. The more usual treatment would be dexamethasone as a temporary measure while arranging cranial radiotherapy predominantly with the intent of relieving symptoms.

Nguyen T, DeAngelis L. Treatment of brain metastases. The Journal of Supportive Oncology 2004; 2(5). http://www.oncologypractice.com/jcso

8. B. Botulism

The enlarged pupils and history of gastrointestinal upset make foodborne botulism the most likely diagnosis. Campylobacter jejuni infection does cause gastrointestinal upset and is associated with both Guillain-Barré syndrome (GBS) and the Miller Fisher variant, which can affect cranial nerves but would not affect the pupil. Epstein Barr virus causes infectious mononucleosis, which is rarely associated with meningitis and cranial nerve palsies. Patients would be pyrexial in the acute phase.

Diphtheria can cause pupillary paralysis but is rare in developed countries due to mass immunization. It presents with inflammation of the pharynx or skin and dissemination of the toxin leads to systemic involvement with progressive cranial nerve involvement and a sensorimotor peripheral neuropathy. Diagnosis is made via throat swab and treatment is with immediate administration of diphtheria antitoxin and antibiotic treatment. Anthrax is caused by inhaling or ingesting the spores of the gram-positive Bacillus anthracis, which can cause pulmonary and gastrointestinal toxicity as well as a severe haemorrhagic meningitis. There is a prolonged interval between exposure and presentation, making diagnosis difficult.

Botulism is caused by the anaerobic gram-positive rod, Clostridium botulinum. Classically, this may be from ingestion of contaminated food such as out-of-date tinned food. However, in the UK it is more commonly seen in drug users using contaminated needles via the subcutaneous route ('skin popping') causing wound botulism. The toxin acts at the peripheral neuromuscular and autonomic nerve junctions by irreversibly binding to the pre-synaptic membrane inhibiting acetylcholine release. The incubation period is 48 hours, following which patients remain apyrexial and develop an acute gastrointestinal illness with cranial neuropathies, descending flaccid paralysis, and autonomic disturbance including pupillary paralysis. Respiratory and cardiac involvement may also rarely occur. Diagnosis is obtained by detecting microbes in food, serum, or stool. Nerve conduction studies are normal but show incremental response with rapid repetitive stimulation mimicking Lambert–Eaton myasthenic syndrome. Management is supportive with recovery dependent on the emergence of new nerve terminals. Important differentials include the Miller Fisher variant of Guillain–Barré syndrome and myasthenia gravis, which are discussed elsewhere.

Botulism. Public Health England. https://www.gov.uk/topic/health-protection

9. A. A decrement in the amplitude of the compound muscle action potential to repetitive nerve stimulation at 3 Hz

Nerve conduction and electromyography (EMG) can be helpful in making the diagnosis acutely, particularly as antibody results can take several weeks to come back. In particular, it can be helpful in distinguishing between myasthenia gravis (MG) and Lambert–Eaton myasthenic syndrome (LEMS), which clinically can be challenging. Repetitive stimulation is one of the most useful tests to demonstrate the neuromuscular junction dysfunction.

MG is an autoimmune disorder caused by antibodies to acetylcholine receptors (AchR) on the post-synaptic membrane at the neuromuscular junction. Seventy-five percent of patients with MG have AchR antibodies and, of the 25% who are seronegative, 50% will have antibodies to muscle-specific kinase, which typically has a bulbar weakness presentation. There is a bimodal pattern of onset with peaks in young women and elderly men. Clinically, it presents with fatiguable weakness in the ocular, cranial nerve, limb, or truncal musculature. This will manifest as fatiguable visual blurring, diplopia, asymmetrical ptosis, jaw claudication, hypomimia, neck drooping, slurred speech, breathlessness, and proximal limb weakness, which worsens towards the end of the day. Examination will reveal fatiguability on repetitive or sustained activity. Ophthalmoplegia does not fit the pattern of a single cranial neuropathy and is best tested by sustained up gaze for one minute to elicit fatiguability. Important causes of MG exacerbations include inter-current illnesses and medications such as aminoglycoside antibiotics, beta-blockers, and phenytoin. Diagnosis is based on clinical, laboratory, and electrophysiological investigations. The Tensilon test has fallen out of favour due to contraindications in the elderly and those with cardiac conduction defects, except in cases where a diagnosis is urgently required in the absence of nerve-conduction study availability. It consists of giving a bolus of edrophonium and assessing for transient improvement in symptoms and signs. Nerve conduction tests using repetitive stimulation at a rate of 3 Hz cause a decrement in the compound muscle action potential (CMAP) amplitude of >15% and is reproducible. Management is symptomatic in the first instance with anticholinesterase therapy, most commonly pyridostigmine. In the first couple of weeks of therapy, propanthaline—an antimuscarinic—is given to combat side effects from excessive stimulation of nicotinic acetylcholine stimulation. Should symptomatic treatment be inadequate then disease-modifying therapy should be instigated, initially with corticosteroids and then with steroid-sparing agents such as azathioprine. Fifteen percent of patients have a thymoma, which is benign in 90%. Resection in those with hyperplasia can lead to remission within five years in 50%.

LEMS is a rare disorder caused by voltage-gated calcium channel antibodies on the presynaptic terminal of the neuromuscular junction, which impairs acetylcholine release. Presentation is similar to MG, except patients are usually older than 40. They present with fatigue; the limbs affected more so than the ocular or bulbar muscles. Reflexes are reduced or absent, but after a short period of sustained effort they become brisker, demonstrating post-tetanic potentiation. Approximately 50% of cases are associated with malignancy, most commonly small cell lung cancer; however, this may not become apparent until many years after the onset, necessitating the need for thorough investigation and close follow-up. Investigations reveal serum antibodies to voltage-gated calcium channels. Nerve-conduction studies reveal a small CMAP with a decremental response to repetitive stimulation at low frequency but an increment following sustained high frequency (i.e. 30 Hz) stimulation, as in answer D. Treatment is of the underlying cause. Successful treatment of any associated malignancy usually leads to improvement in the condition.

Mallik A Weir. Nerve conduction studies: essentials and pitfalls in practice. *Journal of* Neurology, Neurosurgery *and* Psychiatry 2005; 76: ii23–ii31. doi: 10.1136/jnnp.2005.069138. http://jnnp.bmj.com

10. B. Forced vital capacity

This is a typical presentation of acute inflammatory demyelinating polyradiculoneuropathy (AIDP), more commonly known by its eponym Guillain–Barré syndrome (GBS). It is an autoimmune disease of the peripheral nerves directed against unknown antigens triggered by a preceding infection. It occurs at any age but is more common in the elderly. Two-thirds of patients have had an identifiable infection during the preceding six weeks, which is most commonly respiratory, but if it is gastrointestinal (often due to Campylobacter jejuni), the prognosis is worse. The latency between infection and symptom onset is at least seven days, as this is the time taken for autoimmunity to develop.

The presenting weakness may be proximal, distal, or both, and descending or ascending. The face and bulbar muscles are commonly affected, with the ocular motor nerves affected less frequently. Sensory loss is either in a distal ascending stocking and glove pattern or a dermatomal distribution. Miller–Fisher syndrome is a variant of Guillain–Barré syndrome characterized by the triad of ataxia, areflexia, and ophthalmoplegia and is associated with anti-GQ1b antibodies. There are also AIDP variants, which start with cranial nerve palsies and descending paralysis.

Immediate management is initially directed towards life-threatening complications including respiratory failure, bulbar weakness, and cardiac arrhythmias. Respiratory failure is best monitored using bedside spirometry with serial forced vital capacity (FVC) measurements four times a day in the first instance. The normal value is approximately 4.5 L or 70 mL/kg. Should the records display a decremental pattern, then the frequency of testing should be increased to four hourly; should the FVC drop below 2 L, then recordings should be two-hourly and the case discussed with the ITU team; if the FVC drops below 1.5 L or 20 mL/kg, then the patient should have hourly FVCs and be managed in a high-dependency environment. Once the FVC drops below 1 L or less than 15 mL/kg, respiratory failure is impending and intubation with mechanical ventilation will be required. FEV1 and PEFR have poor sensitivity as they may remain normal even in late stages of GBS. Tachypnoea, hypoxia, and hypercarbia are late signs and may not occur until respiratory failure is impending. Respiratory rate and oxygen saturations are, therefore, poor serial markers of lung function in this scenario.

CSF studies should be performed to exclude infection and typically shows a raised protein level; however, this may be normal during the first week. The white cell count is normal; more than ten cells per microlitre should raise suspicion of an infective or vasculitic diagnosis or associated HIV infection. There is no diagnostic blood test but IgG antibodies to ganglioside GM1 are present in 25% of patients, more often in those with the motor axonal neuropathy subtype. Nerve conduction may be normal during the first few days but then becomes abnormal, showing slowing of motor nerve conduction and partial conduction block. Most cases of GBS should be treated with intravenous immunoglobulin 0.4 g/kg/day for five days or, if contra-indicated (known hypersensitivity or renal failure), with plasmapheresis, instigated as early as possible. Corticosteroids do not help.

Hughes R, Wijdicks E, Barohn R et al. Practice parameter: immunotherapy for Guillain–Barré syndrome. Report of the Quality Standards Subcommittee of the American Academy of Neurology. Neurology 2003; 61(6): 736–740. doi: 10.1212/WNL.61.6.736

11. D. Multiple sclerosis

This history is a typical example of Uhthoff's phenomenon where neurological symptoms are exacerbated by increases in body temperature, typically during exercise or in a hot bath. It is typically associated with multiple sclerosis (MS).

MS can present initially with either transient neurological symptoms or slowly progressive neurological deficits. Eighty-five percent of MS presents in the relapsing remitting form. Patients develop neurological deficits which typically evolve over the course of a few hours or days and persist for a few days or weeks and then resolve.

The inflammation in MS can occur anywhere in the brain or spinal cord. Typical first neurological symptoms of MS include ataxia, monocular visual loss secondary to optic neuritis, diplopia, paraparesis, and sensory disturbance. It is important to note that a diagnosis of MS should not be made after a single episode of CNS inflammation leading to transient neurological symptoms. In this situation, the term 'clinically isolated syndrome' (CIS) is used.

Symptoms may only be apparent or exacerbated when the body temperature rises such as in a hot bath, during an infection, or, as in this case, during exercise (Uhthoff's phenomenon). There may also be a positive sensory disturbance along the spine on flexion of the neck (Lhermitte's sign). However, this can be present in other pathologies affecting the cervical spinal cord.

Useful investigations include an MRI of the brain and spinal cord, lumbar puncture, and evoked potentials. The MRI brain is important for both diagnosis of MS and prognosis after CIS. The MRI typically reveals ovoid high-signal lesions on T2 images with a predilection for the periventricular deep cerebral white matter, corpus callosum, cerebellum, and spinal cord. In the context of CIS, if there is only a solitary characteristic inflammatory lesion then the lifetime risk of MS for that patient is 20%, whereas if there are multiple lesions then it is 80%. CSF examination should be essentially normal apart from the presence of oligoclonal bands (90%). The presence of oligoclonal bands is not of prognostic value in CIS or MS and can be seen in other CNS inflammatory conditions. Lesions within the optic nerves and spinal cord are often poorly seen on MRI but the presence of demyelination in these areas can be detected by finding delay on visual or sensory-evoked potentials respectively.

The diagnosis of relapsing remitting MS requires more than one inflammatory event separated clinically in both time and anatomical location with some supportive investigations such as typical lesions on MRI, neurophysiological evidence of demyelination, and the presence of oligoclonal bands in the CSF. Alternatively, there may be progressive neurological deficits with these supportive features in the case of primary progressive disease.

National Institute for Health and Care Excellence. Clinical Guideline 186. Multiple sclerosis in adults: management 2014.

12. D. Outpatient MRI brain, EEG, and follow-up

Following an unprovoked seizure the risk of recurrence is approximately 50%, therefore commencing anti-epileptic therapy is dependent on many factors and more specific prognostication can be made following further investigations. An urgent outpatient MRI should be performed to assess for structural abnormalities that could precipitate seizure activity. A CT is far inferior to MRI at assessing for medial temporal sclerosis, often a result of paediatric febrile convulsions and a common cause of temporal lobe epilepsy. If the patient has persisting abnormal neurology then an urgent inpatient CT head would be indicated to exclude a space-occupying lesion or intra-cranial bleed. An

EEG may show spike and wave discharges suggestive of a high recurrence rate, although a normal EEG does not aid recurrence prognostication. Lifestyle advice should be given as standard, including abstinence from driving for a minimum of six months or at least until reviewed in neurology clinic, avoidance of unsupervised baths/swimming, heights (e.g. ladders), and precipitating factors such as alcohol, illicit drugs, and inadequate sleep.

National Institute for Health and Care Excellence. Clinical Guideline 137. Epilepsies: diagnosis and management. January 2012.

13. D. Total protein 0.85 g/L (0.15–0.45)

This is a typical presentation of Guillain–Barré syndrome (GBS), which in this case appears to have been triggered by a diarrhoeal illness which is most often associated with Campylobacter infections.

The only abnormality usually detected in the CSF in early stages of GBS is mildly raised total protein. It is important to note, however, that the CSF may be normal in the first few days and a repeat CSF examination is often indicated after an interval of about a week.

Total protein levels significantly higher than this are more commonly seen in conditions such as tuberculous or malignant meningitis.

For more information about GBS, see the answer to question 10.

Hughes R, Wijdicks E, Barohn R et al. Practice parameter: immunotherapy for Guillain–Barré syndrome. Report of the Quality Standards Subcommittee of the American Academy of Neurology. Neurology 2003; 61(6): 736–740. doi: 10.1212/WNL.61.6.736

14. A. Intravenous aciclovir 10 mg/kg

This woman's presentation is of a subacute onset of a generalized disorder of cerebral function or encephalopathy. The pace of onset, headache, fever, and temperature suggest an infective aetiology. The impairment of consciousness and cognition indicate that this is likely to be encephalitis rather than meningitis.

The CSF examination reveals the presence of lymphocytes and a normal CSF glucose which is indicative of a viral aetiology, although other infective agents such as mycobacteria or fungi should also be considered. Any history suggesting possible immunosuppression or exposure to TB should alert the physician to consider these rarer organisms. Care should also be taken to enquire about any history of recent antibiotic use as partially treated bacterial meningitis can present with a lymphocytic CSF.

Any suggestion of encephalitis as a possible aetiology should prompt immediate initiation of intravenous aciclovir to cover for HSV encephalitis. This should not be delayed while waiting for cerebral imaging or CSF results, even if the lumbar puncture is delayed or even impossible to perform. HSV PCR on CSF can be positive even after treatment has been started and MRI features can be pathognomonic.

Immune-mediated encephalitis, such as those associated with voltage-gated potassium channels, NMDA receptors, or thyroid peroxidase antibodies (Hashimoto's encephalitis), should also be considered in this type of presentation, particularly when an infective agent is not identified or treatment is ineffective.

Granerod J, Ambrose H, Davies N et al. Causes of encephalitis and differences in their clinical presentations in England: a multicentre, population-based prospective study. Lancet Infectious Diseases December 2010; 10(12): 835–844.

15. A. Discuss risks with her epilepsy specialist before pregnancy

During pregnancy, seizure frequency increases in 15–30% of patients with a similar proportion improving and 60% remaining seizure-free. There is a 1–2% risk of seizure during labour.

Discontinuation of anti-epileptic drugs (AEDs) may increase the risk of sudden unexpected death in epilepsy (SUDEP) and status epilepticus. The risk of harm to a foetus caused by a generalized convulsive seizure outweighs the increased risk of major congenital malformations (MCM) caused by AED therapy in the majority of cases. All women considering becoming pregnant should be offered folic acid 5 mg od to reduce the risk of MCM, in particular spina bifida, but it does not eliminate the risk.

Sodium valproate is generally avoided in women of childbearing age due to the significant dose-related teratogenicity risk (MCM ~6%, increasing to 9% when daily dose >1,000 mg) and, therefore, if taken during pregnancy it should be prescribed as monotherapy at the lowest effective dose. The risk of MCM in the general population is 2.3%, in epilepsy without AEDs is 3.5%, on one AED is 3.7%, increasing to 6% with two or more AEDs. MCM risk with lamotrigine is 3.2%, increasing to 5.4% in daily doses >200 mg and carbamazepine MCM risk is 2.2%, increasing to 3.3% in daily doses >1,000 mg. The newer AEDs such as levetiracetam and lacosamide have insufficient data to accurately predict MCM risk in pregnancy.

NICE guidance states that epileptic patients who become or wish to become pregnant should be reviewed by their neurologist to discuss treatment options to enable them to make an informed decision.

National Institute for Health and Care Excellence. Clinical Guideline 137. Epilepsies: diagnosis and management. January 2012.

16. D. Intravenous magnesium sulphate

This is the first-line treatment for eclampsia. Pre-eclampsia is defined as new hypertension presenting after 20 weeks with significant proteinuria (urinary protein:creatinine ratio >30 mg/mmol or 24-hour urine collection result > 300 mg protein) and complicates approximately 5% of pregnancies. It is usually asymptomatic but can present with visual blurring, headache, and swelling of the face or limbs. There is no known cure except for parturition, which occurs via caesarean section or by induction of labour after 37 weeks. Hypertension is treated with beta-blockers, usually labetalol, in the first instance. Eclampsia is when pre-eclampsia is associated with seizures. In randomized controlled trials, magnesium has been shown to be the most effective seizure preventative medication and should be administered as an intravenous dose of 4 g followed by an infusion of 1 g/hour for 24 hours. Urine output, deep tendon reflexes, respiratory rate, and oxygen saturation should be monitored during administration of magnesium to look for magnesium toxicity. Up to 44% of eclampsia happens after delivery, so women with pre-eclampsia should be closely monitored.

National Institute for Health and Care Excellence. Clinical Guideline 107. Hypertension in pregnancy: diagnosis and management. August 2010.

The Eclampsia Trial Collaborative Group. Which anti-convulsant for women with eclampsia? Evidence from the Collaborative Eclampsia Trial. Lancet 1995; 345 (8963): 1455–1463.

17. A. No cough reflex to bronchial stimulation or gag reflex to pharyngeal stimulation

Brain death is diagnosed in three stages. Firstly, the cause of coma must be from irremediable brain damage of known aetiology. Secondly, reversible causes of coma must be excluded, including drugs, hypothermia, and metabolic disturbance. Thirdly, all brainstem reflexes must be absent. This consists of:

- pupils are fixed, dilated, and do not respond to sharp changes in light intensity
- no corneal reflex
- no vestibular-ocular reflex and no eye movements when 50 mL of ice cold water is injected over one minute into each external auditory meatus in turn (calorific reflex test)

- no gag reflex or cough reflex to bronchial stimulation by placing a suction catheter past the trachea
- no response to supraorbital pressure
- no spontaneous respiratory effort when disconnected from mechanical ventilation and the PaCO$_2$ is allowed to reach 6.65 kPa

Simpson P, Bates D, Bonner S et al. A Code of Practice for the Diagnosis and Confirmation of Death. Academy of Medical Royal Colleges. 2008. http://www.aomrc.org.uk

18. E. Prednisolone 60 mg

Although the onset of these symptoms is quite acute and this gentleman has known cerebrovascular risk factors, the diagnosis and management rest on whether this is an upper motor neurone or lower motor neurone facial palsy.

The part of the facial nerve nucleus that supplies the forehead and periocular muscles receives innervation from both cerebral hemispheres and, therefore, these muscles are usually unaffected by causes of an acute upper motor neurone facial palsy such as stroke.

Therefore, this facial palsy, which includes weakness of eye closure and a positive Bell's phenomenon, is likely to be related to facial nerve or facial nucleus pathology. In absence of other brainstem signs, facial nerve pathology is most likely. The speed of onset of this facial weakness makes the likely aetiology either an idiopathic Bell's palsy or an ischaemic microvascular facial nerve palsy but this cannot be determined either clinically or radiologically. Therefore, treatment for presumed Bell's palsy should be initiated.

Treatment with steroids within 72 hours of onset of symptoms has been shown to increase the likelihood of a full recovery. One recommended regime is 60 mg oral prednisolone for five days, followed by a reduction of 10 mg every day thereafter. There is no evidence for using antiviral agents in this condition despite the fact the likely aetiology is thought to be viral.

Lockhart P, Daly F, Pitkethly M et al. Antiviral treatment for Bell's palsy (idiopathic facial paralysis). The Cochrane Collaboration. John Wiley & Sons Ltd, 2010. DOI: 10.1002/14651858.CD001869.pub4

Salinas R, Alvarez G, Daly F et al. Corticosteroids for Bell's palsy (idiopathic facial paralysis). The Cochrane Collaboration. John Wiley & Sons Ltd, 2010. doi: 10.1002/14651858.CD001942.pub4. http://onlinelibrary.wiley.com

19. D. Pulsed methylprednisolone

This woman has symptoms consistent with an episode of optic neuritis with typical subacute onset, reduced acuity, impaired colour vision, and painful eye movements. While MS is not the only possible diagnosis, her previous history makes it the most likely diagnosis. Other possibilities include neuromyelitis optica and neurosarcoidosis.

Even if there had been no previous neurological history, optic neuritis may warrant treatment. Although there is no evidence that steroids change the eventual outcome in terms of visual acuity, they can reduce pain and speed up recovery. This is similar to the situation with treatment of MS relapses in general; treatment with a pulse of high dose iv methylprednisolone (1 g daily for three days) or oral methylprednisolone (500 mg daily for five days) speeds recovery but does not effect eventual neurological outcome or have any impact on the likelihood of further relapses. In view of the potential significant side effects of steroids, they are reserved for use only in significant disabling relapses.

Prior to treatment, it is important to exclude the presence of an inter-current infection, which is a common trigger for relapses in MS. If present, these can be treated and the steroids given either in parallel or after treatment depending on the severity of the infection.

As this woman has potentially had two inflammatory episodes separated in time and space, she is likely to have a diagnosis of MS if her MRI and lumbar puncture results are compatible. She does, therefore, need onward referral back to her neurologist for consideration of starting disease-modifying treatments such as interferon beta or glatiramer. These drugs have been shown to reduce frequency of relapses but have no role in acute relapses or optic neuritis.

Optic Neuritis Study Group. The clinical profile of optic neuritis. Experience of the Optic Neuritis Treatment Trial. Optic Neuritis Study Group. Archives of Ophthalmology December 1991; 109(12): 1673–1678.

20. C. MRI lumbar spine

Claudication is pain or weakness in the legs that increases with exertion and is relieved by rest. Peripheral vascular disease will cause intermittent claudication characterized by calf pain on exertion, relieved by rest. The treatment is modifying reversible risk factors for atherosclerosis and arterial bypass graft surgery. Lumbar spinal canal stenosis causing neurogenic claudication presents in a similar way; however, patients tend to experience weakness or heaviness more commonly than pain in their legs on exertion, with a feeling of them giving way. Classically, the claudication is eased by a flexed posture such that cycling can be unaffected, yet walking may be very limited. For the same reason, walking uphill is often easier than walking downhill. Leg weakness and muscle stretch reflex loss may be exercise-dependent; therefore, patients should be examined after a period of walking. Vascular claudication is more likely if there is deterioration with increased muscular activity, it does not vary with posture, and is associated with trophic skin changes.

National Institute for Health and Care Excellence. Interventional Procedure Guideline 365. Interspinous distraction procedures for lumbar spinal stenosis causing neurogenic claudication. November 2010.

21. E. Phenytoin level

Phenytoin has a narrow therapeutic range, is subject to predominantly first-order pharmacokinetics, and has many drug interactions. This means in practice that only small changes in dose or minor drug interactions can lead to large changes in serum drug concentration and, therefore, either drug toxicity or subtheraputic levels causing breakthrough seizures. In this case, the trimethoprim has lead to phenytoin toxicity.

Acute phenytoin toxicity typically leads to ataxia, nystagmus, ophthalmolplegia, confusion, and, sometimes, seizures. Longer-term use of phenytoin may lead to many side effects even at non-toxic doses including cerebral atrophy, gum hypertrophy, coarsening of facial features, neuropathy, and osteoporosis. In view of this, while phenytoin is often the drug of choice in an acute setting, there should always be a plan either to withdraw the drug when it is no longer required or to switch to a more suitable long-term maintenance AED.

UK National Poisons Information Service. Guideline for phenytoin poisoning. Commissioned by Public Health England. http://www.toxbase.org

22. A. Intravenous immunoglobulin

This patient requires treatment for presumed Guillain–Barré syndrome (GBS).

Once their condition has become severe enough to impair mobility, patients should be treated first line with intravenous immunoglobulin (IVIG). This has been shown to speed up recovery and to reduce the chances of patients requiring artificial ventilation. Plasmapheresis is equally effective but less easily accessible in the emergency setting.

It should be noted that immunoglobulin is a pooled blood product and patients should be consented regarding this with regard to adverse reactions and the possibility of transmission of blood-borne infectious agents not currently screened for. Since the outbreak of new variant CJD in the UK, IVIG is not made from blood from UK blood donors.

There is no role for steroid treatment in GBS.

This patient has an FVC of 2 L, which is not sufficient to warrant any form of artificial ventilation. However, he should be closely monitored with four-hourly FVC monitoring and early involvement of the intensive care team if there are signs of deterioration.

For more information about GBS, see the answer to question 10.

Hughes R, Wijdicks E, Barohn R et al. Practice parameter: immunotherapy for Guillain–Barré syndrome. Report of the Quality Standards Subcommittee of the American Academy of Neurology. Neurology 2003; 61(6): 736–740. doi: 10.1212/WNL.61.6.736

23. E. Vitamin K and prothrombin complex concentrate

A deep intracerebral haemorrhage (ICH) in the basal ganglia is typical for a hypertension-related ICH. The major risk in this situation is of further haemorrhage expansion, which often occurs early after an ICH and occurs more commonly in patients on warfarin. The priority is to reverse the effects of the warfarin as quickly as possible with vitamin K and prothrombin complex concentrate.

The deep location of the haemorrhage, the patient's age, and the fact that he is on warfarin would be against any benefit being derived from neurosurgical intervention. The STICH II trial has shown that early neurosurgical intervention may be beneficial in some patients with superficial ICH without intraventricular haemorrhage.

This patient may also benefit from acute lowering of his BP to a target of <140 mmHg systolic, using an agent such as iv labetalol (INTERACT 2 trial).

Other roles for neurosurgical intervention include insertion of an external ventricular drain for the treatment of hydrocephalus complicating intraventricular haemorrhage and evacuation of cerebellar haematomas causing impaired consciousness due to brainstem compression.

Although there is a high mortality associated with this presentation and the prognosis for this patient is that he is likely to be left with a significant disability, this is not universal and palliative care at this early stage would not be appropriate unless it was in accordance with the known prior wishes of the patient.

Mendelow A, Gregson B, Rowan E, et al. for the STICH II Investigators. Early surgery versus initial conservative treatment in patients with spontaneous supratentorial lobar intracerebral haematomas (STICH II): a randomised trial. Lancet 2013; 382: 397–408.

Anderson C, Heeley E, Huang Y et al. for the INTERACT 2 investigators. Rapid blood-pressure lowering in patients with acute intracerebral hemorrhage. New England Journal of Medicine 2013; 368(25): 55–65. doi: 10.1056/NEJMoa1214609

24. D. Place a naso-gastric tube and convert the medications to soluble forms

Patients with Parkinson's disease admitted to hospital for other medical or surgical problems are often treated by staff unfamiliar with managing Parkinson's disease.

Missing dopaminergic medications will result in an exacerbation of symptoms causing immobility, rigidity, or rarely neuroleptic malignant syndrome with mental status change, rigidity, raised creatinine kinase, fever, and dysautonomia.

Co-beneldopa (Madopar) comes in capsules and, therefore, cannot be crushed and given via a naso-gastric tube as it will significantly alter drug release and metabolism. However, dispersible forms exist which can be replaced like for like in terms of dose to achieve the same therapeutic effect; however, no controlled release dispersible preparation is available. If the patient had been taking co-careldopa (Sinemet), which comes in tablets, this can be crushed and given via a naso-gastric tube; however, the night-time controlled-release preparation cannot be crushed and should be replaced by a crushed standard-release co-careldopa. If the patient was nil-by-mouth and a nasogastric tube could not be tolerated then the dopamine agonist rotigotine can be used, as it is a transdermal patch. This can also be used as an alternative to other dopamine agonists if no oral or nasogastric route is available.

Derry C, Shah K, Caie, et al. Medication management in people with Parkinson's disease during surgical admissions. Postgraduate Medicine Journal June 2010; 86 (1016): 334–337.

25. E. Monoamine oxidase B inhibitor

Levodopa is the most potent and effective symptomatic treatment for Parkinson's disease (PD). It is given in combination with a peripheral decarboxylase inhibitor (carbidopa or benserazide) which prevents peripheral metabolism. The most common examples are co-careldopa (Sinemet) and co-beneldopa (Madopar). It is absorbed from the small bowel and crosses the blood–brain barrier by active diffusion, competing with other amino acids. Some patients find large protein meals can inhibit the effect of a dose and therefore ingest medications 30 minutes before meals. A typical starting regime would be half a tablet of 25/100 co-careldopa or co-beneldopa (25 is the dose of peripheral decarboxylase inhibitor in mg and 100 is the dose of levodopa in mg) tds. Tablets are scored so halving the dose is straightforward. After two weeks, the dose can be doubled. Following this the medication is titrated according to patient response with changes no sooner than fortnightly. Patients usually tolerate up to 1 g/day of levodopa before side effects, especially dyskinesia, prevent further increases. Levodopa and dopamine agonists stimulate dopaminergic chemoreceptors causing nausea and vomiting, which is prevented by giving domperidone, a peripheral dopamine antagonist, during the first two weeks of treatment. Following this a tolerance to nausea and vomiting develops.

Catechol-O-methyl transferase (COMT) inhibitors block the conversion of levodopa to 3-O-methyldopa, its principle metabolite and, therefore, extend the elimination half-life and duration of effect of levodopa. They can act peripherally (entacapone) or both centrally and peripherally (tolcapone). A combined preparation is also available called Stalevo (co-careldopa and entacapone).

Monoamine oxidase B (MOA-B) inhibitors such as selegiline and rasagiline prevent dopamine metabolism to homovanillic acid. They tend to be used alone in early disease and are safe to combine with levodopa.

Dopamine agonists stimulate dopamine receptors directly. They work well but are less effective than levodopa and have a similar side effect profile of dyskinesia and fluctuations but less marked. The preparations can be given orally (ropinerole, pramipexole), by transdermal patch (rotigotine) or by subcutaneous injection (apomorphine). The main limitation of using dopamine agonists over other anti-Parkinsonian medication is the risk of impulse control disorders characterized by hypersexuality, hyperphagia, and pathological gambling or shopping.

The Parkinson's Study Group. A controlled trial of rasagiline in early Parkinson's disease: the TEMPO Study. Archives of Neurology 2002; 59(12): 1937–1943.

The Parkinson's Study Group. A randomized placebo-controlled trial of rasagiline in levodopa-treated patients with Parkinson's disease and motor fluctuations. The PRESTO study. Archives of Neurology 2005; 62: 241–248.

Rascol O, Brooks D, Melamed E et al. Rasagiline as an adjunct to levodopa in patients with Parkinson's disease and motor fluctuations (LARGO, Lasting effect in Adjunct therapy with Rasagiline Given Once daily, study): a randomised, double-blind, parallel-group trial. Lancet 2005; 365: 947–954.

26. C. Entacapone

The best-choice drug and timing of initiation of medication in Parkinson's disease (PD) remains unclear. There is no evidence that any PD treatment slows the progress of PD or is disease-modifying.

The treatment is symptomatic and, therefore, not usually started until the symptoms affect the patient's quality of life, although delaying therapy may lead to physical complications such as frozen shoulder, which is a common presentation of PD. There have been concerns that starting medication earlier, particularly using levodopa, might predispose to earlier development of complications such as dyskinesia. However, this is now thought to be less of a concern, particularly if the dose of levodopa is kept low.

In practice, treatment can be initiated with either levodopa, a dopamine agonist or a MAO-B. The choice of drug should be individualized. The symptomatic effects of MAO-B inhibitors are quite small and, therefore, they are only suitable for mild disease or as an adjunctive treatment. Dopamine agonists are generally avoided in patients with a history of obsessive behaviour or gambling and in the elderly due to the increasing recognition of significant side effects, including impulse control disorders associated with the use of dopamine agonists. In elderly patients, it is prudent to start on levodopa straightaway as long-term complications are outweighed by efficacy and tolerability.

The only option that cannot be used as the initial treatment is a COMT inhibitor, as it has no effect in the absence of levodopa.

National Institute for Health and Care Excellence. Clinical Guideline 35. Parkinson's disease in over 20s: diagnosis and management. June 2006.

27. B. High-flow oxygen

Cluster headache is the commonest of the trigeminal autonomic cephalgias. It is strictly unilateral but can switch sides. The pain is generally retro-orbital and extremely severe and stabbing. The duration of attacks is typically between 15 and 180 minutes, shorter than typical migraine attacks and longer than the other autonomic cephalgias. There are usually associated features such as ptosis, miosis, tearing, and unilateral rhinorrhoea. These autonomic features can also occur in migraine but, in contrast to migraine patients with cluster headache, are typically restless and agitated in contrast to migraineurs who prefer to stay still as movement exacerbates migraine.

Cluster headaches are typically thought to occur at the same time every day, often at night. However, they can occur several times per day and at unpredictable times. They often occur in clusters lasting several weeks, which can occur several years apart.

Treatment is divided into abortive and preventative treatment. Abortive treatments include high-dose subcutaneous sumatriptan and high-flow 100% oxygen. The oxygen must be delivered via a high-flow oxygen regulator in order to achieve the required concentration. Nasal lidocaine is also occasionally used.

There are also treatments that can terminate a cluster such as oral prednisolone at high dose and then tapering or verapamil at increasing doses with ECG monitoring or in combination.

Verapamil can also be used as a long-term preventative treatment as can lithium, methysergide, or topiramate.

National Institute for Health and Care Excellence. Clinical Guideline 150. Headaches in over 12s: diagnosis and management. September 2012.

28. D. Monitor closely for signs of recovery

The resistance to eye opening and purposeful movements out of keeping with her apparent GCS suggests that this patient is not post-ictal.

This suggests non-epileptic attack disorder (NEAD), which is a broad term which defines the diagnosis by what the problem is not, rather than what it is. The advantage of using this term is that it pragmatically divides patients or events for the physician into those who require anti-epileptic medication and those who do not. It also makes no assumptions regarding the underlying psychiatric aetiology; for example, this could be dissociative, somatization, factitious disorder, malingering, or Munchausen's syndrome. This typically presents with female predominance and in younger patients; however, in middle-aged and older patients the male:female ratio is equal and often accompanied by a history of health anxiety. Movements during a NEAD event are a form of severe tremor rather than clonic movements; typically, there is no isolated 'tonic' phase. Patient descriptions typically lack detail, especially of prodromal symptoms. Patients with epilepsy make much more effort to describe the nature of the warning. One reason for the reluctance of patients with NEAD events to talk about their attacks is that if they have had a prodrome; typically, of rising anxiety with sympathetic symptoms, they either cannot or do not want to remember or discuss it.

In patients diagnosed with intractable epilepsy, approximately 30% will have co-morbidity with NEAD and approximately 20% will have NEAD only. In cases of diagnostic difficulty, video EEG is the gold standard. In patients with epilepsy and NEAD, it is ideal to record typical events for both diagnoses on video telemetry. It is important to note that a normal surface ictal EEG does not exclude epilepsy as a deep frontal focus may not be picked up.

Features which *help* differentiate epilepsy from NEAD are outlined in Table 8.1.

Table 8.1 Table showing distinguishing features of non-epileptic attack disorder versus epilepsy.

Distinguishing feature	NEAD	Epilepsy
Duration over five minutes	common	rare
Gradual onset	common	rare
Fluctuating course	common	rare
Eyes closed	common	rare
Resisting eye opening	common	very rare
Incontinence	common	common
Opisthotonus	occasional	very rare
Cyanosis	rare	occasional
Lateral tongue bite	rare	occasional
Respiration	typically increased	can cease

Reproduced from Postgraduate Medical Journal, 81, Mellers JDC, 'The approach to patients with "non-epileptic seizures"', copyright (2005) with permission from BMJ Publishing Group Ltd.

Mellers J. The diagnosis and management of dissociative seizures. 2007. http://www.e-epilepsy.org.uk

29. B. Her chance of inheriting the Huntington's gene is 50%

Huntington's disease (HD) is an autosomal dominant neurodegenerative disorder caused by a CAG repeat expansion in the gene coding for the protein *huntington*. On normal chromosomes, there are 10–28 repeat copies but in HD there are 36–121 copies with increased CAG repeat lengths resulting in earlier disease onset. Generally, the CAG expansion increases in size when passing through successive generations such that genetic anticipation occurs, whereby subsequent generations experience increasingly earlier onset and more severe disease. In this case, it is impossible to correctly determine the son's chances of HD without knowing the status of the patient or the child's father.

If the patient is symptomatic and the test is diagnostic then it should be performed by the reviewing clinician. In patients who are asymptomatic and wish to be screened for a disease, they ought to be reviewed by a medical geneticist who has the expertise and support to council them on the risks and benefits prior to genetic testing.

The Huntington's Disease Association. A Guide to Huntington's Disease for General Practitioners and the Primary Health Care Team. St Andrew's Healthcare. 2014. http://www.hda.org.uk

Broholm J et al. Guidelines for the molecular genetics predictive test in Huntington's disease. Neurology 1994; 44: 1533–1536.

30. C. Intravenous vitamin B + C compound (Pabrinex®) two pairs three times daily

Wernicke–Korsakoff syndrome is due to an acquired nutritional deficiency of thiamine (vitamin B1) rather than a direct toxic effect of alcohol. Thiamine stores are relatively small with a large daily turnover and, therefore, deficiency can occur within 2–3 weeks of low intake. It is an important co-enzyme in glucose and lipid metabolism, amino acid modification, and neurotransmitter synthesis. Therefore, deficiency leads to impaired cerebral function by a number of mechanisms. Wernicke's encephalopathy is characterized by the triad of ataxia, ophthalmoplegia, and confusion, although it is important to note that only two features are required to make the diagnosis. If Wernicke's is recurrent or left untreated it will progress to Korsakoff's syndrome, a progressive and severe amnestic syndrome which is incompletely reversible. There is profound retrograde and anterograde amnesia with confabulation (fabrication of events) in an effort to disguise the memory defect. Surprisingly, outside of working memory, other cognitive domains are usually well preserved. Treatment for either syndrome is with urgent parental thiamine usually given as the vitamin B + C compound (Pabrinex®), two pairs, tds for 48 hours and then dependent on clinical need. Rapid diagnosis and treatment confers a complete recovery in Wernicke's; however, in Korsakoff's, only mild improvement can be expected while approximately 25% will display no recovery whatsoever.

National Institute for Health and Care Excellence. Clinical Guideline 100. Alcohol use disorders; diagnosis and management of physical complications. June 2010.

31. A. Dix–Hallpike test

This woman has transient vertigo triggered by head movement. In particular, the history of vertigo triggered by turning over in bed is classic of benign paroxysmal positional vertigo (BPPV).

BPPV is caused by loose otoconia (calcium crystals) in the endolymph of the semi-circular canals causing abnormal stimulation of the vestibular nerve on head movement. The commonest canal to be effected is the posterior canal. The Dix–Hallpike test involves lying the patient backwards quickly with the head turned 30 degrees to one side and extended. When positive, it induces torsional nystagmus when the head is turned towards the affected ear. This test only tests the posterior canal.

The Epley manoeuvre is a treatment for BPPV which is thought to help move the otoconia from the posterior semi-circular canal into the utricle.

The head thrust test is a test of impaired vestibular function. The examiner passively turns the patients head to one side while asking the patient to focus on the examiner's nose. This tests the vestibular-ocular reflex. In normal vestibular function, the patients eyes remain fixed on the examiner's nose, even when very fast movements are made. In vestibular impairment, the eyes move with the head and there is then a corrective saccade to bring the eyes back to the examiner's nose when the head is turned towards the affected ear.

Romberg's test is a test for impaired proprioception or sensory ataxia. In a positive test, the patient loses their balance when asked to close their eyes while standing. Patients with cerebellar ataxia are equally unsteady with eyes open or closed.

The tilt-table test would be helpful only for diagnosing disorders of blood pressure control.

Shenoy A. Guidelines in practice: therapies for benign paroxysmal positional vertigo. Continuum (Minneap Minn). 2012; 18(5 Neuro-otology): 1172–1176. doi: 10.1212/01.CON.0000421627.43063.79

32. E. Vestibular neuronitis

The presence of horizontal nystagmus in the absence of any other neurological signs suggests a vestibular origin of the acute symptoms in this case. A posterior circulation vascular event would be likely to be associated with other signs of cerebellar dysfunction or other cranial nerve palsies.

The preceding probable viral illness and the persistence of the symptoms suggest a viral vestibular neuronitis as the cause of her vertigo rather than benign paroxysmal positional vertigo (BPPV) (see answer to question 31).

There are also none of the additional features that would suggest Ménière's disease such as unilateral deafness, severe nausea, and a pressure sensation in the ear.

Shenoy A. Guidelines in practice: therapies for benign paroxysmal positional vertigo. Continuum (Minneap Minn). 2012; 18(5 Neuro-otology): 1172–1176. doi: 10.1212/01.CON.0000421627.43063.79

Macleod D, McAuley D. Vertigo: clinical assessment and diagnosis. British Journal of Hospital Medicine 2008; 69 (6): 330–334.

33. A. Enterovirus

The presentation is in keeping with mild meningitis indicated by the flu-like prodrome, headache, neck stiffness, photophobia, and low-grade pyrexia. Additional features could include myalgia, malaise, nausea, vomiting, and a positive Kernig's sign. Clinically, bacterial meningitis tends to present more aggressively than viral and is associated with greater complications which can cause focal neurology, cranial neuropathies, and decreased consciousness. The two aetiologies cannot be differentiated on clinical grounds alone, requiring further diagnostic investigation with a lumbar puncture (see Table 8.2). In viral meningitis, serum inflammatory markers are usually normal but can be raised. CSF and serum can be sent for viral PCR to isolate the specific pathogen with the most common cause being enterovirus followed by echovirus and coxsackie A and B. The prognosis is good with spontaneous recovery being the norm within 1–2 weeks. Treatment is, therefore, supportive.

Table 8.2 Table comparing CSF results in normal patients and those with viral, bacterial, tuberculous, and fungal cerebral infections.

	Normal	Viral	Bacterial	Tuberculous	Fungal
Appearance	colourless	clear	turbid	transparent	clear
Pressure	5–20 cm	normal/mildly increased	increased	increased	normal/mildly increased
White cells/mm^3	<5	5–1,000	100–60,000	5–1,000	20–500
Polymorphs	none	<50%	>80%	<50%	<50%
CSF:serum glucose	75%	75%	<40%	<50%	<80%
Protein (g/L)	<0.4	0.4–0.9	>0.9	>1	>0.4
Culture positive		<50% PCR	<80%	50–80%	25–50%

Data from *Journal of Infection*, 2012, Solomon, T. et al., 'Management of suspected viral encephalitis in adults – Association of British Neurologists and British Infection Association National Guidelines', 64, pp. 347–373. Published by Elsevier Ltd on behalf of The British Infection Association.

Standards Unit, Microbiology Services, Public Health England. UK Standards for Microbiology Investigations, Investigation of Viral Encephalitis and Meningitis. Clinical Guidance G4, issue 2.3. 2014. https://www.gov.uk/topic/health-protection

34. D. 1,000 mg phenytoin intravenously over 20 minutes

Generalized convulsive status epilepticus is defined as a generalized convulsion lasting 30 minutes or longer, or repeated tonic–clonic convulsions occurring over a 30-minute period without recovery of consciousness between each seizure. Blood should be taken for blood gases, glucose, renal and liver function, calcium and magnesium, full blood count, clotting, and AED levels. If the cause of status is uncertain, it is often useful to take 5 mL of serum and 50 mL of urine to be saved for future analysis, such as toxicology. Other investigations depend on the clinical circumstances and may include brain imaging and lumbar puncture. Once the airway, breathing, and circulation have been assessed and stabilized, the next step is aimed at seizure cessation. Lorazepam is initially given at a dose of 0.1 mg/kg up to a 4 mg bolus and if this is ineffective it can be repeated once more at a 10-minute interval. If seizure termination is refractory to benzodiazepines then phenytoin can be given at a dose of 15 mg/kg. Because of the risk of local toxicity, intravenous phenytoin should be injected slowly directly into a large vein through a large gauge cannula, at a rate not exceeding 50 mg per minute with the patient on cardiac monitoring due to the risk of ventricular arrhythmia. Should the patient develop refractory status then immediate referral to ITU is warranted for seizure suppression via general anaesthesia. In the interim, a second AED can be loaded intravenously using either sodium valproate or levetiracetam. A prolonged convulsive state leads to insurmountable metabolic demands on the body, which eventually progress to metabolic acidosis and cerebral hypoglycaemia.

National Institute for Health and Care Excellence. Clinical Guideline 137. Epilepsies: diagnosis and management. January 2012.

35. B. Ischaemic stroke

This patient has symptoms and signs consistent with lateral medullary syndrome. With the acute onset of these symptoms, the most likely cause is an ischaemic stroke. Typically, this is caused by occlusion of the posterior inferior cerebellar artery (PICA). As this artery usually arises from the vertebral artery, it is often seen as a consequence of ipsilateral vertebral artery occlusion or dissection.

The typical clinical features are an ipsilateral Horner's syndrome, ataxia, facial sensory loss, and contralateral spinothalamic sensory loss below the neck. There may also be associated dysphagia due to involvement of the more medial medullary cranial nerve nuclei.

Horner's syndrome is a useful clinical sign in acute stroke. It is caused by disruption of the sympathetic nerve supply to the eye anywhere along its course from the hypothalamus, through the lateral brain stem and spinal cord, and then into the cervical sympathetic chain at the level of C8. The sympathetic nerves then follow the carotid and ophthalmic arteries to reach the pupil.

Horner's syndrome can be seen either in carotid dissection in the neck or in the lateral medullary syndrome. In carotid dissection it can be an isolated finding or associated with symptoms of anterior circulation ischaemic events due to distal emboli.

Day GS, Swartz RH, Chenkin J et al. Lateral medullary syndrome: a diagnostic approach illustrated through case presentation and literature review. CJEM 1 March 2014; 16(2): 164–170.

36. C. Motor neurone disease

The cardinal feature of this presentation which points to motor neurone disease (MND) is the presence of both upper and lower motor neurone signs within the same body segment and an absence of sensory involvement.

Motor neurone disease can present in any body area including upper limb, lower limb, or bulbar segments. It may be symmetrical or more rarely strikingly asymmetrical such as in the monomelic variety with progressive weakness of one limb. Bulbar onset MND has the worst prognosis due to early dysphagia and respiratory muscles involvement.

The presentation can initially be with predominantly upper, lower, or mixed motor neurone deficits. With disease progression, typically there are signs of both upper and lower motor neurone degeneration; however, pure lower motor neurone (progressive muscular atrophy) or upper motor neurone (primary lateral sclerosis) forms exist. Although previously thought to be a pure motor disorder, there is increasing evidence of more widespread deficits particularly with respect to cognitive deficits. Only 5% of patients have a familial form of the disease inherited in an autosomal dominant fashion.

Due to the insidious nature of the disease, patients with undiagnosed MND can present on the acute medical take with complications such as pneumonia, respiratory failure, falls, or unexplained severe weight loss and inability to self-care.

There is no single test for MND. The diagnosis relies on clinical features of progressive motor neurone signs spreading over time from one body segment to another. The diagnosis can be supported by the presence of moderately elevated serum CK levels and evidence on nerve conduction studies and EMG of lower motor neurone degeneration. However, in early disease and upper motor neurone predominant disease, these tests may be normal. There should also be absence of an alternative cause for the signs such as cervical myelopathy on MRI cervical spine.

Management of motor neurone disease is predominantly supportive multidisciplinary care aimed at prevention of medical complications and helping patients remain independent for as long as possible—in particular, speech and language therapy, with use of artificial methods of feeding if appropriate, and use of non-invasive ventilation. The only drug known to slow down the progress of the disease is riluzole, which on average prolongs life by a few months.

Talbot K, Turner MR. 'Amyotrophic lateral sclerosis', Oxford textbook of neuromuscular disorders. Edited by Hilton-Jones D and Turner MR. Oxford: OUP, 2014.

37. D. Nerve-conduction studies

This patient is likely to have ulnar nerve palsy with a typical distribution of sensory loss and weakness of abductor digiti minimi and flexor digitorum profundus to the fourth and fifth digits leading to the weakness of grip. There may be a clawed posture of the fourth and fifth digits with extension at the metacarpophalangeal joint and flexion at the interphalangeal joints. The likely aetiology of this ulnar nerve palsy is entrapment in the cubital tunnel at the elbow. This patient would be more susceptible to nerve entrapment syndromes due to the diabetes. However, although the symptoms are confined to the ulnar nerve it is always important to examine the rest of the peripheral nervous system for the presence of other nerve palsies in case this is, in fact, mononeuritis multiplex, which would raise the possibility of other more serious underlying causes such as vasculitis.

Nerve-conduction studies should be able to confirm the diagnosis of ulnar neuropathy and also potentially localize the lesion within the course of the ulnar nerve. They would also be able to detect whether there is more generalized large-fibre peripheral neuropathy or any evidence of other subclinical focal neuropathies.

The main differential here is with a C8 radiculopathy, which could cause a sensory deficit in a similar distribution but typically splitting of sensory loss on the ring finger is not seen and it would not cause weakness of abductor digiti minimi.

Although the onset of symptoms is quite acute, the distribution of weakness is too focal to have been caused by a central lesion such as a stroke. Stroke can cause isolated hand weakness when the cortical hand area is affected in isolation but then all finger movements would be affected and often there is more severe loss of hand function and dexterity than would be expected from the degree of weakness.

Radial nerve palsies with weakness of finger and wrist extension are also occasionally mistaken for stroke, particularly because the sensory symptoms and signs are often minor or absent.

The treatment for entrapment neuropathies including ulnar nerve entrapment or the more common carpal tunnel syndrome is very similar. Often, conservative management with avoidance of pressure on the nerve (i.e. avoid leaning on the elbow or wear wrist splints at night for carpal tunnel syndrome) can be sufficient. If not, then surgical procedures can be considered such as carpal tunnel release surgery or ulnar nerve transposition procedures.

Simon NG, Kiernan MC. 2014. 'Mononeuropathy', Oxford textbook of neuromuscular disorders. Edited by Hilton-Jones D and Turner MR. Oxford: OUP, 2014.

Stewart JD. The variable clinical manifestations of ulnar neuropathies at the elbow. Journal of Neurology, Neurosurgery and Psychiatry 1987; 50(3): 252–258.

38. C. Driving must cease

The DVLA guidance states that:

'The minimum field of vision for safe driving is defined as a field of at least 120° on the horizontal measured using a target equivalent to the white Goldmann III4e settings; the extension should be at least 50° left and right. In addition, there should be no *significant* defect in the binocular field which encroaches within 20° of fixation above or below the horizontal meridian.

This means that homonymous or bi-temporal defects, which come close to fixation, whether hemianopic or quadrantanopic, are not normally accepted as safe for driving'.

The visual field examination that is required to determine whether vision is sufficient to allow driving is a binocular Esterman visual field performed on equipment such as a Humphrey visual field analyser.

Patients with vision only in one eye may drive as long as they meet the visual acuity standards. Patients with any form of diplopia must not drive.

Detailed regulations for more complex field defects are available in the DVLA guidance.

Driver & Vehicle Licensing Agency. For medical practitioners: At a glance guide to the current medical standards of fitness to drive. November 2014 Edition (including August 2015 amendments) www.gov.uk/government/publications/at-a-glance.

39. C. Central retinal vein occlusion

All of the options can cause sudden severe painless loss of vision in one eye, although vitreal haemorrhage and retinal detachment rarely cause visual loss of this severity. The fundal appearance in this case is typical for retinal vein occlusion leading to increased venous pressure within the eye and, therefore, to optic nerve swelling and venous haemorrhage.

Retinal detachment is usually associated with visual distortion and/or positive visual phenomena (photopsia). For a retinal detachment to cause this severity of visual loss it would be likely to be involving the macula and may be visible on simple fundoscopy. However, retinal detachment is best detected by slit-lamp examination and is important not to miss.

In a vitreous haemorrhage of this severity, blood within the vitreous will obscure the view of the retina on fundoscopy.

In amaurosis fugax and central retinal artery occlusion, the fundus may be normal or there may be generalized retinal pallor and visible reduction of filling of retinal arteries, and occasionally visible emboli within an arterial branch.

Kennard C. 'Visual Pathways', Oxford textbook of medicine. Edited by Warrell D, Cox T, Firth J. 5th edition. Oxford: OUP, 2010.

40. E. Treatment with dexamethasone led to a significantly reduced risk of 26% of recurrence of acute severe migraine headache within 72 hours compared with placebo

The aim of the meta-analysis was to investigate the effects of treatment with dexamethasone when compared with placebo on the recurrence of acute severe migraine headache. The purpose of the meta-analysis was to combine the sample estimates of the treatment effect (relative risk of recurrence of acute severe migraine headache within 72 hours of treatment with dexamethasone compared with placebo) from those trials identified to give a total overall estimate of the population parameter, thereby reducing a large amount of information to a manageable quantity. The results of the meta-analysis were presented in the forest plot (see Figure 8.4). On the forest plot, the seven trials included in the meta-analysis are identified by the name of the principal author on the left-hand side. For each trial, the relative risk of recurrence of acute severe migraine headache within 72 hours of treatment with dexamethasone compared with placebo and the associated 95% confidence interval are shown on the right-hand side and represented graphically in the centre. For each trial the group size and number of participants experiencing a recurrence of acute severe migraine headache within 72 hours are shown for the dexamethasone group in the second column, and placebo group in the third column. For each trial, the relative risk is represented graphically by a square and its associated 95% confidence interval by the horizontal line. The size of each square is directly proportional to the sample size of the study. The total overall effect is represented by a diamond; the centre of the diamond equals the total overall effect whereas the extremes equal the limits of the confidence interval. The vertical line in the centre of the graph is the 'line of no effect'—that is, a relative risk of 1.0, which represents no difference in risk between the dexamethasone and placebo treatment groups in the risk of recurrence of acute severe migraine headache within 72 hours of treatment.

The total overall estimate for the outcome of recurrence of acute severe migraine from treatment with dexamethasone compared with placebo was given as the relative risk (RR) = 0.74 (95% CI 0.60 to 0.90). A relative risk of 1.0 (unity) would imply the risk of recurrence of acute severe migraine with dexamethasone was equal to that for placebo. The forest plot is read from left to right. As indicated on the forest plot, a relative risk less than 1.0 favours dexamethasone—that is, the risk of recurrence of acute severe migraine is reduced following treatment with dexamethasone. A relative risk greater than 1.0 favours placebo—that is, the risk of recurrence of acute severe migraine is increased following treatment with dexamethasone. Therefore, based on the total overall estimate, the risk of recurrence of acute severe migraine from treatment with dexamethasone was reduced by 26% compared with placebo. The reduction in risk is derived by subtracting the observed relative risk of 0.74 from unity (1.0), resulting in 0.26 (i.e. 26%).

The reduction in risk of recurrence of acute severe migraine from treatment with dexamethasone compared with placebo is statistically significant at the 5% level because the 95% confidence does not include unity (1.0) (Sedgwick, 2012).

Sedgwick P. Confidence intervals and statistical significance: rules of thumb. *BMJ* 2012; 345: e4960.

Sedgwick P. Meta-analyses: heterogeneity and subgroup analysis. *BMJ* 2013a; 346: f4040.

Sedgwick P, Marston L. Meta-analyses: standardised mean differences. *BMJ* 2013b; 347: f7257.

Sedgwick P. How to read a forest plot in a meta-analysis. *BMJ* 2015; 351: h4028.

chapter 9

MUSCULOSKELETAL MEDICINE

QUESTIONS

1. **A 28-year-old woman was admitted to the acute medical unit. She was 34 weeks pregnant, and presented with a four-week history of sore throat, evanescent rash, night sweats, flitting joint pain and stiffness, and fevers of up to 40.0°C, which tended to occur in the early evening. The rash was noted to worsen when her temperature was elevated.**

   On examination, she had bilateral submandibular and inguinal lymphadenopathy, a quiet pericardial rub, mild splenomegaly, a vague macular rash over the trunk with Koebner's phenomenon, and painful knee and wrist movements, but no synovitis or joint effusions. In the week after admission, her symptoms continued with no change.

   ```
   Investigations:
     white cell count              16.6 × 10⁹/L   (4.0-11.0)
     neutrophil count              12.2 × 10⁹/L   (1.5-7.0)
     serum C-reactive protein      144 mg/L       (<10)
     plasma viscosity              1.95 mPa/s     (1.50-1.72)
     antinuclear antibodies:       negative
     rheumatoid factor             9 kIU/L        (<30)
     serum lactate dehydrogenase   550 U/L        (10-250)

     CT scan of chest, abdomen, and pelvis: mild splenomegaly,
       inguinal lymphadenopathy
   ```

   Which investigation is most likely to lead to a diagnosis?
   A. Antistreptolysin antibody
   B. Echocardiogram
   C. Lymph node biopsy
   D. Serum ferritin
   E. Skin biopsy

2. A 34-year-old man was sent to the outpatient clinic with a six-month history of problems with his left hand and forearm. He was experiencing episodes of tingling and numbness in his left hand, pain in the hand extending up to the forearm, and had noticed that his hand occasionally felt cold and turned white and then blue. He had been dropping objects at work, where he was a toolmaker. He was a left-handed non-smoker.

   What would be the most appropriate investigation at this stage?
   A. CT scan of the thoracic aorta and branches
   B. Isotope bone scan
   C. MR scan of the cervical spine
   D. MR scan of the left brachial plexus
   E. Nerve-conduction studies

3. A 68-year-old man was admitted to the acute medical unit with severe central crushing chest pain of sudden onset. Over the previous six months he had lost 10 kg of weight unintentionally, had frequent episodes of sinusitis, muscle pains in his thighs, and numbness in his feet and ankles.

   He had a six-year history of poorly controlled asthma. He was a retired dockworker and had stopped smoking ten years ago and had a 25-pack-year smoking history.

   His ECG showed a heart rate of 80 beats per minute, sinus rhythm, QRS axis + 10°, PR interval 180 ms, QRS complexes 0.14 mm wide and a dominant R wave in V_1.

   ```
   Investigations:
      serum troponin T           449 ng/L              (<14)
      white cell count           34 × 10⁹/L            (4.0-11.0)
      eosinophil count           26.9 × 10⁹/L          (0.04-0.40)
      serum C-reactive protein   74 mg/L               (<10)

      echocardiogram:            normal
      coronary angiography:      minor coronary artery atheroma
      chest X-ray:               normal
   ```

   What is the most likely diagnosis?
   A. Eosinophilic granulomatosis with polyangiitis (Churg Strauss syndrome)
   B. Eosinophilic fasciitis
   C. Hypereosinophilic syndrome
   D. Polyarteritis nodosa
   E. Sarcoidosis

4. A 19-year-old student awoke with pain in the right shoulder of sudden onset. There had been no history of trauma. Two days later she developed pain, swelling, and dusky blue discolouration of the right hand, wrist, and forearm. She smoked 15 cigarettes per day and took a combined oral contraceptive pill.

On examination, there was reduced movement of the right shoulder limited by pain, and mild tenderness of the biceps. The right hand, wrist, and forearm were cool, mottled, swollen, and exquisitely tender to superficial touch. Peripheral pulses were palpable.

```
Investigations:
    serum C-reactive protein                      6 mg/L        (<10)
    serum creatine kinase                         81 U/L        (24-170)

    Doppler ultrasound right arm:                 normal
    ultrasound scan right shoulder:               normal
    X-rays right hand, wrist, and shoulder:       normal
```

What is the most appropriate treatment in this situation?
A. Gabapentin
B. Intravenous morphine
C. Lidocaine patches
D. Sodium valproate
E. Venlafaxine

5. A 56-year-old man was referred to the TIA clinic with a four-week history of progressive left-sided headache, general malaise, lethargy, and two episodes of amaurosis fugax within the previous 48 hours. He had a history of hypertension and smoked ten cigarettes per day, with a 40-pack-year smoking history.

On examination, he had a thickened, red, tender left temporal artery, moderate temporal scalp tenderness, and mild bilateral expiratory wheeze.

```
Investigations:
    white cell count                    13.5 × 10⁹/L      (4.0-11.0)
    neutrophil count                    11.7 × 10⁹/L      (1.5-7.0)
    serum C-reactive protein            81 mg/L           (<10)
    plasma viscosity                    2.07 mPa/s        (1.50-1.72)
    serum alkaline                      163 U/L           (45-105)
      phosphatase
```

What is the most appropriate type of steroid treatment at this stage?
A. Intramuscular methylprednisolone 120 mg for three days
B. Intravenous methylprednisolone 1 g for three days
C. Oral dexamethasone 8 mg twice a day
D. Oral prednisolone 40 mg per day
E. Oral prednisolone 60 mg per day

6. A 62-year-old man presented with pain, swelling, and discolouration of the right elbow of sudden onset. There was no history of trauma. He had mild symptoms of systemic upset. In the past, he had experienced episodes of incapacitating pain in his feet. He admitted to previous 'significant' alcohol intake and had hypertension.

On examination, he had a temperature of 37.8°C and painful swelling over the right elbow (see Figure 9.1).

Investigations:

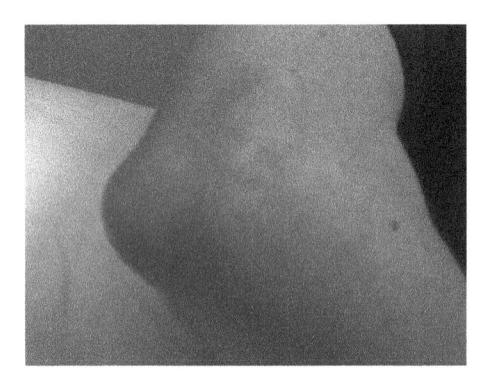

Figure 9.1 Painful swelling over elbow.

```
serum C-reactive protein        96 mg/L              (<10)
serum creatinine                144 µmol/L           (60-110)
estimated glomerular            41 mL/min            (>60)
  filtration rate
serum urate                     0.44 mmol/L          (0.23-0.46)
rheumatoid factor               6 kIU/L              (<30)

aspirate left olecranon bursa:
appearance:                     white
gram stain:                     negative
crystals:                       negatively birefringent
                                crystals
```

What is the most appropriate treatment in this case?
A. Allopurinol
B. Diclofenac
C. Flucloxacillin
D. Prednisolone
E. Tramadol

7. A 36-year-old man presented to the outpatient clinic with a six-week history of right-knee pain and swelling. He played football regularly, but could not recall sustaining an injury. The knee was constantly painful and occasionally felt like it was going to 'give way', although it had never actually done so. He had a seven-year history of plaque psoriasis.

On examination, there was a moderate warm effusion of the right knee, with flexion limited to 0–70°. McMurray's test was negative.

What is the most appropriate investigation?
A. Colourflow ultrasound scan of the knee
B. Contrast MR scan of the knee
C. Synovial fluid analysis
D. Three-phase isotope bone scan
E. Weight-bearing X-ray of the knee

8. A 34-year-old woman was referred to the outpatient clinic with a six-month history of fatigue, joint pain, gritty eyes, and dryness of the mouth. On examination, she had a positive Schirmer's test, mild parotid swelling, and tenderness of the small joints of the hands, but no synovitis.

```
Investigations:
    haemoglobin                117 g/L                    (115-165)
    white cell count           3.6 × 10⁹/L                (4.0-11.0)
    plasma viscosity           1.96 mPa/s (1.50-1.72)
    rheumatoid factor          450 kIU/L                  (<30)
    antinuclear antibodies:    positive 1 in 160
    serum immunoglobulin G     27.9 g/L                   (6.0-13.0)
```

Which test will most effectively confirm the diagnosis?
A. Anti-cyclic citrullinated peptide antibody
B. Anti-double-stranded DNA antibody level
C. Salivary gland biopsy
D. Serum complement C4
E. Ultrasound scan of the parotid glands

9. **A 74-year-old woman was admitted with a productive cough and was diagnosed with community-acquired pneumonia. Twenty-four hours after admission, she complained of severe right wrist pain and swelling. She had no previous medical history.**

    Investigations:

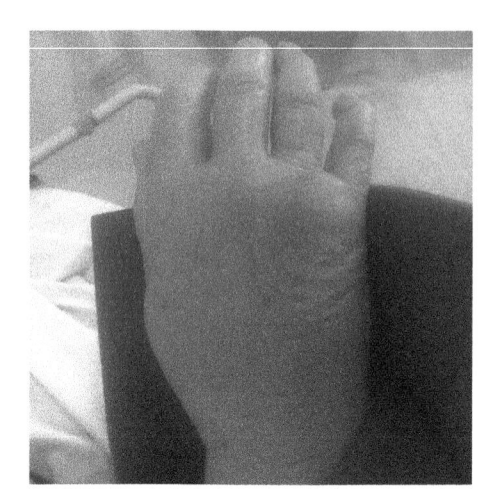

    Figure 9.2 Wrist.

    ```
    serum C-reactive protein    265 mg/L    (<10)
    rheumatoid factor            18 kIU/L    (<30)
    ```

    What is the most likely diagnosis?
    A. Acute gout
    B. Acute pseudogout
    C. Osteoarthritis
    D. Rheumatoid arthritis
    E. Septic arthritis

10. A 63-year-old man with a 35-year history of rheumatoid arthritis was seen urgently in the outpatient clinic. Over the previous six months, he had developed progressive swelling of the legs, weight gain, and immobility. He was currently taking methorexate 20 mg per week, folic acid 10 mg per week, prednisolone 5 mg per day, and diclofenac 50 mg twice a day. He had had monthly injections of sodium aurothiomalate for 12 years until a year ago.

On examination, his blood pressure was 126/72 supine, there was moderate hepatosplenomegaly, and he had pitting oedema to a level of the lower abdominal wall. There was no evidence of active synovitis.

```
Investigations:
  Haemoglobin                    11.7 g/L       (130-180)
  serum creatinine               216 µmol/L     (60-110)
  estimated glomerular           26 mL/min      (>60)
    filtration rate
  serum albumin                  23 g/L         (37-49)
  24-hr urinary total protein    2.7 g          (<0.2)

  chest X-ray: small bilateral pleural effusions
  echocardiogram: good left-ventricular function
  ultrasound scan of the abdomen: moderate enlargement of the
    liver and spleen
```

What is the likely cause of the current problems?

A. AA amyloidosis
B. Diclofenac-induced renal failure
C. Lymphoma
D. Rheumatoid vasculitis
E. Sodium aurothiomalate-induced nephrotic syndrome

11. **A 65-year-old woman with a ten-year history of rheumatoid arthritis was admitted to the acute medical unit with a three-week history of progressive breathlessness and a non-productive cough. She was currently taking methotrexate 15 mg weekly and adalimumab 40 mg fortnightly.**

Investigations:

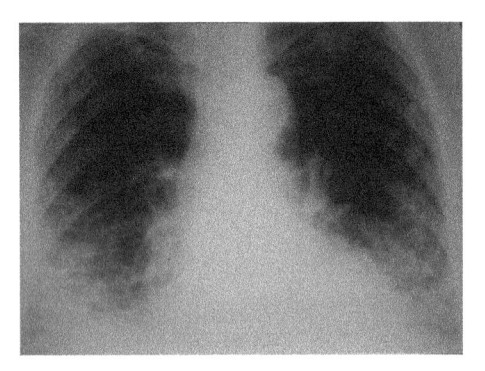

Figure 9.3 Chest X-ray.

haemoglobin	126 g/L	(115–165)
white cell count	16.6 × 10^9/L	(4.0–11.0)
neutrophil count	12.2 × 10^9/L	(1.5–7.0)
serum C-reactive protein	63 mg/L	(<10)
pO$_2$ on air	7.2 kPa	(11.3–12.6)

What is the most likely diagnosis?

A. Cardiogenic pulmonary oedema
B. Legionella pneumonia
C. Methotrexate pneumonitis
D. Pneumocystis jiroveci pneumonia
E. Pulmonary tuberculosis

12. A 35-year-old man was seen in ambulatory care with a ten-day history of feeling generally unwell, with fevers, painful red eyes, a painful rash (Figure 9.4) on his legs, and painful swelling of his ankles. He was a keen scuba diver who helped to clean the aquarium at the local zoo on a regular basis.

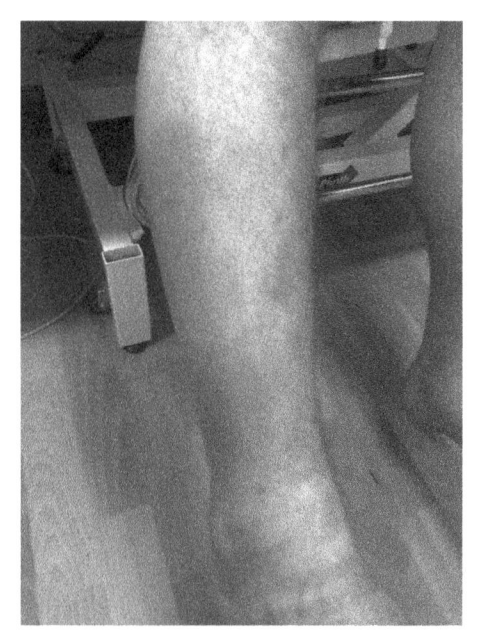

Figure 9.4 Lower limb rash.

What is the most appropriate investigation?
A. Antistreptolysin titre
B. Chest X-ray
C. Interferon-gamma release assay
D. Rheumatoid factor
E. Throat swab

13. A 34-year-old woman was admitted as an emergency by her GP to the acute medical unit. She had a two-day history of a sore throat, headache, fever, joint pain, and a rash. On examination, she had a temperature of 38.7°C, pulse 108 beats per minute, and blood pressure 99/54 mmHg supine. She had a widespread, non-blanching petechial rash. There was no evidence of neck stiffness or photophobia, and Kernig's sign was negative. She had a large, painful hot effusion of the left knee.

```
Investigations:
    white cell count               18.9 × 10⁹/L      (4.0-11.0)
    neutrophil count               14.4 × 10⁹/L      (1.5-7.0)
    serum C-reactive protein       351 mg/L          (<10)
    serum creatinine               126 µmol/L        (60-110)
    estimated glomerular           41 mL/min         (>60)
      filtration rate
    platelet count                 90 × 10⁹/L        (150-400)
    synovial fluid:

    appearance: turbid
    white cell count: 36,000/mL                      (<200)
    gram stain: gram-negative diplococci
```

What is the most likely causative organism?
A. Moraxella catarrhalis
B. Moraxella osloensis
C. Neisseria gonorrhoeae
D. Neisseria meningitidis
E. Staphylococcus aureus

14. A 75-year-old man presented with nine months of progressive lower-back pain. The pain radiated from the lower back to both calves and was worsened by walking; he was able to walk approximately 100 m before the pain occurred, and found that stopping and resting relieved the pain, allowing him to resume walking until the pain occurred again. On examination, extension of the lumbar spine reproduced the symptoms.

What is the most appropriate investigation to confirm the diagnosis?
A. CT angiogram of the aorta
B. CT scan of the lumbo-sacral spine
C. MR scan of the lumbo-sacral spine
D. Nerve-conduction studies
E. X-ray lumbo-sacral spine

15. A 47-year-old woman was admitted with a 24-hour history of acute breathlessness. She had a three-month history of progressive weakness, 8 kg weight loss, and progressive dysphagia. She was a non-smoker.

On examination, her temperature was 38.4°C, pulse 96 beats per minute, and blood pressure 136/65 mmHg. Auscultation revealed coarse inspiratory crackles at the right base and mid zone. She had grade 4/5 weakness of the proximal muscles of the upper and lower limbs. There were no other abnormalities.

```
Investigations:
    white cell count            16.0 × 10⁹/L        (4.0-11.0)
    neutrophil count            13.6 × 10⁹/L        (1.5-7.0)
    serum C-reactive protein    103 mg/L            (<10)
    serum creatine kinase       5285 U/L            (24-170)

    chest X-ray: consolidation right lower lobe
```

Which of the following is most likely to be helpful in making a specific diagnosis?

A. Anti-double-stranded DNA antibodies
B. Anti-nuclear antibodies
C. Anti-smooth muscle antibodies
D. Anti-synthetase antibodies
E. Rheumatoid factor

16. **A 72-year-old woman was admitted to the acute medical unit via her GP with a two-week history of pain and swelling of the left leg. She had a four-year history of pain, stiffness and swelling of the hands, wrists, knees, ankles, and feet, for which her GP had been treating her with oral steroid therapy (prednisolone, between 7.5 mg/day and 15 mg/day) for the last three years. Her current dose was 10 mg/day.**

    On examination, she had a temperature of 37.6°C; there was synovitis of the joints of the hands and wrists; non-tender lumps over the elbows; significant pain and limited movement of the left hip (flexion to 50°), and tender, erythematous swelling of the distal left thigh and calf.

    Investigations:

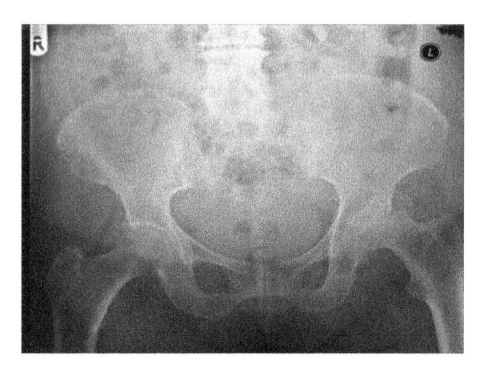

    Figure 9.5 X-ray of the pelvis.

white cell count	14.2 × 10⁹/L	(4.0–11.0)
neutrophil count	12.0 × 10⁹/L	(1.5–7.0)
serum C-reactive protein	45 mg/L	(<10)
plasma viscosity	1.81 mPa/s	(1.50–1.72)
rheumatoid factor	238 kIU/L	(<30)
anti-cyclic citrullinated peptide antibodies	126	(<20)

    Doppler USS left leg: venous thrombus left femoral vein

    What is the most likely cause of the left hip pain?
    A. Avascular necrosis
    B. Osteoarthritis
    C. Rheumatoid arthritis
    D. Septic arthritis
    E. TB arthritis

17. A 27-year-old woman was seen on the acute medical unit with abdominal pain, vomiting, and fevers. She had a history of systemic lupus erythematosus (SLE). Her medication at admission was hydroxychloroquine 200 mg twice a day, prednisolone 5 mg/day, azathioprine 75 mg twice a day, ibuprofen 400 mg as required, and codeine phosphate 30 mg as required.

On examination, her temperature was 37.8°C, pulse 115 beats per minute, blood pressure 85/65 mmHg supine, and respiratory rate 24 breaths per minute. There was tenderness of the epigastrium, but no masses were palpated and bowel sounds were normal.

```
Investigations:
   white cell count              15.0 × 10⁹/L      (4.0-11.0)
   neutrophil count              13.4 × 10⁹/L      (1.5-7.0)
   serum C-reactive protein      114 mg/L          (<10)
   serum creatinine              96 µmol/L         (60-110)
   estimated glomerular          55 mL/min         (>60)
     filtration rate
   serum amylase                 2453 U/L          (60-180)
   lactate                       4.2 mmol/L        (0.5-1.6)
   serum complement C3           67                (65-190)
   serum complement C4           18                (15-50)
```

What is the most likely diagnosis?
A. Azathioprine-induced pancreatitis
B. Codeine-induced pancreatitis
C. Glucocorticoid-induced pancreatitis
D. Ibuprofen-induced pancreatitis
E. Systemic vasculitis secondary to systemic lupus erythematosus (SLE)

18. **A 29-year-old Pakistani woman was admitted to the acute medical unit with increasing breathlessness, chest pain, and fevers. She was two months post-partum, having delivered her third child after an uneventful pregnancy. She had a previous history of Behçet's disease and took colchicine 500 mcg twice a day.**

   On examination, her pulse was 110 beats per minute and blood pressure 105/55 mmHg supine. She was centrally cyanosed and had distension of the veins in her neck and on her chest wall. Her heart sounds were soft but normal.

   ```
   Investigations:
     serum C-reactive protein    45 mg/L           (<10)
     platelet count              167 × 10⁹/L       (150–400)
     prothrombin time            14 s              (11.5–15.5)

     CT pulmonary angiogram: superior vena cava venous
     thrombosis, extending into the right atrium; small bilateral
       pleural effusions
   ```

   Which of the following is the most appropriate treatment?
   A. Aspirin
   B. Intravenous heparin
   C. Intravenous methylprednisolone
   D. Streptokinase
   E. Warfarin

19. **A 62-year-old man presented to the ambulatory care clinic with increasing neck pain, stiffness, and reduced movement.**

    Investigations:

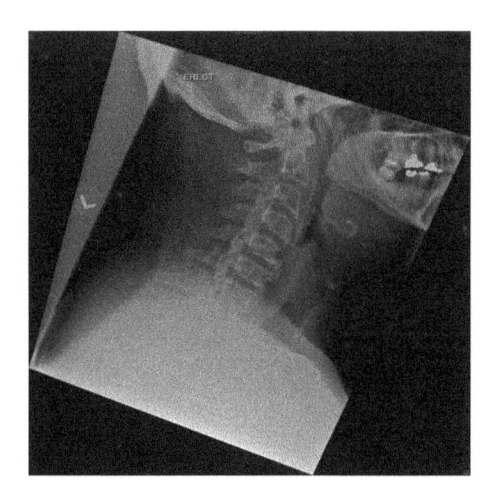

    Figure 9.6 C-spine X-ray.

    ### What is the most likely diagnosis?
    A. Ankylosing spondylitis
    B. Calcific tendonitis
    C. Osteoarthritis
    D. Paget's disease
    E. Rheumatoid arthritis

20. A 69-year-old woman was referred to the ambulatory care clinic with a six-week history of progressive pain and swelling of her left lower leg. She had a history of Paget's disease of the left tibia, which had previously been treated with two courses of oral bisphosphonates.

    On examination, she was afebrile; examination of the left leg revealed a 6 cm × 4 cm warm, tender raised area in the proximal tibia.

    ```
    Investigations:
        white cell count              10.8 × 10⁹/L      (4.0-11.0)
        serum C-reactive protein      18 mg/L           (<10)
        plasma viscosity              1.87 mPa/s        (1.50-1.72)
        serum alkaline phosphatase    630 U/L           (45-105)
        serum lactate dehydrogenase   550 U/L           (10-250)

        Doppler USS left leg: no evidence of deep vein thrombosis
    ```

    Which investigation is most likely to lead to a diagnosis?
    A. CT of the thorax and abdomen
    B. MRI of the left tibia
    C. Ultrasound of the left tibia
    D. Whole body isotope bone scan
    E. X-ray of the left tibia

21. A 26-year-old businesswoman was admitted to the acute medical unit with a 24-hour history of atraumatic acute severe pain in the left wrist. She had a two-year history of episodic acute joint pain affecting differing small joints, occurring approximately every four to five months, and being completely well between episodes.

    On examination, she had a temperature of 36.4°C. The left wrist was mildly warm and tender, but not swollen.

    ```
    Investigations:
        white cell count              8.9 × 10⁹/L       (4.0-11.0)
        neutrophil count              6.6 × 10⁹/L       (1.5-7.0)
        serum C-reactive protein      17 mg/L           (<10)
        serum urate                   0.27 mmol/L       (0.19-0.36)
        rheumatoid factor             6 kIU/L           (<30)

        X-ray left wrist: normal
    ```

    What is the most likely diagnosis?
    A. Gout
    B. Palindromic rheumatism
    C. Rheumatoid arthritis
    D. Septic arthritis
    E. Systemic lupus erythematosus

22. **A 26-year-old nursery schoolteacher was admitted to the acute medical unit via her GP with a two-day history of severe pain and swelling of both hands and feet. She had recently had a coryzal illness, headaches, and malaise.**

    On examination, she had a temperature of 37.3°C. Cardiorespiratory examination was normal, and there was no rash. She had moderate polyarticular synovitis of the metacarpophalangeal joints of both hands, and tenderness of the metatarsophalangeal joints of both feet.

    ```
    Investigations:
      haemoglobin                128 g/L           (115-165)
      white cell count           9.4 × 10⁹/L       (4.0-11.0)
      neutrophil count           6.1 × 10⁹/L       (1.5-7.0)
      serum C-reactive protein   55 mg/L           (<10)
      plasma viscosity           1.89 mPa/s        (1.50-1.72)
      rheumatoid factor          26 kIU/L          (<30)

      X-rays of hands and feet: normal
    ```

    What is the most likely diagnosis?
    A. Mycoplasma pneumoniae arthritis
    B. Parvovirus B19 arthritis
    C. Rheumatoid arthritis
    D. Rubella arthritis
    E. Systemic lupus erythematosus

23. **A 62-year-old man was seen in the ambulatory care clinic. He had progressive back pain and reported areas of ulceration after minor trauma when gardening.**

Investigations:

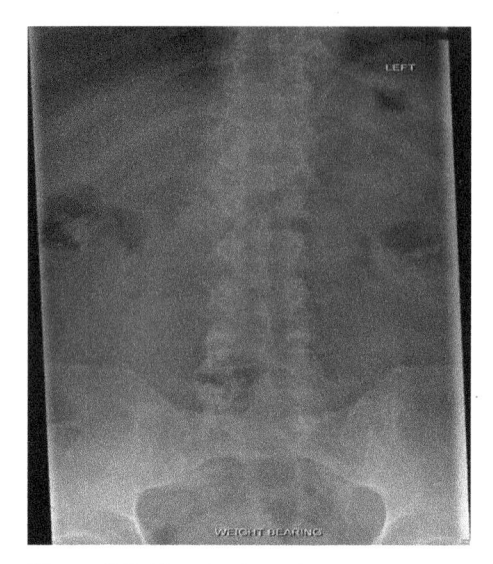

Figure 9.7 X-ray lumbar spine.

```
haemoglobin              127 g/L          (130-180)
white cell count         12.9 × 10⁹/L     (4.0-11.0)
serum albumin            32 g/L           (37-49)
serum C-reactive protein 31 mg/L          (<10)
```

What is the most likely unifying cause?

A. Crohn's disease
B. Multiple myeloma
C. Rheumatoid arthritis
D. Systemic lupus erythematosus (SLE)
E. Type I diabetes mellitus

24. A 68-year-old man was admitted to the acute medical unit with a history of progressive unilateral loss of vision and headaches. Over the previous 12 months, he had experienced episodic ear pain, redness of his eyes, and progressive loss of hearing. He also reported early morning stiffness and pain in his hands.

On examination, he had a saddle-shaped nose, floppy auricular cartilage, bilateral episcleritis, and tender, non-swollen small joints of the hands. Visual acuity was 6/6 in the right eye and 6/12 in the left eye.

```
Investigations:
  haemoglobin                 115 g/L           (130-180)
  white cell count            12.9 × 10⁹/L      (4.0-11.0)
  neutrophil count            9.4 × 10⁹/L       (1.5-7.0)
  serum C-reactive protein    142 mg/L          (<10)
  plasma viscosity            2.04 mPa/s        (1.50-1.72)
```

What is the most likely diagnosis?

A. Giant-cell arteritis
B. Granulomatosis with polyangiitis
C. Relapsing polychondritis
D. Rheumatoid arthritis
E. Systemic lupus erythematosus

25. A 75-year-old man was admitted to the acute medical unit following a fall. He was complaining of persistent left-shoulder girdle pain radiating to the upper arm.

On examination, he was unable to abduct his left shoulder beyond 20°. There was no swelling, discolouration, or tenderness. Peripheral pulses were palpable. There was no obvious neurological abnormality, but examination was limited by pain in the left shoulder.

```
Investigations:
  serum troponin T                          <14 ng/L      (<14)
  serum creatinine                          251 µmol/L    (60-110)
  estimated glomerular filtration rate      28 mL/min     (>60)
  serum C-reactive protein                  8 mg/L        (<10)
```

What is the next most appropriate investigation?

A. ECG
B. MRI cervical spine
C. Repeat troponin T
D. Ultrasound scan left shoulder
E. X-ray left shoulder

26. A 43-year-old Indian call-centre worker was seen in the ambulatory care clinic with a two-month history of worsening chest pain. She had a previous history of treated hypothyroidism and asthma, and was taking thyroxine 75 mcg once daily. Further questioning revealed a 12-month history of widespread pain.

On examination, there was evidence of spasm and tenderness of the trapezius muscle bilaterally. There was no other muscle tenderness or weakness. Cardiorespiratory examination was normal.

```
Investigations:
    serum C-reactive protein            3 mg/L          (<10)
    serum creatine kinase               675 U/L         (24-170)
    serum Troponin T                    <14 ng/L        (<14)
    serum-corrected calcium             2.15 mmol/L     (2.20-2.60)
    serum phosphate                     0.85 mmol/L     (0.8-1.4)
    serum alkaline phosphatase          175 U/L         (45-105)
    serum thyroid-stimulating hormone   3.6 mU/L        (0.4-5.0)

ECG: normal
```

What is the most appropriate investigation?

A. Anti-nuclear antibody assay
B. Electromyogram (EMG)
C. MRI of the upper-limb muscles
D. Open muscle biopsy
E. Serum 25-OH-cholecalciferol level

chapter 9

MUSCULOSKELETAL MEDICINE

ANSWERS

1. D. Serum ferritin

The most likely diagnosis is adult-onset Still's disease. This is a variant of systemic-onset juvenile idiopathic arthritis that is characterized by chronic polyarthritis in association with a systemic inflammatory illness.

The patient has a fever of unknown origin, fulfilling the three criteria:

- an illness of more than three weeks' duration
- a temperature >38.3°C (101°F) on several occasions
- a failure to reach a diagnosis despite one week of inpatient investigation

The key abnormalities are: fevers >39°C; evanescent rash; arthralgia; sore throat; splenomegaly and lymphadenopathy; raised white blood cells and CRP; evidence of pericarditis; and negative rheumatoid and anti-nuclear factors.

Significantly elevated serum ferritin levels are often seen in adult-onset Still's disease; the reasons for this finding are not clear, but it is thought to be more likely to be due to cytokine-induced synthesis by the reticuloendothelial system or of hepatocyte damage with increased release, and not related to iron metabolism.

There are various diagnostic criteria used to make a diagnosis of adult-onset Still's disease:

Yamaguchi

Five or more criteria; at least two are major.

Major criteria:

- Temp of >39°C for >one week
- WBC >10 with >80% neutrophils
- Typical rash
- Arthralgia >two weeks

Minor criteria:

- Sore throat
- Lymph node enlargement
- Splenomegaly
- Liver dysfunction (high AST/ALT)
- Negative ANA, RF

Data from *Journal of Rheumatology*, 19.3, 1992, Yamaguchi M et al., 'Preliminary criteria for classification of adult Still's disease', pp. 424–430.

Cush

All of:

- Fever >39°C
- Arthralgia or arthritis
- Rheumatoid factor <1:80
- ANA< 1:100

And two of:

- WBC count >15,000
- Still's rash
- Pleuritis or pericarditis
- Hepatomegaly, splenomegaly, or lymphadenopathy

Data from *Arthritis & Rheumatology*, 2005, 30.2, Cush JJ et al., 'Adult-onset still's disease'.

Yamaguchi M et al. Preliminary criteria for classification of adult Still's disease. Journal of Rheumatology 1992; 19(3): 424–430.

Cush JJ et al. Adult-onset Still's disease. Arthritis & Rheumatology 2005; 30: 2.

2. E. Nerve-conduction studies

The diagnosis is carpal tunnel syndrome—a condition due to an entrapment neuropathy affecting the median nerve in the carpal tunnel in the wrist.

It is most prevalent among middle-aged women, and is associated with a variety of conditions: wrist injuries (e.g. Colles' fractures); rheumatoid arthritis and other inflammatory arthritides (which may cause synovitis or tenosynovitis of the wrist); diabetes mellitus; thyroid disease (especially hypothyroidism); peri-menopausal state; renal dialysis; acromegaly; and amyloidosis. Repetitive activities and professions involving vibrating tools may also increase the risk of carpal tunnel syndrome.

Although often bilateral, it may be unilateral, usually involving the dominant hand. Symptoms include numbness, tingling, pain (which may extend proximally as far as the elbow), and weakness. Autonomic symptoms (colour and temperature changes) may lead to the clinical picture being confused with Raynaud's phenomenon, which may also lead to symptoms of pain and numbness after significant vasospasm.

Examination reveals a variety of possible abnormalities: muscle weakness and wasting (especially abductor and flexor pollicis brevis); sensory change (affecting the palmar aspect of the thumb, index, middle, and radial aspect of the ring finger); and positive provocation tests of the median nerve in the carpal tunnel (Tinel's and Phalen's).

Nerve-conduction studies show typical changes of slowing of conduction in the median nerve within the carpal tunnel. Other conditions which can sometimes be mistaken for carpal tunnel syndrome include thoracic outlet syndrome, cervical spondylosis/disc disease, and peripheral neuropathies (e.g. due to diabetes).

Mallik A, Weir AI. Nerve conduction studies: essentials and pitfalls in practice. Journal of Neurology, Neurosurgery and Psychiatry 2005; 76: ii23–ii31. doi: 10.1136/jnnp.2005.069138; http://jnnp.bmj.com

3. A. Eosinophilic granulomatosis with polyangiitis (Churg Strauss syndrome)

The diagnosis is eosinophilic granulomatosis with polyangiitis (EGPA), formerly known as Churg–Strauss syndrome. It is a vasculitic condition which affects small- and medium-sized arteries and veins.

The 1990 American College of Rheumatology (ACR) diagnostic criteria for the diagnosis of Churg–Strauss syndrome are (four out of six needed):
- Asthma
- Eosinophilia of more than 10% in peripheral blood
- Paranasal sinusitis
- Pulmonary infiltrates (may be transient)
- Histological proof of vasculitis with extravascular eosinophils
- Mononeuritis multiplex or polyneuropathy

Patients may experience a variety of symptoms:
- General symptoms: malaise, fatigue, weight loss, fever, myalgia
- Pulmonary disease: asthma (which may precede vasculitis by many years), cough, haemoptysis
- Sinus/nasal disease
- Arthralgia
- Cutaneous lesions: nodules, urticaria, ischaemia
- Cardiac disease: myocarditis, pericarditis, heart failure, myocardial infarction
- Gastrointestinal disease: gastritis, colitis, bleeding, abdominal pain
- Peripheral neuropathy: often mononeuritis multiplex

Investigations may show:
- Eosinophilia
- Anaemia
- Raised inflammatory response (ESR, CRP, plasma viscosity)
- Abnormal renal function/urine microscopy with renal involvement
- Antineutrophil cytoplasmic antibodies (ANCA): present in about 40% of patients, mostly perinuclear (p) ANCA (often antimyeloperoxidase positive)
- Elevated serum IgE levels

Reproduced from Masi AT et al., 'The American College of Rheumatology 1990 criteria for the classification of Churg–Strauss syndrome (allergic granulomatosis and angiitis)' Arthritis & Rheumatology, 2010, 33, pp. 1094–1100, with permission from John Wiley and Sons. Copyright © 1990 American College of Rheumatology.

Masi AT et al. The American College of Rheumatology 1990 criteria for the classification of Churg–Strauss syndrome (allergic granulomatosis and angiitis). Arthritis & Rheumatology 2010; 33: 1094–1100.

4. A. Gabapentin

The diagnosis is complex regional pain syndrome. This condition has many other names, including 'reflex sympathetic dystrophy'. It is a condition which involves disproportionate pain and neurovascular responses following some noxious stimulus. It may occur at any age and affects women more than men.

Key symptoms are:
- Pain
- Vascular abnormalities (discolouration, oedema, temperature changes, sweating abnormalities)
- Altered sensation (including allodynia, hyperalgesia, and hypoaesthesia)
- Altered motor function (spasm, weakness, tremors, dystonia)
- Dystrophic changes (skin, nails, hair, muscle, and bone)

The diagnosis is made by a combination of clinical assessment, radiology (X-ray, isotope bone scan, and MR scan) and thermography.

Management of patients involves a variety of strategies:
- Physical and occupational therapy
- Medication
  - Opioids
  - Antidepressants e.g. TCAs, SSRIs, others (venlafaxine)
  - Anticonvulsants e.g. gabapentin, pregabalin, sodium valproate
  - Others e.g. ketamine, baclofen, lignocaine patches
- Interventional procedures
  - Sympathetic/regional blockade
  - Dorsal column stimulators
  - Sympathectomy (chemical/surgical)
- Physical therapies
  - Mirror therapy
- Clinical psychology support

With the extent of the problem in this case, topical therapy would be difficult and so systemic therapy with an agent such as gabapentin would be most appropriate. The use of opioid analgesia would be reasonable, but would not deal with the underlying neuropathic basis to the condition.

Goebel A, Barker C, Turner-Stokes L et al. Complex regional pain syndrome in adults: UK guidelines for diagnosis, referral and management in primary and secondary care. Royal College of Physicians. London. 2012.

5. B. Intravenous methylprednisolone 1 g for three days

The diagnosis is giant cell arteritis (GCA). The combination of a new unilateral temporal headache, constitutional symptoms, an abnormal temporal artery, scalp tenderness, and transient visual disturbance in a man over 50 years old would be compatible with a diagnosis of complicated GCA. Other possible symptoms include scalp pain, fevers, symptoms of polymyalgia rheumatica, chest/throat pain, and jaw/tongue claudication. Additional signs include visual field/pupillary defects, retinal abnormalities (pallor, haemorrhages, arterial occlusion), upper cranial nerve palsies, and abnormalities in the upper limb pulses.

5% of patients with GCA do not demonstrate an inflammatory response. A temporal artery biopsy (TAB) should be considered, but treatment should not be delayed whilst waiting for a biopsy, especially with visual symptoms. TAB is only positive in approximately 70% of patients even without steroids, due to the nature of the 'skip' lesions in the artery. Steroids will affect the results of the TAB, but results may remain positive for several weeks.

The British Society for Rheumatology (BSR) Guidelines on the treatment of GCA recommend that complicated GCA (i.e. where visual loss is impending or threatened) treatment should be 500 mg–1 g intravenous methylprednisolone for three days and then oral prednisolone 60 mg per day. Where visual loss has occurred, the starting dose of prednisolone is 60 mg per day. In uncomplicated GCA, the starting dose of prednisolone is 40–60 mg per day.

Dasgupta B, Borg F, Hassan N et al. BSR and BHPR Guidelines for the management of giant cell arteritis. British Society for Rheumatology. 2010.

MUSCULOSKELETAL MEDICINE | ANSWERS

6. D. Prednisolone

The diagnosis is acute gouty olecranon bursitis. Olecranon bursitis may be caused by a variety of conditions:

- sepsis
- crystal deposition disease (gout and pseudogout)
- rheumatoid arthritis
- trauma

Acute gout may be associated with systemic symptoms, including fevers. It can affect a variety of tissues, including joints, tendon sheaths, and bursae.

The finding of negatively birefringent crystals in fluid is the gold-standard test to diagnose gout. The serum uric acid may be normal in approximately 30% of cases of acute gout (and will then become elevated several weeks after the acute episode has settled).

Treatment of acute gout includes the use of non-steroidal anti-inflammatories (NSAIDs) (which should be avoided in this case with the finding of significant renal impairment), colchicine, simple analgesia (which is ineffective at treating the inflammatory component of the condition), and steroids (which can be oral, intralesional, intramuscular, or intravenous). Allopurinol should not be commenced during an acute episode of gout, but instead a minimum of 4–6 weeks after the acute episode has settled.

Jordan K, Cameron J, Snaith M. BSR & BHPR in Rheumatology Guideline for the Management of Gout. 2007.

7. B. Contrast MR scan of the knee

The key differential diagnoses are psoriatic arthritis (PsA) and mechanical knee pain. Synovial fluid analysis may suggest inflammatory disease such as PsA, but is not specific. The history of problems is likely to be too short for x-rays to show changes of PsA and will not be helpful with mechanical knee pain. Isotope bone scans may show inflammatory changes, but these would not be specific, and some inflammatory change may be seen after injuries. Ultrasound scans may show some changes of PsA, such as synovitis, enthesitis, and tenosynovitis, but will miss other changes of PsA such as bone marrow oedema, and will not help with mechanical knee pain. Contrast (gadolinium)-enhanced MR scans will differentiate between PsA and mechanical knee pain, readily showing the pathology in either condition. This technique is a significant advance in the diagnosis of a variety of inflammatory joint diseases, including PsA and other sero-negative arthritides, as well as rheumatoid arthritis.

Coakley G, Mathews C, Field M et al. BSR & BHPR, BOA, RCGP and BSAC guidelines for management of the hot swollen joint in adults. Rheumatology 2006; 45: 1039–1041. doi: 10.1093/rheumatology/kel163a

8. C. Salivary gland biopsy

The diagnosis is primary Sjögren's syndrome. Sjögren's syndrome may be primary or secondary, when it occurs in association with a variety of connective tissue diseases (e.g. systemic lupus erythematosus (SLE), rheumatoid arthritis, systemic sclerosis, cryoglobulinaemia, polyarteritis nodosa).

Sicca symptoms involve exocrine glands (tear glands, salivary glands, and vagina). Schirmer's test is a non-specific test which will show reduced tear production. Parotitis is a common finding in Sjögren's syndrome, and ultrasound scans will show typical changes in a proportion of people.

Primary Sjögren's syndrome may be diagnosed by a variety of tests, including serological tests; antibodies against SSA/Ro are found in approximately 75% of patients with primary Sjögren's and 15% of patients with secondary Sjögren's. Antibodies against SSA/Ro are also present in 50% of patients with systemic lupus erythematosus (SLE) and are sometimes found in healthy individuals, and can therefore not be used in isolation to diagnose primary Sjögren's syndrome. Antibodies against SSB/La are present in 40–50% of patients with primary Sjögren's and in 15% of patients with SLE.

Salivary gland biopsy is the most definitive way of confirming the diagnosis of primary Sjögren's syndrome—sections will show a typical lymphocytic infiltrate.

Rheumatoid factor (RF) is a generic term that refers to autoantibodies (which can be IgG/A/D/E/M) which target the Fc fragment of IgG. Primary Sjögren's is associated with a polyclonal gammopathy, and positive RF tests are seen in approximately 50% of patients. Anti-cyclic citrullinated peptide antibody (anti-CCP) levels are characteristically elevated in rheumatoid arthritis, although they can be elevated in other conditions such as SLE. The anti-citrullinated protein antibody (ACPA) level was added to the 2010 American College of Rheumatology (ACR)/European League Against Rheumatism (EULAR) diagnostic criteria for rheumatoid arthritis. ACPA may be present in the early presentation of rheumatoid arthritis when the rheumatoid factor is negative. A positive ACPA level makes rheumatoid arthritis more likely.

Hakim A, Clunie G, Haq I. Oxford handbook of rheumatology. Third edition. Chapter 12: Sjögrens syndrome. Oxford: Oxford University Press. 2011.

9. B. Acute pseudogout

The diagnosis is acute pseudogout. It is due to the presence calcium pyrophosphate dihydrate crystals within the joint/bursa/tendon sheath. The condition may present in a similar manner to gout, with an acute onset of mono- or polyarthritis. It may occur spontaneously, or can be precipitated by acute illness, such as infection. The commonest joints affected are the knees, shoulders, wrists, ankles, and elbows. It can cause a marked fever, and acute confusion in the elderly. Investigations show an acute inflammatory response. X-rays may show chondrocalcinosis. Joint fluid aspiration is diagnostic with positively birefringent calcium pyrophosphate dihydrate crystals.

Management of acute attacks is with non-steroidal anti-inflammatory drugs (NSAIDs), steroids, and joint-fluid aspiration. There is no role for allopurinol.

It may be associated with prior trauma or surgery, hyperparathyroidism, haemochromatosis, hypophosphatasia, hypomagnesemia, and ageing.

Hakim A, Clunie G, Haq I. Oxford handbook of rheumatology. Third edition. Chapter 7: The crystal arthropathies. Oxford: Oxford University Press. 2011.

10. A. AA amyloidosis

The diagnosis is AA (inflammatory) amyloidosis. This occurs as a consequence of a variety of rheumatological diseases (as well as acute and chronic infections and some malignancies):

- Rheumatoid arthritis (RA)
- Juvenile inflammatory arthritis
- Ankylosing spondylitis
- Psoriasis and psoriatic arthritis
- Adult-onset Still's disease
- Behçet disease (1–2% in Turkey)
- Familial Mediterranean fever (up to 100%)
- Reactive arthritis (0.3%)
- Osteomyelitis

It typically affects the liver, spleen, and kidneys.

Clinical presentation includes:

- Renal failure or nephrotic syndrome
- Weakness, weight loss, and peripheral oedema

- Constipation, diarrhoea, gastrointestinal bleeding, abdominal fullness or mass
- Cardiac failure, peripheral neuropathy, and carpal tunnel syndrome are late features

Hakim A, Clunie G, Haq I. Oxford handbook of rheumatology. Third edition. Chapter 18: Miscellaneous conditions. Oxford: Oxford University Press. 2011.

11. C. Methotrexate pneumonitis

The diagnosis is methotrexate-induced pneumonitis. This occurs in approximately 1–5% of patients taking methotrexate. It can occur any time after starting the drug, and at varying doses. High-resolution CT scan of the thorax will show typical changes. Cessation of methotrexate, high-dose steroids, and supportive treatment are the mainstay of treatment. Pneumonitis is also seen rarely with leflunomide and sodium aurothiomalate (gold).

Other pulmonary disease in rheumatoid arthritis includes:

- Pleural disease—especially pleural effusions
- Rheumatoid nodules
- Interstitial lung disease (non-specific interstitial pneumonia (NSIP), organizing pneumonia, bronchiolitis obliterans, organizing pneumonia, diffuse alveolar damage)
- Airways involvement (bronchiolitis obliterans, bronchiectasis)
- Pulmonary infections (greater risk of tuberculosis and opportunistic infections, especially with anti-TNF therapy).

National Institute for Health and Care Excellence. Clinical Guideline 79. Rheumatoid arthritis in adults: management. February 2009.

Chakravarty K, McDonald H, Pullar T et al. BSR/BHPR guideline for disease modifying anti-rheumatic drug (DMARD) therapy in consultation with the British Association of Dermatologists. Rheumatology 2008: 1–16. doi: 10.1093/rheumatology/kel216b

12. B. Chest X-ray

Figure 9.4 demonstrates erythema nodosum, which is likely to be caused by sarcoidosis (Löfgren syndrome).

Erythema nodosum may be caused by a number of different conditions:

- Bacterial infections: streptococcus, tuberculosis, yersinia, mycoplasma, salmonella, and campylobacter
- Fungal infections: coccidioidomycosis, histoplasmosis, blastomycosis
- Drugs: sulphonamides, gold, sulphonylureas, oral contraceptive pill
- Inflammatory bowel disease
- Lymphoma
- Sarcoidosis: Löfgren syndrome consists of erythema nodosum, hilar lymphadenopathy, fever, arthritis, and uveitis
- Behçet's disease
- Pregnancy

Mycobacterium marinum is an organism which is found in fresh and salt water and causes infection when the organism penetrates broken skin. It may cause a variety of cutaneous lesions and septic arthritis, tenosynovitis, and bursitis. It may occasionally cause a false positive interferon-gamma release assay.

Hakim A, Clunie G, Haq I. Oxford handbook of rheumatology. Third edition. Chapter 18: Miscellaneous conditions. Oxford: Oxford University Press. 2011.

13. D. Neisseria meningitidis

The diagnosis is septic arthritis secondary to meningococcal septicaemia.

Pre-disposing factors for septic arthritis include:

- Age >60
- Diabetes/sickle cell/immunoparesis
- Intravenous drug use/indwelling vascular lines/invasive procedures
- Pre-existing joint disease
- Prosthetic joints
- Intra-articular injection

Septic arthritis is polyarticular in 20% of cases, and the knee is the most commonly affected joint in adults. The primary presentation of septic arthritis is not always the affected joint.

Common causative organisms include:

- Staphylococcus
- Streptococcus
- Gram negative bacilli
- Haemophilus
- Neisseria
- Tuberculosis
- Lyme

Joint aspiration (before antibiotics) and microscopy/culture is the gold-standard investigation to make a diagnosis of septic arthritis.

Gonococcal infection will usually present with macular, pustular, and papular lesions, rather than petechial lesions; the rash has often settled by the time that joint symptoms have developed.

Coakley G, Mathews C, Field M et al. BSR & BHPR, BOA, RCGP and BSAC guidelines for management of the hot swollen joint in adults. British Society for Rheumatology. 2006.

14. C. MR scan of the lumbo-sacral spine

The symptoms are typical of lumbar canal stenosis. Neurogenic claudication may affect either or both legs with variable neurological symptoms, including numbness, weakness, and tingling. The pain is often relieved by flexion movements of the lumbar spine, such as sitting down. Symptoms may be mistaken for vascular claudication, which is an entirely different problem.

While X-ray and CT scans provide useful imaging of the lumbar spine which may confirm the diagnosis, false positive and false negative CT scan results may occur. MR scans will show definitive changes of lumbar canal stenosis with very few false positive scans. Nerve-conduction studies may show changes of lumbar canal stenosis and differentiate from other causes (e.g. peripheral neuropathy) but are not as reliable.

Hakim A, Clunie G, Haq I. Oxford handbook of rheumatology. Third edition. Chapter 20: Back pain. Oxford: Oxford University Press. 2011.

15. D. Anti-synthetase antibodies

The diagnosis is aspiration pneumonia secondary to dysphagia caused by polymyositis. The other key differential diagnosis is dermatomyositis. The lack of dermatological abnormalities makes dermatomyositis less likely, but not impossible (up to 40% of patients diagnosed with dermatomyositis have no evidence of myositis at presentation, and only have cutaneous disease).

A number of autoantibodies are seen with both polymyositis and dermatomyositis; however, many of these are not disease-specific. Rheumatoid factor is seen in at least 50% of cases of polymyositis, whilst anti-nuclear antibodies (ANA) are seen in approximately 30% of cases. Anti-double-stranded DNA antibodies are more specific for systemic lupus erythematosus (SLE). Anti-smooth muscle antibodies are seen in autoimmune hepatitis.

Antibodies in myositis can be divided into those which are *specific* for myositis, and those which are *associated* with myositis.

Myositis-specific antibodies are targeted against three types of proteins:

1. Transfer ribonucleic acid (tRNA) synthetases: whilst a number of antibodies have been described, the main one is the Anti-Jo-1 antibody, which is seen in 25–30% of all patients with polymyositis. Patients who are Anti-Jo-1 positive tend to have interstitial lung disease, arthritis (non-deforming) and fevers.
2. Nuclear Mi-2 protein: these are seen in approximately 20% of patients with myositis, and are more specific for dermatomyositis.
3. Signal recognition peptide (SRP): anti-SRP antibodies are seen in approximately 5% of patients with polymyositis, and are associated with poor response to treatment and a poor prognosis.

Myositis-associated antibodies are seen in up to 50% of patients with myositis. They are typically seen in other connective tissue diseases. Examples include anti-PM/Scl antibodies (seen in polymyositis/systemic sclerosis overlap disease), and anti-Ku antibodies, seen in overlap myositis/connective tissue diseases.

Hakim A, Clunie G, Haq I. Oxford handbook of rheumatology. Third edition. Chapter 14: Idiopathic inflammatory myopathies: polymyositis and dermatomyositis. Oxford: Oxford University Press. 2011.

16. A. Avascular necrosis

The most likely cause of the left hip pain is avascular necrosis (AVN) of the hip; in this case, secondary to prolonged high-dose steroid therapy.

It is, in general, more prevalent in men. AVN may be idiopathic, but there are a number of predisposing/associated conditions: these include corticosteroid use (or Cushing's disease), chronic alcohol abuse, systemic lupus erythemtosus (SLE) (greater prevalence in women), anti-phospholipid syndrome, sickle cell disease and other haemoglobinopathies, infection, post-trauma, hyperlipidaemia, gout, renal failure/post-renal transplant, pregnancy, malignancies (primary or secondary), decompression sickness (Caisson disease), and bisphosphonate therapy.

AVN may be asymptomatic, being diagnosed as a coincidental finding on radiological investigations, but most commonly presents with pain of the affected area. The hip is the most typically affected area, but the carpal bones, talus, femur, metatarsals, mandible, and humerus are also well recognized sites of AVN.

The diagnosis is made radiologically, MRI being the most sensitive investigation; X-ray, CT, and isotope bone scan can all be used. Treatment is initially medical (rest, analgesia, treat underlying causes) and then surgical (bone decompression, bone graft, osteotomy, joint replacement).

Aldridge J, Urbaniak J. Avascular necrosis of the femoral head: etiology, pathophysiology, classification, and current treatment guidelines. American Journal of Orthopedics July 2004; 33(7): 327–332.

17. A. Azathioprine-induced pancreatitis

The most likely diagnosis is azathioprine-induced pancreatitis. The list of drugs which may cause pancreatitis is long, of which several are used in rheumatology. Azathioprine is one of the most frequent causes of drug-induced pancreatitis. The dose of glucocorticoids needed to cause pancreatitis is usually higher than in this case.

The following rheumatological drugs may cause pancreatitis:
- Azathioprine
- Colchicine
- Cyclophosphamide
- Ciclosporin
- Gold
- Methotrexate
- Mycophenolate
- Sulfasalazine
- Anti-TNF therapy

Additionally, the following drugs commonly used in rheumatology may also cause pancreatitis:
- Codeine
- Non-steroidal anti-inflammatory drugs
- Paracetamol

Trivedi C, Pitchumoni C. Drug-Induced pancreatitis: an update. Journal of Clinical Gastroenterology 2005; 39 (8): 709–716.

18. C. Intravenous methylprednisolone

Vascular manifestations of Behçet's disease may involve any type of vessel (arterial, venous, and capillary) of any size. Arterial disease is more common in men, and may lead to aneurysm formation, which, if found in the pulmonary arterial system, may be fatal. Venous disease commonly manifests as superficial thrombophlebitis, but thromboses may also occur in a variety of vessels, causing a variety of complications (e.g. superior vena cava obstruction or Budd Chiari syndrome). Vasculitis in Behçet's disease can affect vessels of any size in a wide range of sites.

The main cause of venous thrombosis in Behçet's disease is inflammation of the vessel wall; venous thrombus tends to be adherent to vessel walls and rarely embolizes (the incidence of pulmonary emboli in Behçet's disease is much less than that of venous thrombosis). As a result, the key treatment is immunosuppression; this may initially involve corticosteroids, which should be used alongside agents such as azathioprine, cyclophosphamide, or ciclosporin. For resistant or recalcitrant disease, agents such as infliximab, interferon-alpha, or rituximab may be necessary. Studies show that the risk of recurrent venous thrombosis is much less in Behçet's disease patients who are treated with immunosuppressant therapy.

There is no significant evidence for the use of anticoagulation, antiplatelet, or antifibrinolytic therapy for acute venous disease in Behçet's disease.

EULAR Standing Committee for Clinical Affairs. EULAR recommendations for the management of Behcet disease. Annals of the Rheumatic Diseases 2008; 67: 1656–1662.

19. A. Ankylosing spondylitis

The X-ray shows anterior-flowing syndesmophytes, which are formed when ossification of the outer fibres of the annulus fibrosis (fibrocartilage and fibrous tissue) leads to bridging of the corners of one vertebra to another. These findings are classically seen in spondyloarthritides (SpA), which include enteropathic, psoriatic and reactive SpA, as well as ankylosing spondylitis.

Other imaging modalities, which are very useful in the diagnosis of SpA, include MRI using fat-saturating techniques such as short tau inversion recovery (STIR) or MRI with gadolinium enhancement.

Hakim A, Clunie G, Haq I. Oxford handbook of rheumatology. Third edition. Chapter 8. The spondyloarthropathies. Oxford University Press. 2011.

20. B. MRI of the left tibia

The most likely diagnosis is osteosarcoma of the left tibia, secondary to Paget's disease. In Britain, Paget's disease affects approximately 2% of adults over 55, rising to 5–8% of the over 80s. Osteosarcoma is a rare complication of Paget's disease, affecting less than 1% of all patients; symptoms of pain and swelling can develop over weeks or months, and most commonly affect the pelvis, femur, tibia, humerus, and skull. Metastatic disease to the chest is well recognized, but may have minimal symptoms.

Various imaging modalities can be used to investigate for possible osteosarcoma; X-ray, and CT may suggest the diagnosis, but false negatives may occur; isotope bone scans may not be able to differentiate between osteosarcoma and active Paget's disease. MRI scanning is the most reliable non-invasive diagnostic test. Biopsy of a suspicious lesion is the gold standard.

Treatment involves surgical excision and chemotherapy. The prognosis is worse with multifocal/metastatic disease, with five-year survival rates of approximately 50% for those patients undergoing surgery and chemotherapy.

Hakim A, Clunie G, Haq I. Oxford handbook of rheumatology. Third edition. Chapter 16. Metabolic bone diseases and disorders of collagen. Oxford: Oxford University Press. 2011.

21. B. Palindromic rheumatism

The diagnosis is palindromic rheumatism. This is a migratory inflammatory arthritis characterized by episodic joint inflammation. The majority of episodes are monoarticular, but may occasionally be oligo or polyarticular, affecting a variety of small joints. Episodes occur with varying frequency and have an onset over several hours up to 1–2 days. Each episode may last for up to 14 days, and symptoms of pain can be severe. Systemic symptoms such as fever are not typical, and bloods may show a mild inflammatory response.

Approximately one-third of patients with palindromic rheumatism go on to develop rheumatoid arthritis. Treatment for the condition includes non-steroidal anti-inflammatory drugs (NSAIDs), corticosteroids, antimalarial drugs (chloroquine and hydroxychloroquine), sulfasalazine, methotrexate, and ciclosporin.

There are a number of conditions which may present in this way; these include crystal arthritides such as gout (highly unlikely in a premenopausal woman with no other history), reactive arthritis, systemic lupus erythematosus, and sarcoidosis.

The absence of rheumatoid factor does not in itself exclude a diagnosis of rheumatoid arthritis. Rheumatoid factor is not specific for rheumatoid arthritis. The anti-citrullinated peptide antibody (ACPA) has a greater specificity and sensitivity for rheumatoid arthritis.

National Institute for Health and Care Excellence. Clinical Guideline 79. Rheumatoid arthritis in adults: management. February 2009.

22. B. Parvovirus B19 arthritis

The most likely diagnosis is parvovirus B19 arthritis. Parvovirus B19 infection has also been called 'erythema infectiosum' or 'Fifth disease'. It is a single-stranded DNA virus. Parvovirus B19 infection is very common, often occurring in outbreaks, especially in settings such as schools and nurseries; non-immune adults who work in such settings are particularly susceptible to infection.

Typical symptoms of the infection include fever, malaise, headache, myalgia, nausea, and coryzal symptoms, which typically begin five to seven days after initial infection. Approximately one week later, the classical 'slapped cheek' rash appears; this is, however, uncommon in adults, which can often lead to under-diagnosis. Parvovirus infection may, especially in adults, be asymptomatic. Complications of the infection include arthritis and, more rarely, myocarditis, vasculitis, and meningoencephalitis. Parvovirus infections can precipitate significant haematological complications in those with pre-existing disease (e.g. haemoglobinopathies).

Parvovirus arthritis is most commonly seen in adult women with acute infection: patients develop an acute symmetrical arthritis affecting the small joints of the hands and feet. It will typically last for one to three weeks, but in a small number of people may be prolonged, lasting for months; there are, however, no long-term sequelae. Parvovirus arthritis may cause an occasional, transient false positive rheumatoid factor result, reflecting the immune response to the viral infection.

Treatment is according to symptoms: simple analgesia, non-steroidal anti-inflammatory drugs (NSAIDs) and, occasionally, low-dose corticosteroids have all been used.

Hakim A, Clunie G, Haq I. Oxford handbook of rheumatology. Third edition. Chapter 17. Infection and rheumatic disease. Oxford: Oxford University Press. 2011.

23. A. Crohn's disease

The diagnosis is Crohn's disease, causing enteropathic spondyloarthritis and pyoderma gangrenosum.

The X-ray shows evidence of fused sacroiliac joints, indicating previous sacroilitis and syndesmophytes, which does not occur in the other listed conditions but is seen in enteropathic sponyloarthritis due to either Crohn's disease or ulcerative colitis.

Pyoderma gangrenosum is seen in association with a number of conditions, including inflammatory bowel disease, rheumatoid arthritis, haematological disorders (types of leukaemia, monoclonal gammopathy), hepatic disease (chronic active hepatitis, primary biliary cirrhosis), and connective tissue diseases (SLE and Sjögren's syndrome).

Hakim A, Clunie G, Haq I. Oxford handbook of rheumatology. Third edition. Chapter 8. The spondyloarthropathies. Oxford: Oxford University Press. 2011.

24. C. Relapsing polychondritis

The diagnosis is relapsing polychondritis. It is a progressive, inflammatory systemic disorder of predominantly cartilaginous tissue. It typically affects the ears, nose, and throat, resulting in problems such as sensorineural hearing loss, the classical 'floppy ears' (resulting from loss of auricular cartilage), and changes in the nasal structure. Arthritis is common, and is typically a non-deforming involving the small joints. Involvement of respiratory tissue, particularly within the trachea, leads to problems such as stridor and breathlessness. A number of ocular problems may occur, notably reduced visual acuity, episcleritis, scleritis, and conjunctivitis. There are numerous cardiovascular and central nervous system features which may occur.

Many of the features of relapsing polychodritis are similar to granulomatosis with polyangiitis (formerly known as Wegener's granulomatosis). Relapsing polychondritis may be associated with a number of other conditions, such as rheumatoid arthritis, diabetes, systemic lupus erythematosus (SLE), and mixed connective tissue disease.

There are several possible diagnostic criteria which may be used, such as the McAadam criteria, which requires three of six of the following features:

- Bilateral auricular chondritis
- Non-erosive seronegative inflammatory polyarthritis
- Nasal chondritis
- Ocular inflammation
- Respiratory tract chondritis
- Audiovestibular damage

Treatment involves the use of corticosteroids and immunosuppressants, such as cyclophosphamide, azathioprine, methotrexate, and ciclosporin. Anti-TNF therapy has been used for more resistant cases.

McAdam L, O'Hanlan M, Bluestone R et al; Relapsing polychondritis: prospective study of 23 patients and a review of the literature. Medicine (Baltimore) 1976; 55(3): 193–215.

25. D. Ultrasound scan left shoulder

The most likely problem is a post-traumatic rotator cuff tear. The clinical examination is highly suggestive of this, with a limited range movement and pain, but no tenderness. X-ray may suggest a rotator cuff tear (with a loss of the acromio-humeral distance), but ultrasound scanning gives a more accurate image of the actual rotator cuff and the extent of any injury.

Hakim A, Clunie G, Haq I. Oxford handbook of rheumatology. Third edition. Chapter 19. Common upper limb musculoskeletal lesions. Oxford: Oxford University Press. 2011.

26. E. Serum 25-OH-cholecalciferol level

The diagnosis is osteomalacia due to vitamin D deficiency, causing a myopathy.

Osteomalacia is the failure of osteoid bone to calcify in adulthood. The commonest cause is vitamin D deficiency, which has a prevalence of approximately 14% in the UK as a whole, but as high as 90% in the South Asian population (although not all people are symptomatic).

Osteomalacia can cause a variety of musculoskeletal symptoms, including generalized or localized bone pain/tenderness, and painful proximal muscle weakness, often affecting the pelvic girdle more than the shoulder girdle.

Biochemical abnormalities are as previously outlined. Other investigations for a myopathy (MRI, EMG, and muscle biopsy) show non-specific, non-diagnostic abnormalities.

Replacement therapy can be given orally or parenterally.

Hakim A, Clunie G, Haq I. Oxford handbook of rheumatology. Third edition. Chapter 16. Metabolic bone diseases and disorders of collagen. Oxford: Oxford University Press. 2011.

chapter 10

ONCOLOGY AND PALLIATIVE CARE

QUESTIONS

1. A 56-year-old man was receiving palliative chemotherapy with cisplatin and pemetrexed for right-sided malignant mesothelioma. He presented to the emergency department with worsening right-sided chest pain. The pain was 8/10 in severity and on further questioning there was a sensation of burning associated with it. A chest X-ray showed thickening of the pleura in the right hemithorax consistent with the known diagnosis of mesothelioma. He was taking two tablets of co-codamol 30/500 every six hours to relieve the pain. His eGFR was 90 mL/min.

   What is the next best step in the management of the patient's pain?
   A. Stop co-codamol 30/500 and start normal release oral morphine (e.g. oramorph) 5 mg every six hours with normal release oral morphine 5 mg hourly PRN
   B. Stop co-codamol 30/500 and start normal release oral morphine 10 mg every four hours with normal release oral morphine 10 mg hourly PRN and consider starting a neuropathic agent (e.g. gabapentin)
   C. Stop co-codamol 30/500 and start normal release oral morphine 10mg every four hours with normal release oral morphine 5 mg hourly PRN and consider starting a neuropathic agent (e.g. gabapentin)
   D. Stop co-codamol 30/500 and start sustained release oral morphine 10 mg every 12 hours
   E. Switch co-codamol 30/500 to tramadol 50 mg po qds and consider starting a neuropathic agent (e.g. gabapentin)

2. A 63-year-old woman was admitted to the acute medical unit with a two-month history of weight loss, increasing shortness of breath, lethargy, and, more recently, headaches and speech problems. She smoked 20 cigarettes per day and had no significant past medical history. She was not on any regular medication. Her GP had been investigating her and blood results performed last week were as follows.

   ```
   Investigations:
     haemoglobin          140 g/L           (130-180)
     white cell count     6.0 × 10⁹/L       (4.0 - 11.0)
     platelet count       330 × 10⁹/L       (150-400)
     serum sodium         130 mmol/L        (137-144)
     serum potassium      4.0 mmol/L        (3.5-4.9)
     serum urea           6.8 mmol/L        (2.5-7.0)
     serum creatinine     112 µmol/L        (60-110)
   ```

On examination, there was lymphadenopathy in the right supraclavicular fossa. On auscultation, there was reduced air entry in the right lung field. On palpation, there was hepatomegaly. The patient was euvolaemic. Neurological examination revealed some word finding difficulties and dysarthria. A chest X-ray showed a bulky right hilum highly suggestive for malignancy.

While awaiting an urgent CT of the chest, abdomen, and pelvis, the patient had a self-terminating tonic–clonic seizure lasting approximately 45 seconds. Her Glasgow Coma Score (GCS) returned to 14/15 and her neurological examination was as before. The biochemistry laboratory telephoned the ward with the following admission blood results.

```
Investigations:
  haemoglobin                      138 g/L            (130-180)
  white cell count                 7.9 × 10⁹/L        (4.0-11.0)
  platelet count                   360 × 10⁹/L        (150-400)
  serum sodium                     125 mmol/L         (137-144)
  serum potassium                  4.2 mmol/L         (3.5-4.9)
  serum urea                       6.9 mmol/L         (2.5-7.0)
  serum creatinine                 100 µmol/L         (60-110)
  serum bilirubin                  <5 µmol/L          (1-22)
  serum alkaline phosphatase       100 U/L            (45-105)
  serum alanine aminotranferase    45 U/L             (5-35)
```

On the basis of these results, more tests including thyroid function, serum and urine osmolality, urinary sodium, serum uric acid, and short synacthen test were performed and were in keeping with a diagnosis of the Syndrome of Inappropriate Antidiuretic Hormone secretion (SIADH).

What is the next best step in management?

A. Continue diagnostic work up including CT of head, chest, abdomen and pelvis, biopsy, and start appropriate anti-cancer treatment as soon as possible
B. Fluid restriction (e.g. 750 mL/24 hours), consider demeclocyline po 300 mg bd or vasopressin–receptor antagonist if no response to this, and perform CT of head, chest, abdomen, and pelvis
C. Fluid restriction (e.g. 750 mL/24 hours), urea 30 g po per 24 hours, and CT of head, chest, abdomen, and pelvis
D. Intravenous infusion of 3% saline, aiming to raise the serum sodium level by 0.5–1 mmol/L per hour to a maximum of 8–10 mmol/L in the first 24 hours and CT of head, chest, abdomen, and pelvis
E. Intravenous infusion of 3% saline, aiming to raise the serum sodium level by 1–2 mmol/L per hour to a maximum of 8–10 mmol/L in the first 24 hours and CT of head, chest, abdomen, and pelvis

3. **A 52-year-old woman attended the emergency department with a 24-hour history of unsteady gait and difficulty mobilizing.** She had seen her **GP** twice over the past two months with increasing pain in the lower back that was now only partially controlled with co-codamol. On examination, she had power 4/5 in the right leg and 3/5 in the left, reflexes were normal, and plantars downgoing. She had a palpable bladder and admitted to passing urine more frequently. She had previously been diagnosed with breast cancer at the age of 47 and received adjuvant chemotherapy and tamoxifen. She had no other past medical history of note.

   What is the most appropriate next test?
   A. CT scan of head
   B. MR scan of the lumbar sacral spine
   C. MR scan of the whole spine
   D. Plain X-ray of the lumbar spine
   E. CT scan of the whole spine

4. **A 66-year-old man presented with a two-week history of headache, dyspnoea, and facial swelling.** He gave a history of 7 kg unintentional weight loss over the last six months and occasional night sweats. He was a smoker with a history of smoking 20 cigarettes per day for 50 years.

   On examination, he had superficial venous distension over the neck, arms, and chest. His pulse was 100 beats per minute, blood pressure 134/91 mmHg, and oxygen saturation 95% on air. A chest **X-ray** showed a widened mediastinum and a right lung shadow.

   Contrast enhanced **CT** showed superior vena cava obstruction.

   He was started on dexamethasone 8 mg bd.

   What is the most appropriate next step?
   A. Referral to the cardiothoracic surgeons for resection
   B. Referral to the clinical oncologist for radiotherapy
   C. Referral to the interventional radiologist for CT-guided biopsy
   D. Referral to the interventional radiologist for insertion of a stent
   E. Referral to the oncologist for chemotherapy

5. **A 59-year-old woman, recently diagnosed with breast cancer, presented to the emergency department nine days after her first cycle of adjuvant FEC (fluorouracil, epirubicin, and cyclophosphamide) chemotherapy. She described fatigue and over the last 12 hours she had four episodes of diarrhoea. On her thermometer at home she had recorded a temperature of 38.5°C.**

   On examination, she felt clammy and was clinically dehydrated. Her temperature was 37.4°C and blood pressure was 95/60 mmHg. Abdominal palpation found generalized tenderness with no guarding. Bowel sounds were normal.

   An urgent full blood count, kidney and liver function tests, C-reactive protein, and blood culture were ordered. Intravenous fluids were started.

   What is the most appropriate initial management?
   A. Commence broad-spectrum intravenous antibiotics (e.g. piperacillin–tazobactam) pending the blood result
   B. Commence oral metronidazole pending the blood results
   C. Request a surgical review of her abdomen
   D. Request an urgent abdominal CT scan
   E. Wait for blood results before starting broad-spectrum intravenous antibiotics (e.g. piperacillin–tazobactam)

6. **A 69-year-old man with non-small cell lung cancer was referred by his GP to the acute medical unit with a five-day history of confusion. His wife told you that he had received radiotherapy to the lung four months ago. His appetite had been poor and he was complaining of constipation. He had started taking morphine sulphate modified release 30 mg twice daily two weeks ago for back pain.**

   On examination, he was disorientated. He had no focal neurological signs. He was clinically dehydrated, pulse 96 beats per minute and regular, and blood pressure 114/68 mmHg.

   His GP had checked his blood tests earlier in the day.

   ```
   Investigations:
       haemoglobin                      98 g/L              (130-180)
       white cell count                 9.0 × 10⁹/L         (4.0-11.0)
       platelet count                   420 × 10⁹/L         (150-400)
       serum sodium                     132 mmol/L          (137-144)
       serum potassium                  4.8 mmol/L          (3.5-4.9)
       serum corrected calcium          3.7 mmol/L          (2.20-2.60)
       serum urea                       11.6 mmol/L         (2.5-7.0)
       serum creatinine                 123 µmol/L          (60-110)
       calculated creatinine clearance  63 mL/min
       serum albumin                    26 g/L              (37-49)
   ```

   What is the most likely diagnosis?

   A. Brain metastases
   B. Hypercalcaemia
   C. Opiate toxicity
   D. Spinal cord compression
   E. Urinary tract infection

7. A 74-year-old man received his first cycle of palliative chemotherapy with carboplatin and gemcitabine yesterday for the treatment of metastatic squamous cell carcinoma of the lung with bone and liver metastases. He was given the following antiemetic regime 30 minutes before the chemotherapy: ondansetron 8 mg orally and dexamethasone 8 mg orally.

He presented to the emergency department 18 hours after chemotherapy with a 12-hour history of nausea and vomiting. He had reduced oral intake and had vomited six times. He had been taking dexamethasone 4 mg orally twice daily and domperidone 10 mg orally three times daily regularly at home but could no longer keep the tablets down without vomiting.

On examination, he had decreased skin turgor and dry mucous membranes.

His temperature was 37.0°C, pulse 102 beats per minute, blood pressure 105/82 mmHg, and respiratory rate 16 breaths per minute.

```
Investigations:
   haemoglobin          132 g/L           (130-180)
   white cell count     9.8 × 10⁹/L       (4.0-11.0)
   neutrophil count     3.2 × 10⁹/L       (1.5-7.0)
   serum urea           12 mmol/L         (2.5-7.0)
   serum creatinine     109 µmol/L        (60-110)
```

He was admitted for intravenous fluid therapy and for symptom control.

What would be the most appropriate management in addition to intravenous fluids?

A. Increase domperidone to 20 mg orally tds and inform the acute oncology service of patient's admission

B. Increase oral domperidone to 20 mg tds and start metoclopramide 10 mg intravenously tds

C. Stop domperidone and start fosaprepitant 150 mg intravenously and inform the acute oncology service of patient's admission

D. Stop domperidone and start ondansetron 8 mg intravenously twice a day and inform the acute oncology service of patient's admission

E. Switch to intravenous domperidone 20 mg tds, start cyclizine 50 mg intravenously tds, and inform the acute oncology service of patient's admission

8. An 86-year-old woman presented to the acute medical unit having collapsed at home. She described breathlessness and intermittent vaginal bleeding over the past four weeks, which had become more persistent over the last three days. Her haemoglobin was 65 g/L (115–165) and a chest X-ray showed coin-like lesions throughout both lung fields.

   She received a three unit transfusion of packed red cells and a CT scan of thorax and abdomen was performed. This showed a large pelvic mass arising from the uterine cervix and invading the base of the bladder. There were enlarged para-aortic lymph nodes and multiple lung metastases. The gynaecologists reviewed her and a biopsy was taken and vaginal packing placed.

   Overnight, she continued to have further fresh bleeding per vagina. Repeat haemoglobin the next day was 70 g/L (115–165). Her temperature was 36.0°C, pulse 82 beats per minute, and blood pressure 110/70 mmHg.

   What is the most appropriate management?

   A. Refer to gynaecologist for emergency hysterectomy
   B. Refer to oncologist for consideration of chemotherapy
   C. Refer to oncologist for consideration of palliative radiotherapy
   D. Refer to radiologist for consideration of embolization
   E. Tranexamic acid

9. **A 24-year-old plumber presented to the emergency department with a one-week history of shortness of breath on exertion and a two-day history of cough.**

   On examination, he was apyrexial, pulse was 90 beats per minute and regular, blood pressure 105/72 mmHg, respiratory rate 16 breaths per minute, and oxygen saturation 92% on air.

   Investigations:

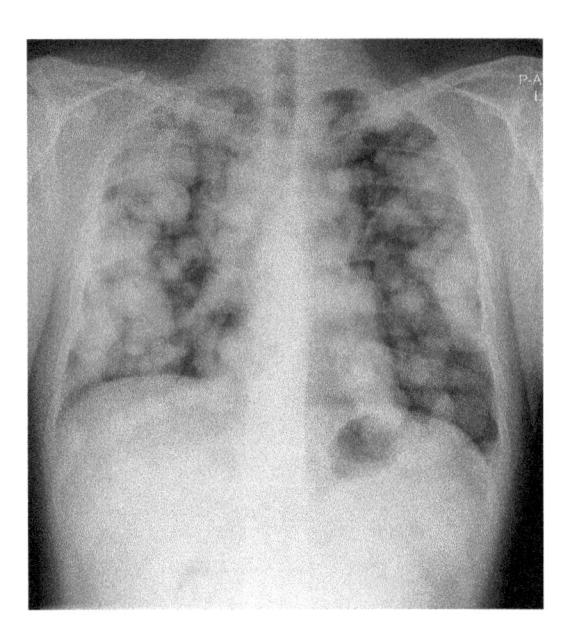

   Figure 10.1 Chest X-ray on admission.

   What is the most likely diagnosis?
   A. Germ cell cancer
   B. Non-Hodgkin's lymphoma
   C. Pulmonary embolism
   D. Renal cell cancer
   E. Small-cell lung cancer

10. A 76-year-old woman with a past medical history of renal cancer was referred by her GP to the acute medical unit with back pain and urinary retention. Compression of the spinal cord was suspected and an MR scan of the whole spine was performed. This showed an isolated bone metastasis at the T11 vertebra with compression of the cord at this level and a distended bladder. The patient was given analgesia and a urinary catheter was placed.

    What is the most appropriate next step in management?
    A. Dexamethasone 8 mg and refer to the acute oncologist for review
    B. Dexamethasone 16 mg and refer to the clinical oncologist for radiotherapy
    C. Dexamethasone 16 mg and refer to the spinal surgeon for consideration of surgery
    D. Dexamethasone 16 mg and refer to the radiologist for a biopsy
    E. Dexamethasone 96 mg and refer to the clinical oncologist for radiotherapy

11. A 65-year-old woman underwent a right hemicolectomy for a T3N1M0 adenocarcinoma of the caecum eight weeks ago. During her post-operative recovery, she was seen in the oncology clinic and a course of adjuvant oral capecitabine chemotherapy was recommended to reduce her risk of recurrence. Six hours after taking the second dose of tablets, the patient developed tightness in the retrosternal/epigastric area and became more short of breath. She called for an ambulance and arrived in the emergency department. The patient was given aspirin 300 mg orally and fondaparinux 2.5 mg subcutaneously.

    On examination, her temperature was 37.3°C, pulse rate 108 beats per minute, blood pressure 110/65 mmHg, and oxygen saturation 99% on room air. Cardiovascular and respiratory examinations were unremarkable.

    ```
    Investigations:
      CXR - normal
      ECG - sinus rhythm, rate 105, no ischaemic changes
      FBC, U&Es, LFTs - normal

      Troponin on arrival     <14 ng/L         (<14ng/L)
      Troponin 12 hours       <14 ng/L         (<14ng/L)
    ```

    The patient's pain and shortness of breath completely resolved within a few hours and a repeat ECG showed sinus rhythm rate 80 with no ischaemic changes.

    What would be the most appropriate management?
    A. Admit the patient, continue the capecitabine tablets, and refer to cardiology for coronary angiography
    B. Admit the patient, stop the capecitabine tablets, and organize a CTPA to exclude pulmonary embolism
    C. Send the patient home, advise her to stop the capecitabine tablets, and inform the acute oncology service/oncology team to follow up the patient
    D. Send the patient home with gaviscon and tell her to continue the capecitabine tablets as her cancer treatment must not be interrupted
    E. Send the patient home with gaviscon, stop the capecitabine tablets, arrange outpatient OGD, and inform the acute oncology service/oncology team to follow up the patient

chapter 10

ONCOLOGY AND PALLIATIVE CARE

ANSWERS

1. B. Stop co-codamol 30/500 and start normal release oral morphine 10 mg every four hours with normal release oral morphine 10 mg hourly PRN and consider starting a neuropathic agent (e.g. gabapentin)

By taking two tablets of co-codamol 30/500 every six hours, the patient is taking 240 mg of codeine per 24 hours, which is equivalent to 24 mg of oral morphine per 24 hours. Therefore, the regular equivalent oral morphine doses, excluding PRN doses, for option A and D (each equivalent to 20 mg oral morphine per 24 hours) would be a lower equivalent dose of oral morphine than the patient is already taking in co-codamol 30/500. Details for opiate conversion doses are available in the 'prescribing in palliative care' section of the British National Formulary.

By switching from co-codamol 30/500 to 10 mg normal release oral morphine every four hours, the patient will start to receive 60 mg oral morphine in 24 hours, which is an increase on the 24 mg equivalent oral morphine dose per 24 hours that they were receiving on co-codamol. The PRN dose should be one-sixth of the 24-hour dose of normal release oral morphine and this can be given up to a maximum of one-hourly. Answer C is not the best option as the PRN dose is one-twelfth of the 24-hour dose of normal release oral morphine. Answer E is incorrect, as the patient needs an increase in analgesia from step 2 to step 3 on the WHO pain ladder.

Adjuvant analgesics are drugs which are analgesic in some painful conditions, but their primary indications are for something other than pain (e.g. antidepressants and anticonvulsants). They should be considered at each step on the pain ladder. In this case, it appeared that there was a neuropathic element producing the sensation of burning and this is commonly seen in mesothelioma, as pain may be due to tumour infiltration of the intercostal nerves, or a previous procedure such as a thoracotomy.

WHO Pain Ladder. http://www.who.int/cancer/palliative/painladder/en/

Abrahm JL. Palliative care for the patient with mesothelioma. Seminars in Thoracic and Cardiovascular Surgery 2009; 21: 164–171.

2. B. Fluid restriction (e.g. 750 mL/24 hours), consider demeclocyline po 300 mg bd, or vasopressin–receptor antagonist if no response to this, and perform CT of head, chest, abdomen, and pelvis

SIADH is the most frequent cause of euvolaemic hyponatraemia and, out of all malignancies, the risk is highest in small-cell lung carcinoma. Assessment of the chronicity of the condition is important to guide the management, as in the acute setting (where the condition is known to have developed within 48 hours) rapid correction of low sodium is warranted with the risk of osmotic demyelination being low. This is in contrast to chronic SIADH or if the duration of hyponatraemia is unclear, as rapid correction of serum sodium in these situations carries a higher risk of osmotic demyelination.

In this scenario, blood results from one week ago revealed hyponatraemia, indicating that this is chronic hyponatraemia. Therefore, answer E would possibly result in serum sodium levels being corrected too quickly. It is suggested for cases of acute severe hyponatraemia with symptoms such as seizure and coma that the serum sodium levels should be raised by 1–2 mmol per litre per hour. Experts believe that serum sodium levels should not be raised by more than 8–10 mmol per litre within the first 24 hours of treatment. In chronic settings or in cases where the duration of hyponatraemia is unclear, but the patient is symptomatic, a lower rate of serum sodium correction is advised (e.g. 0.5–1.0 mmol per litre per hour). In this scenario, it is unlikely that the seizure was a consequence of the hyponatraemia with the serum sodium level of 125 mmol/L, as neurological sequelae of hyponatraemia occur more commonly when serum sodium is <115 mmol/L. For this patient, the diagnosis of small-cell lung cancer should be considered and, therefore, the risk of brain metastases is considerable (approximately 10% of small-cell lung cancer patients present with brain metastases at time of diagnosis and more than 50% of patients with small-cell lung cancer will develop symptomatic brain metastases during their remaining lifetime). The seizure could have resulted from undiagnosed brain metastases and, hence, imaging of the brain is warranted in addition to the chest, abdomen, and pelvis. Answer D was not felt to be the next best step in management because of the chance of the seizure being more likely related to the existence of brain metastases than the serum sodium level and the risk of osmotic demyelination even with a slow infusion of 3% saline.

Urea to promote an osmotic diuresis is poorly tolerated and, therefore, is no longer commonly used (answer C). Most cases of SIADH caused by malignant disease resolve with effective antineoplastic therapy, and even though the need for a diagnosis is important, more urgent and definitive management of this patient's hyponatraemia is warranted in the first instance, as it may take a few days to confirm a tissue diagnosis that will guide appropriate antineoplastic therapy (answer A).

In patients with no symptoms attributable to chronic hyponatraemia, fluid restriction is the cornerstone of therapy. The degree of fluid restriction is based on levels of urinary and plasma electrolytes (Table 10.1).

Table 10.1 General Recommendations for Employment of Fluid Restriction and Predictors of the Increased Likelihood of Failure of Fluid Restriction

General recommendations:
- Restrict all intake that is consumed by drinking, not just water.
- Aim for a Fluid restriction that is 500 mL/d below the 24-hour urine volume.
- Do not restrict sodium or protein intake unless indicated.

Predictors of the likely failure of fluid restriction:
- High urine osmolality (>500 mOsm/kg H_2O).
- Sum of the urine Na^+ and K^+ concentration exceeds the serum Na^+ concentration.
- 24-hour urine volume <500 mL/day.
- Increase in serum Na^+ concentration <2 mmol/L/day in 24–48 hours on a fluid restriction of ≤1 L/day.

D = day; H_2O = water; K = potassium; kg = kilogram; L = liter; mL = millilitre; mmol = millimole; mOsm = milliosmole; Na = sodium.
Reproduced from The American Journal of Medicine, Verbalis J. G et al., 'Diagnosis, Evaluation, and Treatment of Hyponatremia: Expert Panel Recommendations', 126, 10, pp. 1–42, Copyright (2013), with permission from Elsevier.

Demeclocycline reduces urinary osmolality and increases serum sodium levels, but its effects can be variable and a side effect can be nephrotoxicity, and therefore it may be best considered after failure of fluid restriction to increase serum sodium levels. Vaptans are vasopressin receptor antagonists and are a more recent option for treating SIADH. They have been shown to be more effective than fluid restriction alone in the management of hyponatraemia and are increasingly being used in clinical practice.

Ellison DH, Berl T. The syndrome of inappropriate antidiuresis. The New England Journal of Medicine 2007; 356: 2064–2072.

Newman S, Hansen H. Frequency, diagnosis, and treatment of brain metastases in 249 consecutive patients with bronchogenic carcinoma. Cancer 1974; 33: 492–496.

Gheorghiade M et al. Vasopressin V_2 Receptor Blockade with Tolvaptan versus fluid restriction in the treatment of hyponatraemia. American Journal of Cardiology 2006; 97(7): 1064–1067.

Verbalis, JG, Goldsmith JR, Greenburg A, et al. Diagnosis, Evaluation, and Treatment of Hyponatremia: Expert Panel Recommendations. The American Journal of Medicine (2013) 126, S1–S42.

3. C. MR scan of the whole spine

Metastatic spinal cord compression (MSCC) is defined as compression of the dural sac and its contents by an extradural mass. It is a medical emergency. Neurological status at the time of diagnosis correlates with prognosis. Given that back pain is a common presenting symptom, it can be challenging to determine which patients have a serious spinal process underlying their symptoms. The key is to have a high index of suspicion in those with a previous history of malignancy and new onset back or neck pain. Education of patients at risk of metastatic spinal cord compression is recommended in National Institute for Health and Care Excellence (NICE) guidelines.

Bone metastases are common in patients with cancer and the most common site is the spinal column. It is estimated that 5–10% of patients with cancer develop MSCC. More than 60% of MSCC occurs in the thoracic spine and 17% of patients have two or more levels of cord compression.

Pain is the most common presenting symptom in patients with spinal metastases. The pain can be local, radicular, or mechanical (with pain on movement suggesting spinal instability). Motor and sensory changes may occur below the level of compression. Autonomic symptoms, including bowel and bladder dysfunction, can occur in 40–60% of patients with metastatic cord compression.

Where cord compression is suspected, urgent MR scan of the whole spine should be performed. Patients unable to have MRI should have a CT scan +/– myelogram.

National Institute for Health and Care Excellence. Clinical Guideline 75. Metastatic spinal cord compression in adults: diagnosis and management. November 2008.

Schiff D. Spinal cord compression. Neurologic Clinics 2003; 21: 67–86, viii.

Levack P, Graham J, Collie D et al. Don't wait for a sensory level—listen to the symptoms: a prospective audit of the delays in diagnosis of malignant cord compression. Clinical Oncology (R Coll Radiol) 2002; 14: 472–480.

Helweg-Larsen S, Sorensen P. Symptoms and signs in metastatic spinal cord compression: a study of progression from first symptom until diagnosis in 153 patients. European Journal of Cancer 1994; 30A: 396–398.

Loblaw DA, Perry J, Chambers A, Laperriere NJ. Systematic review of the diagnosis and management of malignant extradural spinal cord compression: the Cancer Care Ontario Practice Guidelines Initiative's Neuro-Oncology Disease Site Group. Journal of Clinical Oncology 2005; 23: 2028–2037.

4. C. Referral to the interventional radiologist for CT-guided biopsy

80% of superior vena cava obstructions (SVCO) are due to malignancy. The most common malignant cause is non-small-cell lung cancer accounting for around 50% of cases. While SVCO may be asymptomatic, it can cause significant discomfort. The resulting increased venous pressure in the upper body can lead to oedema in the arms, neck, and head. Signs include plethora, cyanosis, and distended subcutaneous vessels. Swelling of the larynx can lead to cough, hoarseness, and dyspnoea. Headache and even coma can result from cerebral oedema.

History should focus on the length of symptoms, previous malignant diagnoses, and recent intravascular procedures. Onset of symptoms is usually gradual and can improve or stabilize with the development of collaterals. Chest X-ray may indicate widening of the mediastinum, but contrast enhanced CT scan is the most useful investigation. Where a malignant cause is suspected a tissue diagnosis should be obtained, as this will determine the most appropriate management of the obstruction and the malignancy.

The patient should be sat upright. Dexamethasone is commonly prescribed and may lead to symptomatic improvement, though the benefits have not been formally studied. In patients with chemosensitive cancers, such as small-cell lung cancers, lymphomas, or germ cell tumours, chemotherapy should be commenced as soon as possible. For patients with a short to medium life expectancy and less chemo-sensitive tumours, or life-threatening symptoms of SVCO, endovascular stenting should be considered. Stenting provides excellent and immediate symptomatic relief in the majority of cases. Radiotherapy is an alternative treatment but symptoms generally take 72 hours to improve and while symptomatic benefit is recorded in more than 60% of patients at two weeks, objective measures only show relief of the obstruction in a minority. Equally, chemotherapy can be used in this setting combined with or after radiotherapy. Surgical bypass grafting is rarely indicated; however, surgery may be the primary treatment of SVCO caused by a thymoma.

Ostler P, Clarke D, Watkinson A, Gaze M. Superior vena cava obstruction: a modern management strategy. Clinical Oncology (R Coll Radiol) 1997; 9: 83–89.

Yellin A, Rosen A,Reichert N, Lieberman Y. Superior vena cava syndrome. The myth—the facts. American Review of Respiratory Disease 1990; 141: 1114–1118.

Rowell N, Gleeson F. Steroids, radiotherapy, chemotherapy and stents for superior vena caval obstruction in carcinoma of the bronchus: a systematic review. Clinical Oncology (R Coll Radiol) 2002; 14: 338–351.

5. A. Commence broad-spectrum intravenous antibiotics (e.g. piperacillin–tazobactam) pending the blood results

Neutropenic sepsis is an acute medical emergency. This patient was nine days post chemotherapy, had symptoms of infection, and had a pyrexia at home. On admission, she was hypotensive and required urgent rehydration and immediate empiric broad-spectrum antibiotics without waiting for results of her full blood count. NICE guidance recommends initial treatment with piperacillin–tazobactam. Routine use of granulocyte colony stimulating factors (GCSF) is not recommended.

Neutropenic sepsis is defined as patients having anticancer treatment whose neutrophil count is 0.5×10^9 per litre or lower and who have either:

- a temperature higher than 38.0°C *or*
- other signs or symptoms consistent with clinically significant sepsis

Neutropenia is more common between days 7 and 14 of a typical 21-day cycle of chemotherapy.

Following initial treatment, the patient should be referred to their oncology team for review. Validated scoring systems (e.g. MASCC (Multinational Association for Supportive Care in Cancer risk index)) may be used to identify patients at low risk of complications from febrile neutropenia who can safely be switched to oral antibiotics and be offered early empiric outpatient treatment.

This patient would have a MASCC score of 18 on initial assessment and inpatient admission for intravenous antibiotics would be recommended.

National Institute for Health and Care Excellence. Clinical Guideline 151. Neutropenic sepsis: prevention and management of in people with cancer patients. September 2012.

6. B. Hypercalcaemia

This patient has a number of possible causes for confusion, although the biochemical profile indicated hypercalcaemia. His symptoms included confusion, anorexia, dehydration, and constipation.

Hypercalcaemia of malignancy is a potentially life-threatening complication of advanced cancer. It is most common in patients with metastatic prostate cancer, breast cancer, multiple myeloma, and non-small-cell lung cancer, although can occur with any cancer. Hypercalcaemia is often, but not always, associated with bone metastases.

Symptoms depend on the level of serum calcium and the rate of onset. They include nausea and vomiting, constipation, anorexia, polyuria and polydipsia, bone pain, lethargy, seizures, and confusion. Clinical signs may include dehydration, hyporeflexia, psychosis, and intestinal ileus. ECG changes can include arrhythmia, short QT, and prolonged PR intervals.

The diagnosis is usually confirmed with an elevated serum calcium. The calcium should be corrected for albumin. One formula that can be used is:

corrected calcium = measured calcium (mmol/L) + [40 − serum albumin (g/L)] × 0.027

Treatment depends on the severity of symptoms and the level of dehydration. Initial management should include intravenous 0.9% sodium chloride, usually 3–5 L/24 hours if dehydrated. Potassium should be corrected as indicated. An intravenous infusion of a bisphosphonate (e.g. pamidronate or zoledronic acid) is usually recommended, after rehydration, if the initial serum calcium is >3.0 mmol/L. The patient's existing medication should be reviewed and, where appropriate, stopped (e.g. calcium supplements, thiazides).

The patient should experience symptomatic improvement within 24 hours, although measured serum calcium may not normalize for 3–7days. Where possible, the underlying cause for the hypercalcaemia should be investigated and appropriate anti-cancer therapy initiated.

Body J. Hypercalcemia of malignancy. Seminars in Nephrology 2004; 24(1): 48–54. doi: org/10.1053/j.semnephrol.2003.08.015

7. D. Stop domperidone and start ondansetron 8 mg intravenously twice daily and inform the acute oncology service of patient's admission

Chemotherapy-induced nausea and vomiting (CINV) is one of the most frequent side effects experienced by patients undergoing chemotherapy. Patients naturally find it distressing and modern drug treatment can successfully control CINV for the majority of patients.

There are different classes of CINV (Table 10.2).

Table 10.2 Classes of CINV.

Acute	Experienced during the first 24-hour period immediately after chemotherapy administration.
Delayed	Nausea & vomiting that occurs more than 24 hours after chemotherapy and may continue for up to six or seven days after chemotherapy.
Anticipatory	Nausea & vomiting that occurs prior to the beginning of a new cycle of chemotherapy. It is either a learned response following CINV on a previous cycle or an anxiety response. It is most common after three to four cycles of chemotherapy where acute or delayed symptoms have been poorly controlled.
Refractory	Nausea & vomiting which persists despite treatment with both standard and rescue therapy.

This patient has acute CINV. The first thing to check is that the patient has been taking the prescribed antiemetic regime regularly if they are feeling nauseous. If this patient hadn't been using oral domperidone regularly, but was still able to keep tablets down, the first step would be to encourage regular oral antiemetic usage. As this patient cannot currently tolerate oral antiemetic medications, an alternative route for drug administration (such as the IV route) is required to control CINV.

The CINV developed despite taking regular oral domperidone. Domperidone and metoclopramide both act on dopaminergic pathways, and therefore should not be used together, as the risk of side effects is increased without additional clinical benefit. Cyclizine is an anti-histamine and anti-cholinergic. Like all anti-cholinergics, it should not be co-prescribed with prokinetics (e.g. metoclopramide or domperidone), since it antagonizes effects on the myenteric plexus in the bowel wall.

Aprepitant is a neurokinin-1 (NK-1) receptor antagonist and has been shown to inhibit emesis induced by chemotherapy agents, such as cisplatin, via central actions. Fosaprepitant is prodrug of aprepitant and is available in IV form. These two drugs are commonly used in the prevention of CINV in chemotherapy regimens with high emetogenic potential, but are not used to treat CINV once it has developed.

For this patient ondansetron (or another 5-HT3 receptor antagonist) is the best option and is particularly effective in controlling acute CINV. It is generally only used for a short period (i.e. two to three days maximum). Common side effects include constipation, dizziness, and headache.

Dexamethasone is helpful for delayed nausea and vomiting and is usually prescribed for one to three days after chemotherapy. This patient should continue with the dexamethasone as prescribed. Acute oncology is a nationwide initiative to improve the care of patients who have been admitted with side effects of anti-cancer treatment. Every Trust with an emergency department is expected to develop an acute oncology service and a patient with CINV should be referred to the service for advice.

Jordan K, Sippel C, Schmoll H. Guidelines for antiemetic treatment of chemotherapy-induced nausea and vomiting: past, present and future recommendations. The Oncologist 2007; 12: 1143–1150.

Leonard P. What is an acute oncology service? British Journal of Hospital Medicine 2011; 72(4): 184–185.

8. C. Refer to oncologist for consideration of palliative radiotherapy

This patient has metastatic disease from a likely cancer of the uterine cervix. Her main symptom is of persistent vaginal bleeding. While it would be appropriate to prescribe tranexamic acid in the first instance, this is unlikely to control the bleeding on its own. The cancer is not curable and treatment should be focused on palliating symptoms. Chemotherapy would not be appropriate and is unlikely to cause haemostasis. Palliative radiotherapy is effective at causing rapid haemostasis and should be well tolerated with manageable side effects.

More than 50% of patients will receive radiotherapy at some point during the treatment of their cancer and it remains the most important non-surgical intervention. External beam radiotherapy is effective in the palliation of patients with symptoms from cancer. Between 40–50% of those receiving radiotherapy are receiving treatment with palliative intent. It is particularly useful in treating pain from bone metastases but can also be used to prevent bleeding. Bleeding from lung, uterine, bladder, stomach, and rectal tumours has been shown to decrease after palliative radiotherapy. Bleeding from ulcerating tumours of the skin can also be rapidly stopped with radiotherapy. The mechanism of haemostasis from external beam radiotherapy is unclear but is thought to relate to damage to the tumour blood vessels.

The aim of palliative radiotherapy is to achieve symptom control as quickly as possible with minimal side effects and disruption to the patient. This can often be delivered as a single treatment, or two to five treatments (fractions) given over one week. For bone metastases, trials have reported an overall response rate of around 60–70%, with a complete response rate of around 30%. The same area can usually be treated more than once but occasionally the maximum dose of radiotherapy has already been delivered and no further treatment is possible.

Roos DE, Fisher RJ. Radiotherapy for painful bone metastases: an overview of the overviews. Clinical Oncology (R Coll Radiol) 2003; 15: 342–344.

9. A. Germ cell cancer

Testicular cancer has an age standardized incidence rate of 7.0 per 100,000 of the UK population with around 2,200 new cases per year in the UK. It is the commonest cancer in men aged 15–44 years with 47% cases diagnosed in men under the age of 35 years. Ninety five percent of testicular tumours are germ cell cancers. These can be further divided into seminomas and non-seminomas. The majority of men will present with a lump or swelling of the testicle. A small proportion will be diagnosed as a result of symptoms from metastatic disease with the most common sites of metastases being the retroperitoneal lymph nodes (causing back pain and abdominal swelling) or the lungs (causing shortness of breath and cough).

Further assessment of this patient should include testicular examination, scrotal ultrasound, CT scan of chest, abdomen and pelvis, serum tumour markers including AFP, HCG, and LDH. He should be referred for urgent oncology review. Initial treatment would be with a platinum-based chemotherapy schedule. Even with extensive metastatic disease, this patient has a potentially curable cancer with five-year survival rates ranging between 50% and 95% depending on the classification of the disease based on the sites of metastases and level of tumour marker expression. The mostly commonly used classification for metastatic disease is the International Germ Cell Consensus Classification.

International Germ Cell Consensus Classification: a prognostic factor-based staging system for metastatic germ cell cancers. International Germ Cell Cancer Collaborative Group. J. Clinical Oncology 1997; 15(2): 594–603.

10. C. Dexamethasone 16 mg and refer to the spinal surgeon for consideration of surgery

Once a diagnosis of metastatic spinal cord compression is confirmed, definitive treatment should start within 24 hours. Patients should be commenced on high-dose steroids (loading dose of dexamethasone 16 mg, then 8 mg bd) with gastric protection. They should be given appropriate analgesia and, if they have bladder dysfunction, a urinary catheter inserted. Trials suggest that in carefully selected patients, surgery followed by radiotherapy may lead to better outcomes. NICE recommends that patients with a prognosis of more than three months, and fit enough for surgery, should be discussed with the spinal surgeons if they have any of the following: spinal cord compression and paraplegia for less than 48 hours, an unstable spine, compression despite previous radiotherapy, radio-resistant tumours, and deteriorating neurological function. The majority of patients will not be suitable for surgery and urgent radiotherapy should be considered and discussed with the clinical oncologist. Chemotherapy may be appropriate primary treatment in some chemosensitive tumours such as lymphoma and small-cell lung cancer.

Graham P, Capp A, Delaney G et al. A pilot randomised comparison of dexamethasone 96 mg vs 16 mg per day for malignant spinal-cord compression treated by radiotherapy: TROG 01.05 Superdex study. Clinical Oncology (R Coll Radiol) 2006; 18: 70–76.

Patchell R, Tibbs P, Regine W et al. Direct decompressive surgical resection in the treatment of spinal cord compression caused by metastatic cancer: a randomised trial. Lancet 2005; 366: 643–648.

11. C. Send the patient home, advise her to stop the capecitabine tablets, and inform the acute oncology service/oncology team to follow up the patient

Capecitabine is a fluoropyrimidine antimetabolite that is converted to fluorouracil (FU) via a complex enzymatic pathway with its final activation preferentially occurring in tumour tissue. Capecitabine is commonly used in the treatment of breast, colorectal, stomach, and oesophageal malignancies. Cardiotoxicity has been reported in 1.2–18% of patients treated with FU and coronary vasospasm has been demonstrated in animal as well as human vascular studies during FU infusion.

Patients with fluoropyrimidine-induced vasospasm usually present with chest pain at rest and ischaemic ECG changes (but not always), and less frequently myocardial infarction, ventricular arrhythmias, and death. Typical presentations and pathophysiologic mechanisms of FU or capecitabine toxicity closely resemble variant angina. It classically manifests as chest pain at rest with ST segment changes caused by focal major coronary artery spasm that typically occurs at the sites of or adjacent to atherosclerotic fatty streaks or fibrous plaques. The main treatment of fluoropyrimidine-induced vasospasm is discontinuation of the drug, as the risk of cardiotoxicity increases with repeated administration. Informing the oncology team is good practice, as changes in the adjuvant treatment of this patient are likely to be necessary.

Jones RL, Ewer MS: Cardiac and cardiovascular toxicity of nonanthracycline anticancer drugs. Expert Review of Anticancer Therapy 2006; 6: 1249–1269.

Jensen SA, Sorensen JB: Risk factors and prevention of cardiotoxicity induced by 5-fluorouracil or capecitabine. Cancer Chemotherapy and Pharmacology 2006; 58: 487–493.

chapter 11

HAEMATOLOGY

QUESTIONS

1. **A 62-year-old woman attended the haematology clinic for assessment of a monoclonal protein of 12g/L. Examination showed no lymphadenopathy or hepatosplenomegaly but assessment of blood pressure showed a postural drop and peripheral oedema was noted. She had a mild normochromic normocytic anaemia.**

   ```
   Investigations:
     haemoglobin                      110 g/L          (130-180)
     white cell count                 7.2 × 10⁹/L      (4.0-11.0)
     platelet count                   230 × 10⁹/L      (150-400)
     serum sodium                     141 mmol/L       (137-144)
     serum potassium                  3.5 mmol/L       (3.5-4.9)
     serum urea                       6.3 mmol/L       (2.5-7.0)
     serum creatinine                 95 µmol/L        (60-110)
     serum-corrected calcium          2.32 mmol/L      (2.20-2.60)

     urinary protein: creatinine ratio    56 mg/mmol   (<30)
     urinary immunofixation showed free lambda light chains

     bone marrow assessment showed 8% plasma cells
   ```

   What is the most likely diagnosis?
   A. AL amyloidosis
   B. Hypertrophic cardiomyopathy
   C. Membranous glomerulopathy
   D. Monoclonal gammopathy of undetermined significance (MGUS)
   E. Multiple myeloma

2. An 18-year-old woman known to have sickle cell anaemia was seen on the acute medical unit. She had multiple previous hospital admissions and reported blood transfusions during some of these. She had chest pains worsening over a couple of days and had become breathless.

On examination, her temperature was 38.7°C. Pulse was 100 beats per minute and blood pressure was 120/85 mmHg. Her oxygen saturation was 94% on 10 litres of oxygen via a reservoir mask.

```
Investigations:
    haemoglobin         70 g/L              (130-180)
    white cell count    12.1 × 10⁹/L        (4.0-11.0)
    platelet count      340 × 10⁹/L         (150-400)
```

Which complication of sickle cell anaemia has occurred?

A. Acute chest syndrome
B. Aplastic crisis
C. Haemolytic crisis
D. Osteomyelitis
E. Pneumonia

3. **A 30-year-old man attended the haematology day unit following self-referral having received his second cycle of carboplatin for testicular seminoma through a peripherally inserted central catheter (PICC line) ten days ago.**

On examination, he had a fever of 38.2°C.

```
Investigations:
    haemoglobin         100 g/L             (130-180)
    white cell count    1.2 × 10⁹/L         (4.0-11.0)
    neutrophil count    0.4 × 10⁹/L         (1.5-7.0)
    platelet count      70 × 10⁹/L          (150-400)
```

What is the most appropriate management?

A. He has a PUO and needs a bone marrow biopsy to investigate for infection
B. He should be prescribed granulocyte colony stimulating factor (G-CSF)
C. He should be risk scored and may be discharged home on empirical oral antibiotics
D. He should stay on a fluroquinolone once recovered from this episode
E. His venous access device should be removed as part of the initial empiric management

4. **A 45-year-old man was admitted to the acute medical unit with pneumonia. On the ward round the venous thromboembolism (VTE) prophylaxis decision made by the admitting junior doctor was reviewed.**

   When preventing VTE in the hospitalized patient, which statement is correct?

   A. Anti-embolism stockings that provide graduated compression and produce a calf pressure of 14–15 mmHg should be used in appropriately identified patients
   B. If there is marking, blistering or discolouration of the skin, particularly over the heels and bony prominences, or if the patient experiences pain or discomfort, fit a pressure dressing inside the stocking over the affected area
   C. Offer anti-embolism stockings but not heparin for VTE prophylaxis to patients who are admitted for acute stroke
   D. Offer anti-embolism stockings but not heparin for VTE prophylaxis to patients with cancer
   E. Patients should be encouraged to wear their anti-embolism stockings during the day and to remove them at night, until they no longer have significantly reduced mobility

5. **A 75-year-old woman was assessed in the ambulatory clinic for a possible deep vein thrombosis (DVT).**

   In a patient with signs and symptoms of a possible DVT, the D-dimer test would not be useful under what circumstances?

   A. The two-level DVT Wells score is 'likely' and the proximal leg vein ultrasound test is negative
   B. The two-level DVT Wells score is 'likely' and the proximal leg vein ultrasound test is negative the following day
   C. The two-level DVT Wells score is 'likely' and the proximal leg vein ultrasound scan is positive
   D. The two-level DVT Wells score is 'likely' and the proximal leg vein ultrasound test is unavailable within four hours
   E. The two level DVT Wells score is 'unlikely'

6. **A 65-year-old woman had been diagnosed with pancreatic cancer. She came into the emergency department with sudden onset of right chest pain, breathlessness, and a small amount of haemoptysis.**

   On examination, she had a temperature of 38.0°C. Her pulse rate was 110 beats per minute with a blood pressure of 150/100 mmHg. She had no calf pain or swelling.

   What is the most appropriate next step in her management?

   A. Chest X-ray
   B. CT scan pulmonary angiogram
   C. D-dimer test
   D. Immediate parenteral anticoagulant therapy
   E. Proximal leg vein scan

7. A 55-year-old man had been diagnosed with an inoperable glioblastoma. He was admitted to the acute medical unit with shortness of breath. A pulmonary embolism was diagnosed, which was treated initially with low molecular weight heparin.

   What is the most appropriate management on discharge?
   A. Low molecular weight heparin is contraindicated in patients with a brain tumour so a direct thrombin inhibitor should be commenced and continued for six months
   B. Low molecular weight heparin should be continued for five days or until the international normalized ratio (INR), adjusted by a vitamin K antagonist, is 2 or above for at least 24 hours, whichever is longer
   C. Low molecular weight heparin should be continued for ten days or until the international normalized ratio (INR), adjusted by a vitamin K antagonist, is 2 or more for at least 24 hours, whichever is longer
   D. Low molecular weight heparin should be continued for six months. At six months, the risks and benefits of continuing anticoagulation should be assessed
   E. Low molecular weight heparin should be continued lifelong

8. A 58-year-old man was referred to the acute medical unit by his GP. The patient attended the GP surgery the previous week, complaining of increased tiredness and aching in his bones. A routine full blood count was sent which showed anaemia, leucocytosis with promyelocytes containing Auer rods, neutropenia, and thrombocytopenia. Overnight, the patient experienced bleeding gums, malaena, and noticed large bruises on his legs. He felt dizzy on standing.

   Which mechanism is active in the complication he has developed?
   A. Activation of anti-inflammatory molecules
   B. An increase in platelet aggregation
   C. Down regulation of expression of adhesion molecules on white blood cells
   D. Rapid fibrin removal due to an increased activity of the fibrinolytic system
   E. Tissue factor-mediated thrombin destruction

9. **A 45-year-old man was admitted to the acute medical unit with haematemesis and melaena. No previous history was available. He required fluid resuscitation and, following an eight-unit red cell transfusion, he was haemodynamically stable.**

```
Investigations:
   haemoglobin                         110 g/L          (130-180)
   white cell count                    10.0 × 10⁹/L     (4.0-11.0)
   platelet count                      80 × 10⁹/L       (150-400)
   prothrombin time                    14.2s            (11.5-15.5)
   international normalized ratio      1.3              (<1.4)
   activated partial                   32s              (30-40)
     thromboplastin time
   thrombin time                       17s              (15-19)
   fibrinogen                          2.1g/L           (1.8-5.4)
```

Which blood product should he be given at this stage?

A. Cryoprecipitate and fresh frozen plasma
B. Fresh-frozen plasma
C. Fresh-frozen plasma and platelets
D. No blood products are indicated
E. Platelets

10. **A 60-year-old woman had become severely breathlessness on the orthopaedic ward. She was receiving the third unit of a red-cell transfusion, following a total hip arthroplasty the previous day. The transfusion had been immediately stopped by the nursing staff. She had a past medical history of hypertension.**

    On examination, her temperature was 37.6°C and she was distressed. Her pulse rate was 110 beats per minute. Her blood pressure was 100/65 mmHg and the jugular venous pressure was not elevated. Her respiratory rate was 28 breaths per minute and her oxygen saturation was 98% on 10 litres of oxygen via a reservoir mask. There were bilateral lung crackles on auscultation.

    Chest X-ray showed bilateral pulmonary infiltrates with bronchoalveolar shadowing.

    What is the best management plan?

    A. Commence broad-spectrum intravenous antibiotics and continue supplemental oxygen and provide supportive care (including airway, ventilation, and haemodynamic support as necessary)
    B. Continue supplemental oxygen and provide supportive care (including airway, ventilation, and haemodynamic support as necessary)
    C. Continue supplemental oxygen, give IV morphine and a loop diuretic, stop the beta blocker, and give supportive care (including airway, ventilation, and haemodynamic support as necessary)
    D. Give intramuscular adrenaline, provide supportive care (including airway, ventilation, and haemodynamic support as necessary), give inhaled bronchodilators, an antihistamine, and corticosteroids
    E. Give paracetamol and restart the transfusion at a slower rate once her temperature falls below 37.5°C

chapter 11

HAEMATOLOGY

ANSWERS

1. A. AL amyloidosis

Light-chain (AL) amyloidosis is the commonest form of systemic amyloidosis. It is associated with an underlying plasma cell dyscrasia from which immunoglobulin light chains accumulate to give accumulation of amyloid in tissues. Diagnostic assessment includes distinguishing other causes of amyloidosis that may be present in an individual with coexisting monoclonal gammopathy of undetermined significance (MGUS) to inform the therapeutic approach.

It is difficult to distinguish hypertrophic cardiomyopathy from cardiac amyloidosis on clinical assessment. ECG typically shows changes of left ventricular hypertrophy in the former and low QRS voltages in the latter. Echocardiography has diagnostic criteria for hypertrophic cardiomyopathy, such as asymmetric septal hypertrophy. Diastolic dysfunction is an early feature in cardiac amyloidosis with other changes in more advanced disease. Cardiac MRI can help distinguish between the two syndromes.

Nephrotic syndrome is a complication of AL amyloidosis and has a similar presentation to membranous glomerulopathy. A renal or other tissue biopsy (rectal or abdominal wall fat aspiration) stained with Congo red would show the typical apple green birefringence of amyloid and light chain clonality may be demonstrable by immunostaining.

MGUS is an asymptomatic condition so cannot be the cause of significant degrees of proteinuria or cardiomyopathy. This diagnosis requires the finding of a monoclonal protein with no associated disease features (of plasma cell myeloma, lymphoma, or AL amyloidosis). There is a 1% per annum risk of progression to haematological malignancies and an increased risk of venous thromboembolism.

Plasma cell myeloma requires the presence of at least two from monoclonal protein in serum or urine, increased plasma cells in the marrow (>10%), and bone lesions. There are typically symptoms of bone pain, anaemia may be marked, hypercalcaemia is present at diagnosis in about half of cases, and renal failure in about one-fifth. Investigations should include FBC, renal function, calcium, serum and urine electrophoresis, (albumin and ß 2-microglobulin form a useful prognostic index for confirmed disease), bone marrow and skeletal survey to assess for lytic bone lesions, compression fractures, and diffuse osteoporosis.

AA amyloidosis occurs due to deposition of protein A (as opposed to immunoglobulin light chain in AL amyloidosis) in conditions with persistent inflammation such as rheumatoid arthritis, bronchiectasis, some malignancies, or familial fever syndromes. There is a different pattern of tissue involvement with liver, spleen, kidneys, and marrow involved in AA but also heart, nerves, skin, tongue, and connective tissues potentially involved in AL.

Gatt ME, Palladini G. Light chain amyloidosis 2012: a new era. British Journal of Haematology March 2013; 160(5): 582–598.

HAEMATOLOGY | ANSWERS

2. A. Acute chest syndrome

Sickling disorders occur in individuals with red cells that contain a sufficient proportion of haemoglobin S to undergo aggregation of deoxyhaemoglobin S. Such conditions include sickle cell disease (HbSS) and haemoglobin SC disease where a chronic haemolytic anaemia is interspersed with acute crises and accumulating sequelae of chronic disease. There is considerable variety in the degree that individuals are affected. Children most commonly have painful (vaso-occlusive) crises or infection whereas chronic manifestations of sickling are seen in adults. Crises may be precipitated by infection, dehydration, acidosis, or deoxygenation. Management in pregnancy requires specialist care.

Acute stroke is an acute complication of vaso-occlusive crisis affecting the brain or spinal cord. Occurrence is more common in children; by mid-forties, a quarter of patients will have had a stroke. Screening with transcranial Doppler has been used to select patients for transfusion regimens to reduce the stroke risk.

Pain is a common component of acute chest syndrome in which are seen fever, leucocytosis, and pulmonary infiltrates. This is a visceral sequestration crisis involving the lungs and is the commonest cause of death in post-pubertal sickle cell patients. Careful monitoring is required with appropriate escalation through management with analgesia, oxygen, hydration, exchange transfusion, and ventilation for respiratory support.

Aplastic crisis occurs as a result of infection, such as with parvovirus or folate deficiency. An acute fall in haemoglobin due to failure of erythrocyte production and recticulocytopenia occurs.

Infection is a major cause of mortality in children and the basis for sickle cell disease screening programmes to allow pneumococcal vaccination and penicillin prophylaxis to be given. In sickle cell disease, sickling leads to splenic infarction in adulthood but in childhood and those with other sickling disorders there may be splenomegaly and even splenic sequestration crisis.

Sickling in bone causes bone infarction which can cause dactylitis in children (hand–foot syndrome) but by adulthood avascular necrosis of femoral or humeral heads may require surgical intervention. Bone infarction increases the risk of osteomyelitis with causative agents including Salmonella and Staphylococcus aureus.

Vaso-occlusive crisis is the most common form of crisis seen in sickle cell disease. Vascular occlusion may lead to infarcts in organs including bone where hips, shoulders, and vertebrae are commonly involved giving the typical presentation with bone pain. Involvement of others organs may be seen—lungs, spleen, liver, central nervous system, and eye where neovascularization should be screened for.

Haemolytic crisis usually occurs as a life-threatening complication of painful vaso-occlusive crisis. There is hyperhaemolysis and fall in haemoglobin for which transfusion support can be extremely challenging.

National Institute for Health and Care Excellence. Clinical Guideline 143. Sickle cell disease: managing acute painful episodes in hospital. June 2012.

3. C. He should be risk scored and may be discharged home on empirical oral antibiotics

This is a young man presenting with a neutropenic fever. Appropriate assessment includes vital signs and clinical examination (including the venous access line site and mouth); followed by assessment of blood count, renal and liver function, blood cultures (central and peripheral), and chest X-ray. Bone marrow assessment is not required.

Granulocyte colony stimulating factor (G-CSF) is not indicated in this setting. In some circumstances, such as severe infection post cytotoxic therapy, it may be used to shorten the duration of neutropenia (or used routinely to mobilize stem cells into the peripheral blood for harvest by leukapheresis).

There is no evidence at this point that the venous access device is the source of infection. It is, therefore, reasonable to leave the device *in situ* pending the outcome of investigations and treatment.

Established risk-scoring systems have been developed to identify patients as relatively low risk of harm from neutropenic sepsis by consideration of factors such as level of neutropenia, likely duration, and evidence of organ dysfunction. A favourable risk assessment may allow outpatient antibiotic therapy with an appropriate regimen.

Unless there is a specific complicating factor for which antibiotic prophylaxis is recommended, there is no indication for fluroquinolone prophylaxis, which may increase the risk of C. difficile infection or emergence of resistant organisms.

National Institute for Health and Care Excellence. Clinical Guideline 151. Neutropenic sepsis: prevention and management in people with cancer. September 2012.

4. A. Anti-embolism stockings that provide graduated compression and produce a calf pressure of 14–15 mmHg should be used in appropriately identified patients

A risk assessment for venous thromboembolism is part of the management of all patients, together with an assessment of the risks of the various potential interventions. Where there is considered to be a significant risk of VTE developing, but there are contraindications to pharmacological preparations, mechanical methods such as class 1 (14–15 mmHg) compression anti-embolism stockings (AESs) may be used.

In contrast to use in control of chronic venous insufficiency, AESs should be used until mobility is regained.

Damage to the skin, abnormal leg shape, impaired sensation, and significant peripheral vascular disease (ankle-brachial pressure index <0.8) may be a caution or contraindication to use of AESs.

Acute stroke, whether haemorrhagic or ischaemic, is a contraindication to pharmacological thromboprophylaxis. Trial data show that mechanical compression with AESs increases the rate of complications without a reduction in the rate of DVT.

Patients with cancer have an increased risk of VTE and are likely to benefit from thromboprophylaxis given in line with a suitable risk assessment.

National Institute for Health and Care Excellence. Clinical Guideline 92. Venous thromboembolism: reducing the risk for patients in hospital. January 2010.

5. C. The two-level DVT Wells score is 'likely' and the proximal leg vein ultrasound test is positive

The two-level DVT Wells score combines ten factors to quantitate the likelihood that symptoms in the leg are due to DVT and stratify further assessment.

A low-risk score where DVT is unlikely should lead to a D-dimer assessment and if that is negative DVT, investigation terminated.

A higher-risk score where DVT is likely should lead to Doppler ultrasound assessment of the leg to look for thrombus. However, if there is likely to be a delay of more than four hours to the scan then a D-dimer is used to guide a decision on administering parenteral anticoagulation. Furthermore, should an ultrasound be negative at initial presentation or when delayed to the following day, assessment of the D-dimer is used to direct care.

A two-level Wells score of likely should lead to an ultrasound of the leg and, if this is positive, DVT is diagnosed and there is no indication to undertake D-dimer testing.

National Institute for Health and Care Excellence. Clinical Guideline 144. Venous thromboembolic diseases: diagnosis, management and thrombophilia testing. June 2012.

HAEMATOLOGY | ANSWERS

6. A. Chest X-ray

Pulmonary embolism (PE) is in the differential diagnosis. However, to apply the two-level Wells score for PE, another cause (such as pneumonia) should be excluded (by history, clinical examination, and chest radiograph) before moving further down the PE diagnostic algorithm. The two-level Wells score for PE may be significantly altered by the chest radiograph finding as 'pulmonary embolism is the most likely clinical diagnosis' gives a score of 3, with a total score of 4 being the threshold of 'PE likely'.

Where PE is suspected and two-level PE Wells score is 'likely', either organize an immediate computed tomography pulmonary angiogram (CTPA) or interim parenteral anticoagulant therapy followed by CTPA, if a CTPA cannot be carried out immediately. Consider a proximal leg vein Doppler ultrasound scan if the CTPA is negative and DVT is suspected. In patients where PE is suspected and two-level PE Wells score is unlikely, undertake a D-dimer test and, if the result is positive, offer either an immediate CTPA or immediate interim parenteral anticoagulant therapy followed by a CTPA, if a CTPA cannot be carried out immediately.

It is suggested that for patients over 40 years of age in whom first idiopathic VTE is diagnosed that investigations for cancer are considered with an abdomino-pelvic CT scan (and a mammogram for women).

National Institute for Health and Care Excellence. Clinical Guideline 144. Venous thromboembolic diseases: diagnosis, management and thrombophilia testing. June 2012.

7. D. Low molecular weight heparin should be continued for six months. At six months, the risks and benefits of continuing anticoagulation should be assessed

The cancers most strongly associated with venous thromboembolism (VTE) when cases are adjusted for disease prevalence, are cancer of the pancreas, ovary, and brain. Overall, cancer has an approximately fourfold risk of thrombosis, which is increased during treatment with chemotherapy to 6.5-fold, so that there is estimated to be an approximate annual incidence of VTE of 1 of 200 in cancer patients.

In cancer patients, clinical trial data show an improved outcome (relative risk reduction of 52%) in terms of recurrence of VTE in patients treated with low molecular weight heparin (LMWH) rather than a vitamin K antagonist in the six months after diagnosis of VTE. Of note, the clinical trial did not use full-dose LMWH for all of the six months, but the dose was reduced to 75% after the four weeks of therapy. In the warfarin arm, there was no evidence that poor INR control was the explanation for more VTE in the warfarin arm. There was no significant difference in the bleeding risk.

Novel oral anticoagulation agents (NOACs), such as apixaban, dabigatran, and rivaroxaban, may be used in the UK for VTE prevention and treatment. None of the NOACs have been tested to show equivalent or better efficacy and safety than LMWH in the treatment of cancer-related VTE.

Khorana AA, McCrae KR. Risk stratification strategies for cancer-associated thrombosis: an update. Thrombosis Research May 2014; 133(Suppl 2): S35–S38.

8. D. Rapid fibrin removal due to an increased activity of the fibrinolytic system

The patient developed a coagulopathy due to underlying acute myelogenous leukaemia (AML). The features described point to acute promyelocytic leukaemia (APL), which accounts for approximately 10–15% of adult cases of AML. Cytogenetically, APL is identified by a translocation between chromosomes 15 and 17, which results in formation of fusion gene between ProMyelocytic Leukemia and Retinoic Acid Receptor Alpha genes. This determines the particular sensitivity of APL to all-trans retinoic acid that dramatically increases the likelihood of early control of the disease and associated coagulopathy with consequent survival, although bleeding haemostasis-related complications remain the major cause of death.

The coagulopathy is caused by the leukaemic cells which express activators of coagulation such as tissue factor (leading to disseminated intravascular coagulation) and fibrinolysis such as annexin II (leading to hyperfibrinolysis), as well as proteases and cytokines. Thrombocytopenia is contributed to by failure of platelet production due to marrow invasion. At presentation, the predominant feature is usually hyperfibrinolysis. Blood-product support and early initiation of all-trans retinoic acid are important.

Kell J, Knapper S, Burnett A. 'Acute myeloid leukaemia', Oxford textbook of medicine. Edited by Warrell D, Cox T, Firth J. 5th edition. Oxford: OUP, 2010.

9. D. No blood products are indicated

Acute hospitals have protocols for emergency presentations such as this where the policy for massive transfusion applies. Decisions on transfusion of blood products should recognize that over-transfusion may be as damaging as under-transfusion by exposing patients to the risk of fluid overload and other complications of transfusion. Do not offer platelet transfusion to patients who are not actively bleeding and are haemodynamically stable. Platelets may be given to those actively bleeding and have a platelet count of less than $50 \times 10^9/L$. Offer fresh frozen plasma to bleeding patients who have either a prothrombin time or activated partial thromboplastin time greater than 1.5 times normal; and cryoprecipitate or fibrinogen concentrate to those with a fibrinogen level of less than 1 g/L. Offer prothrombin complex concentrate to patients who are taking warfarin and actively bleeding. Treat patients who are taking warfarin and whose upper gastrointestinal bleeding has stopped in line with local warfarin protocols. Bleeding in a patient treated with the NOACs may also benefit from intervention with prothrombin complex concentrate, or FEIBA (Factor Eight Bypassing Activity—contains factors II, IX and X, and activated factor VII) or recombinant activated factor VII.

Do not use recombinant factor VIIa as it has no proven place in the management of acute haemorrhage.

Perrotta PL, Han Y, Snyder EL. 2010 'Blood transfusion', Oxford textbook of medicine. Edited by Warrell D, Cox T, Firth J. 5th edition. Oxford: OUP, 2010.

10. B. Continue supplemental oxygen and provide supportive care (including airway, ventilation, and haemodynamic support as necessary)

The management is based on the correct diagnosis, which in this case is transfusion-associated lung injury (TRALI).

In an acute haemolytic transfusion reaction, the patient may express a 'sense of illness'; respiratory distress; rigors; collapse; hypo- or hypertension; urticaria; chest, bone, or muscle pain; and dark urine. The blood transfusion should be stopped immediately. Take sample for FBC, coagulation, renal and liver function, group and save, and blood cultures. Send the blood unit back for investigation. The patient should be resuscitated with normal saline to prevent oliguric renal failure. If the urine output is not adequate, despite fluid resuscitation, forced diuresis may be attempted. Antibiotics should be given if bacterial infection is suspected. Seek intensive care and haematology advice.

TRALI is associated with fever, chills, and left ventricular failure. The central venous pressure (CVP) is not elevated whereas this is the case in fluid overload. Management is similar to that of adult respiratory distress syndrome and can range from supplemental oxygen by facemask for a brief period to mechanical ventilation for a period of days, depending on the severity. Resolution of the syndrome typically occurs within seven days following transfusion.

Mild allergic reactions may be treated with chlorpheniramine and the transfusion restarted when symptoms resolve. Severe reactions cause bronchospasm, angioedema, and abdominal pain. The transfusion should be stopped and retained for investigation as already indicated. Give chlorpheniramine, oxygen, and salbutamol nebulizer. If severe hypotension is present, IM adrenaline should be administered. Normal saline should be given to support the circulation. Future blood units may need to be washed and supplied as a special blood product.

Cardiogenic oedema occurs when the fluid volume or transfusion rate is excessive. Treat for an acute exacerbation of congestive cardiac failure (i.e. give oxygen and diuretics). Volume overload is a particular risk with the use of 20% albumin solution.

If the fever has occurred before completion of the transfusion, then allergic transfusion reaction should be considered and the transfusion should be discontinued until a haemolytic reaction has been ruled out. Once symptoms subside, the patient may be transfused with a new component. The remainder of the implicated component should not be transfused to the patient. An antipyretic, such as paracetamol, may be administered for patient comfort.

Bacterial contamination causes a very severe acute reaction with rapid onset of hyper- or hypotension, rigors, and collapse. The presentation is similar to acute haemolytic transfusion reactions or severe acute allergic reactions. Bacterial contamination of blood components is rare but evidence for it may be obtained from the abnormal appearance of the unit being transfused. Treat in the same way as potential acute haemolytic reaction, and give antibiotics against the likely range of bacteria—this may be achieved by following the local protocol for antibiotic management of neutropenic sepsis (commonly piperacillin/tazobactam).

http://www.transfusionguidelines.org.uk

chapter 12

INFECTIOUS DISEASES AND HIV

QUESTIONS

1. A 22-year-old woman returned two months ago from a four-week trip to Kenya. She took mefloquine as antimalarial prophylaxis, which she stopped on return to the UK, and was up to date with vaccinations against yellow fever, typhoid, rabies, and hepatitis A and B. She had developed fever three days earlier, which was associated with headaches, rigors, and myalgia. On the day of admission she was confused and had profuse watery diarrhoea. She had vomited bile twice in the acute medical unit.

   On examination, she had a temperature of 40°C, pulse 120 beats per minute and regular, and blood pressure 90/50 mmHg. Fundoscopy revealed a small retinal haemorrhage on the left. She had reduced tissue turgor but there was no lymphadenopathy. There was no meningism. Respiratory and abdominal examinations were normal. She weighed 60 kg.

   ```
   Investigations:
      haemoglobin                        102 g/L           (130-180)
      white cell count                   3.8 × 10⁹/L       (4.0-11.0)
      platelet count                     106 × 10⁹/L       (150-400)
      serum sodium                       132 mmol/L        (137-144)
      serum potassium                    3.2 mmol/L        (3.5-4.9)
      serum urea                         11.5 mmol/L       (2.5-7.0)
      serum creatinine                   148 µmol/L        (60-110)
      serum total bilirubin              28 µmol/L         (1-22)
      serum alanine aminotransferase     54 U/L            (5-35)
      serum alkaline phosphatase         120 U/L           (45-105)
      serum glucose                      2.2 mmol/L

      blood film revealed 2% trophozoites of plasmodium falciparum
   ```

   What immediate management is required?

   A. Intravenous artesunate bolus
   B. Intravenous dextrose saline infused over 30 minutes
   C. Intravenous glucose 10% bolus
   D. Intravenous quinine bolus
   E. Intravenous quinine infused over four hours

2. A 32-year-old man presented with a five-day history of fever, severe myalgia, headaches, mild photophobia, and cramping abdominal pain. He had just returned from a two-week holiday in Honduras. He had initially been prescribed trimethoprim two days earlier for a presumed urinary tract infection. Three days before admission he developed large volume watery diarrhoea, but by the day of admission the stool volume had reduced, and he was producing frequent small volumes of liquid stool with mucus and blood.

On examination, his temperature was 39°C. He had mild neck stiffness. Kernig sign was negative. Fundoscopy was normal. Abdominal examination revealed a tender abdomen without guarding. Bowel sounds were active. There was no organomegaly and no masses felt. Rectal examination revealed pink-tinged mucus and an otherwise empty rectum.

```
Investigations:
    haemoglobin                         145 g/L             (130-180)
    white cell count                    7.9 × 10⁹/L         (4.0-11.0)
    neutrophil count                    5.2 × 10⁹/L         (1.5-7.0)
    lymphocyte count                    0.9 × 10⁹/L         (1.5-4.0)
    monocyte count                      1.4 × 10⁹/L         (<0.8)
    eosinophil count                    0.2 × 10⁹/L         (0.04-0.40)
    platelet count                      279 × 10⁹/L         (150-400)
    serum creatinine                    137 µmol/L          (60-110)
    serum total bilirubin               7 µmol/L            (1-22)
    serum alanine aminotransferase      39 U/L              (5-35)
    serum alkaline phosphatase          120 U/L             (45-105)
    serum albumin                       32 g/L              (37-49)

    cerebrospinal fluid appeared clear and colourless
    total protein                       0.28 g/L            (0.15-0.45)
    cell count                          122/µL              (≤5)
    white cell count                    2/µL                (≤5)
    red cell count                      120/µL              (0)
    no organisms seen on direct microscopy
```

What is the most likely diagnosis?
A. Clostridium difficile infection
B. Enterotoxigenic eschericia coli infection
C. Katayama fever
D. Shigella flexneri infection
E. Viral meningitis

3. A 27-year-old man presented with fever, headache, a dry cough, and bloody diarrhoea. Symptoms started eight days ago. Eight weeks earlier he had been on an adventure holiday in Zambia with a group of friends, which involved rafting and visiting a game reserve. A couple of his friends had developed a similar illness.

On examination, he was febrile, and was noted to have an urticarial rash on his trunk. He had a polyphonic wheeze in both lung fields and the tip of his spleen was palpable.

```
Investigations:
    haemoglobin           134 g/L              (130-180)
    white cell count      12.2 × 10⁹/L         (4.0-11.0)
    neutrophil count      6.5 × 10⁹/L          (1.5-7.0)
    lymphocyte count      1.1 × 10⁹/L          (1.5-4.0)
    monocyte count        1.5 × 10⁹/L          (<0.8)
    eosinophil count      3.4 × 10⁹/L          (0.04-0.40)
    platelet count        350 × 10⁹/L          (150-400)
    stool negative for ova, cysts, and parasites
```

What is the pathogen causing the patient's symptoms?

A. Dengue virus
B. Epstein–Barr virus
C. Human immunodeficiency virus (HIV)
D. Leptospira icterohaemorrhagica
E. Schistosoma mansoni

4. A 37-year-old man had been complaining of intermittent itchy swellings on his right wrist and forearm over the last few months lasting two to four days before subsiding; they were sometimes painful. He was otherwise well. He had been working in Nigeria for two years in oil exploration.

Clinical examination was normal.

```
Investigations:
    haemoglobin           142 g/L              (130-180)
    white cell count      9.2 × 10⁹/L          (4.0-11.0)
    neutrophil count      3.5 × 10⁹/L          (1.5-7.0)
    lymphocyte count      2.1 × 10⁹/L          (1.5-4.0)
    monocyte count        1.1 × 10⁹/L          (<0.8)
    eosinophil count      2.1 × 10⁹/L          (0.04-0.40)
    platelet count        310 × 10⁹/L          (150-400)
```

What is the most likely diagnosis?

A. Cysticercosis
B. Guinea worm infection
C. Loa loa infection
D. Onchocerciasis
E. Trichinosis

5. **A 45-year-old man was admitted to the acute medical unit with an 11-day history of a swinging pyrexia associated with profuse sweats, anorexia, and malaise. He had spent the last six months travelling overland through Central America, and returned three weeks ago.**

   Abdominal examination revealed tenderness in the right upper quadrant.

   ```
   Investigations:
     haemoglobin                      122 g/L              (130-180)
     white cell count                 18.2 × 10⁹/L         (4.0-11.0)
     neutrophil count                 15.2 × 10⁹/L         (1.5-7.0)
     platelet count                   460 × 10⁹/L          (150-400)
     serum total bilirubin            18 µmol/L            (1-22)
     serum alanine aminotransferase   36 U/L               (5-35)
     serum alkaline phosphatase       150 U/L              (45-105)
     serum albumin                    28 g/L               (37-49)

     blood culture result was pending

     Chest X-ray showed atelectatic changes in the right lower
        zone with an elevated right hemidiaphragm and small right-
        sided pleural effusion.
     Ultrasound scan of abdomen showed a hypoechoic lesion
        measuring 4 cm in the right lobe of the liver.
   ```

   What test is most likely to provide the diagnosis?
   A. Aspirate from liver lesion
   B. Blood culture
   C. CT scan of thorax
   D. Serology
   E. Stool microscopy

6. A 28-year-old woman presented with fever, anorexia, and vomiting. She had a fleeting macular rash at the outset, and her friends thought that her face appeared a little puffy. During the second week her sore throat intensified, and she was admitted with difficulty in swallowing.

On examination, she looked unwell. She had generalized lymphadenopathy and was noted to have an urticarial rash. She was faintly jaundiced, and her spleen was palpable. Her temperature was 39.5°C.

```
Investigations:
    haemoglobin           141 g/L           (130-180)
    white cell count      9.5 × 10⁹/L       (4.0-11.0)
    neutrophil count      3.5 × 10⁹/L       (1.5-7.0)
    lymphocyte count      4.8 × 10⁹/L       (1.5-4.0)
    monocyte count        0.7 × 10⁹/L       (<0.8)
    platelet count        220 × 10⁹/L       (150-400)

    blood film atypical lymphocytes
    Paul Bunnell is positive
```

Which of these is commonly associated with this condition?

A. Droplet transmission from sneezing
B. Hepatomegaly
C. Infection of T lymphocytes
D. Sarcoma
E. Splenomegaly

7. A 25-year-old woman returned from South Africa where she had been teaching orphaned children for the last year. She had been unwell for six weeks with fevers, night sweats, and a dry cough. She had become increasingly breathless over the last two weeks, which precipitated this admission.

On admission, she had a temperature of 37.9°C. There was dullness to percussion with absence of breath sounds at the right base. The rest of the clinical examination was unremarkable.

Broad-spectrum antibiotics were commenced after a diagnostic aspiration of her pleural effusion was performed, which led to symptomatic improvement.

```
Investigations:
  chest X-ray showed a right pleural effusion
  pleural aspirate: straw coloured fluid
  protein 33 g/L
  lactate dehydrogenase 1059 IU/L
  cells: 1,000 lymphocytes
  auramine stain: negative
  gram stain: negative
  day ten: mycobacterial growth in liquid culture
```

What is the most appropriate course of action?

A. Arrange bronchoalveolar lavage before starting quadruple therapy for tuberculosis.
B. Await further identification before commencing treatment
C. Notify as tuberculosis but await culture sensitivities before commencing therapy
D. Start quadruple antituberculous therapy and notify as tuberculosis
E. Start quadruple antituberculous therapy but await culture confirmation of mycobacterium tuberculosis before notifying

8. A 24-year-old woman returned from a two-week trip to Thailand eight days ago. She had stayed mainly in tourist resorts, but had also travelled to rural areas. She had travelled with her long-term boyfriend and denied any other sexual partners. She became ill four days earlier with fever, headache, and myalgia. She had several presumed insect bites to her arms and legs, and one lesion on her thigh had developed a 9mm black scab-like centre with an erythematous border. The left inguinal nodes were swollen and tender.

She was admitted for further investigations, and commenced empirically on flucloxacillin for presumed infected insect bites. Her headache worsened and she developed a cough. She was also noted to have conjunctival suffusion and splenomegaly. Two days after admission she developed a sparse maculopapular rash with petechial elements mainly on the trunk and proximal limbs.

How did she contract this?

A. Bite from Aedes Egyptii mosquito
B. Bite from a flea
C. Bite from anopheline mosquito
D. Bite from a rat
E. Bite from a trombiculid mite

9. **A 65-year-old Peruvian woman was visiting her daughter in London. She had a grand mal seizure and was brought to the emergency department. On arrival, she was complaining of right hip pain.**

Investigations:

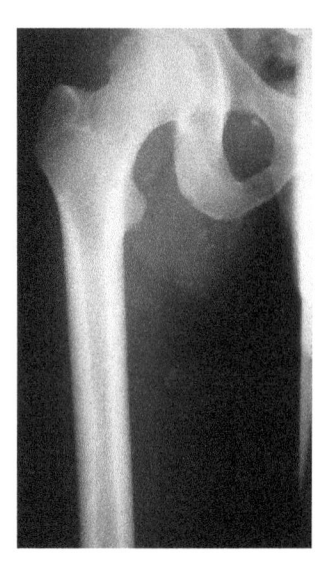

Figure 12.1 X-ray right hip.

What can you tell the daughter about this condition?
A. Her mother acquired this by ingesting food contaminated with human urine
B. Serological tests are not useful in diagnosis
C. She is likely to require lifelong anticonvulsants even with definitive treatment
D. Steroids should be avoided in treating this condition
E. The intermediate host is the pig

10. A 25-year-old cross-country athlete presented with a six-week history of worsening headache and pain across his shoulders that radiated down both arms. Writing had become difficult, and he was unable to button his shirts. He also had word finding difficulties and memory loss over the last six weeks.

Examination of his cranial nerves revealed a partial left-lower motor neurone facial palsy. He had grade 4/5 **MRC** power in all movements in the muscles of his hands. His reflexes were normal and plantars were down going. Inspection of his skin was unremarkable.

```
Investigations:
  MR scan of brain and cervical spine were normal
  chest X-ray was normal
  full blood count, urea, and electrolytes as well as liver
  function tests were all normal
  serum C-reactive protein            15mg/L          (<10)
  serum angiotensin-converting        32 U/L          (25-82)
    enzyme
  cerebrospinal fluid:
  total protein                       0.8 g/L         (0.15-0.45)
  cell count                          160/µL          (≤5)
  white cell count                    160/µL          (≤5)
  red cell count                      0/µL            (0)
  lymphocyte count                    160/µL          (≤3)
  neutrophil count                    0/µL            (0)
  Indian ink stain: negative
  Ziehl-Nielsen stain: negative
  oligoclonal IgG studies: identical bands in serum and CSF
```

What is the most likely diagnosis?

A. Borrelia burgdorferi infection
B. Cryptococcal meningitis
C. Multiple sclerosis
D. Secondary syphilis
E. Tuberculous meningitis

11.
A 19-year-old woman was admitted with diarrhoea, vomiting, and myalgia for the last 24 hours. She was recovering from chickenpox. She had no past medical history.

On examination, she looked unwell with conjunctival suffusion and appeared confused. She had a diffuse blanching erythematous rash with multiple healing chickenpox scabs. A couple of scabs were red and hot. Her temperature was 40.0°C with a pulse of 120 beats per minute. Her blood pressure was 85/40 mmHg.

```
Investigations:
   haemoglobin                       142 g/L          (130-180)
   white cell count                  7.5 × 10⁹/L      (4.0-11.0)
   platelet count                    89 × 10⁹/L       (150-400)
   serum urea                        8.9 mmol/L       (2.5-7.0)
   serum creatinine                  187 µmol/L       (60-110)
   serum total bilirubin             16 µmol/L        (1-22)
   serum alanine aminotransferase    124 U/L          (5-35)
   serum alkaline phosphatase        197 U/L          (45-105)
   serum creatine kinase             508 U/L          (24-170)

   cerebrospinal fluid results were normal
   blood cultures: no growth at 48 hours
```

What is the most likely diagnosis?

A. Chickenpox encephalitis
B. Kawasaki disease
C. Parvovirus infection
D. Staphylococcal toxic shock syndrome
E. Streptococcal infection

12.
A 25-year-old woman presented with a five-day history of a coryzal illness with high fever. She noticed a rash three days ago, appearing behind her ears and on her face. By the second day, the rash had spread to her chest, and on the day she presented it was on her trunk and proximal limbs, and she had developed a chesty cough.

Two weeks earlier her 3-year-old nephew had a similar illness, and was currently an inpatient being treated for pneumonia.

On examination, she had a widespread maculopapular rash. She had marked conjunctivitis, and her face appeared puffy. She had fine crackles in both lung fields.

What is the most likely diagnosis?

A. Measles
B. Mycoplasma pneumonia
C. Parvovirus infection
D. Pharyngoconjunctival fever
E. Rubella

13. **A 14-year-old girl presented with painful blisters in her mouth. She had a fever, anorexia, and a severe headache.**

    On examination, her temperature was 38.1°C. She had shallow ulcers on her tongue, gums buccal mucosa, and chin. She had symmetrical cervical lymphadenopathy in the posterior and anterior triangles. There was no meningism.

    What is the most likely diagnosis?
    A. Chickenpox
    B. Hand, foot, and mouth disease
    C. Herpangina
    D. Periodic fever, aphthous pharyngitis, and cervical adenopathy (PFAPA) syndrome
    E. Primary herpes gingivostomatitis

14. **A 45-year-old man had been working as an aid worker in the Dominican Republic. Two days after he returned to the UK he developed sudden onset watery diarrhoea and had been incontinent of faeces. He was complaining of muscle cramps. He had been symptomatic for eight hours.**

    On examination, he was apyrexial. He had sunken eyes and reduced tissue turgor with cold peripheries. His pulse was 100 beats per minute and thready.

    ```
    Investigations:
      haemoglobin          185 g/L           (130-180)
      white cell count     8.1 × 10⁹/L       (4.0-11.0)
      platelet count       405 × 10⁹/L       (150-400)
      haematocrit          0.61              (0.40-0.52)
    ```

    What does the pathophysiology of this condition include?
    A. Enterocyte chloride channels are closed
    B. Enterocyte sodium chloride co-transport mechanism is inhibited
    C. Metabolic alkalosis is a recognized complication
    D. Pathogen is enteroinvasive
    E. Toxin binds to adenylate cyclase decreasing cyclic AMP

15. **A 24-year-old woman who was usually fit and well presented to the acute medical unit with a six-day history of sore throat and persistent cough associated with tracheitis. She had a severe headache and myalgia. She had noticed some diarrhoea and in the last 24 hours her urine had become dark.**

    On examination, she had a temperature of 40.0°C. Her respiratory rate was 24, and she was noted to have a widespread maculopapular rash with some target lesions. Respiratory examination was normal.

    ```
    Investigations:
       chest X-rays showed bilateral fluffy shadows in both lung
          fields
       blood tests reveal the presence of cold agglutinins
    ```

    What is the treatment of this condition?

    A. Aciclovir
    B. Coamoxiclav
    C. Cotrimoxazole
    D. Doxycycline
    E. Oseltamivir

16. **A 33-year-old woman was admitted with breathlessness and confusion. She became unwell five days ago with fever and myalgia. A day later she developed a vesicular rash, which appeared first on her chest, but spread to her face and limbs. She was 30 weeks pregnant.**

   Investigations:

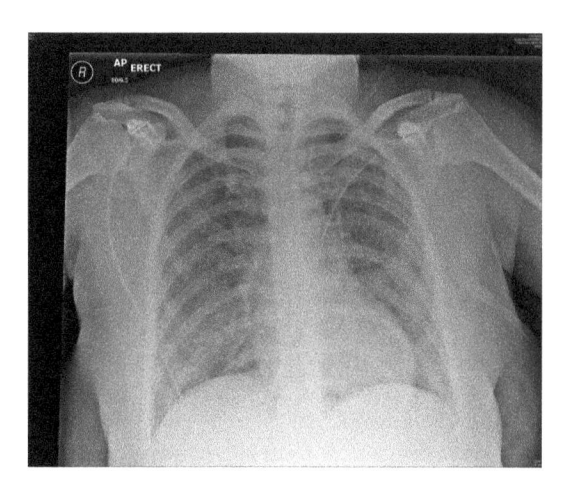

   Figure 12.2 Chest X-ray.

   ```
   arterial blood gases, breathing air:
   PO2      8 kPa     (11.3-12.6)
   PCO2     4 kPa     (4.7-6.0)
   ```

   What could be said about this woman's illness or its management?
   A. Aciclovir should be avoided as she is pregnant
   B. Pregnancy is not likely to influence the evolution
   C. Rash density does not correlate with severity
   D. She should receive broad-spectrum antibiotics
   E. The rash distribution is typically centrifugal

17. A 28-year-old woman from India presented to the dermatology department with a rash consisting of several reddish macules on her face, trunk, and limbs. Some were hypopigmented. Over the previous six months, she had become aware of reduced sensation in both hands and her right foot, and had a trophic ulcer on her right foot. She was noted to have thickened greater auricular and ulnar nerves, reduced sensation to light touch in a glove and stocking distribution beyond the palmar crease on her right hand and fingertips on the left, and the right forefoot. Some of the macules were noted to be anaesthetic.

    What can be said of the likely diagnosis in this lady?
    A. BCG offers no protection
    B. It is highly contagious
    C. It is likely that she caught this from a nine-banded armadillo
    D. The neuropathy would be expected to recover with antibiotic therapy
    E. Steroids can be a useful adjunct to treatment

18. A 37-year-old man who was HIV positive had disengaged from services and stopped all therapy two years ago. He was diagnosed with HIV five years previously and his virus had been well controlled, but he disliked taking regular medication and had stopped his treatment. He had declined the offer to restart HIV therapy nine months previously when admitted with a pneumococcal pneumonia and since then had not answered calls from the HIV team.

    A female ex-partner who had two children of his and had contracted HIV from him informed the team that her children had been introduced to their new 'half-brother' by him; she informed you of where and when he was born.

    What should you do next?
    A. Ask his ex-partner to contact his new partner to inform her of her risk
    B. Carry out investigations and directly contact the new mother
    C. Contact him and ask him to inform her
    D. Inform the index patient of the potential danger to his new partner
    E. Take no action

19. A 25-year-old man attended the ambulatory care clinic complaining of a large joint arthritis.

    What would allow you to exclude Reiter's syndrome?
    A. Conjunctivitis
    B. A negative chlamydia and gonorrhoea test
    C. A negative HLA B27 test
    D. A negative white cell first pass urine dip test
    E. A positive HLA B27 test

20. A 53-year-old Caucasian married man presented via his GP to the acute medical unit with a four-month history of worsening shortness of breath that failed to respond to three courses of antibiotics, whose spectrum covered both typical and atypical pneumonia. His chest X-ray had excluded focal consolidation but demonstrated vague bilateral patchy increased opacification.

    What investigation would you perform next?

    A. Atypical pneumonia antigens in blood
    B. Atypical pneumonia antigens in urine
    C. Bronchoalveolar lavage
    D. HIV test
    E. Serum calcium levels

21. A 17-year-old Caucasian woman presented to the emergency department with lower abdominal pain. On examination, she was tender to palpation over the right iliac fossa. She had an elevated serum white count and negative pregnancy test.

    She underwent an appendectomy. The histology of which was normal. Her pain improved.

    What outpatient investigation should be performed?

    A. Abdominal ultrasound
    B. CT scan of abdomen
    C. Pelvic ultrasound
    D. A sexual-health screen
    E. Test for gonorrhoea

22. A 42-year-old Caucasian man attended his GP surgery for vaccination advice. He felt generally well but reported a two-week history of rash. On examination, there was a faint macular rash that was evenly distributed over his body but also affecting his palms and soles.

    What test should be carried out next?

    A. CMV serology
    B. Contact allergy and food allergy testing
    C. Haematology and biochemistry profile
    D. Skin biopsy
    E. Syphilis serology

23. **A 21-year-old woman presented to the emergency department with a two-day history of genital pain that was followed by the development of multiple discrete genital ulcers over the last 12 hours. She also complained of dysuria, making urination difficult. She felt systemically unwell with a headache but had no neck stiffness or photophobia. Her medical history was unremarkable; she was taking no other medication and had been in a stable relationship with the same partner for six months. He attended with her and reported no history of genital or oral ulceration.**

    On examination, the patient had a mild pyrexia but blood pressure and pulse were normal.

    What do you feel is the most likely diagnosis?
    A. Aphthous ulceration
    B. Behçets disease
    C. Epstein–Barr Virus
    D. Primary herpes simplex
    E. Recurrent herpes simplex

24. **A 45-year-old woman with type 1 diabetes presented to the acute medical unit via her GP with painful oral candida. She grew up in South Africa and moved to the UK ten years ago. She was otherwise fit and well but she admitted to recent poor diabetic control.**

    In addition to enabling improved diabetic control and treating her oral candida empirically, you should also?
    A. No further tests are indicated
    B. Send a charcoal swab for culture
    C. Send a charcoal swab for speciation
    D. Send a mid-stream urine
    E. Test for immune deficiency

25. Researchers investigated the effectiveness of a probiotic drink for the prevention of diarrhoea associated with antibiotic use. A randomized double-blind, placebo-controlled, multicentre study design was used. Intervention was a 100 g (97 mL) probiotic drink containing *Lactobacillus*, twice a day during a course of antibiotics and for one week after the course finished. The placebo group received a long-life sterile milkshake. The primary outcome was occurrence of antibiotic-associated diarrhoea. Participants were adult hospital patients taking antibiotics, recruited from three London hospitals. When participants were recruited, they were allocated to the probiotic drink or placebo group with equal probability. It was reported that consumption of the probiotic drink reduced the incidence of antibiotic-associated diarrhoea.*

Which one of the following best describes how trial participants were assigned to treatment groups?

A. Alternate allocation
B. Cluster random allocation
C. Random allocation
D. Random sampling
E. Systematic allocation

* Data included in this question is from M Hickson et al., 'Use of probiotic *Lactobacillus* preparation to prevent diarrhoea associated with antibiotics: randomised double blind placebo controlled trial', *BMJ*, 2007; 335:80

chapter 12

INFECTIOUS DISEASES AND HIV

ANSWERS

1. C. Intravenous glucose 10% bolus

Malaria is caused by a protozoan parasite, transmitted by the bite of a female Anopheles mosquito. The usual incubation period is 11–28 days depending on the species, but onset can be delayed by antimalarial prophylaxis and malaria can present up to a year after exposure. Five species of malaria affect humans: plasmodium falciparum, plasmodium vivax, plasmodium ovale, plasmodium malariae, and plasmodium knowlesi. Around 5 million cases of malaria occur each year, with 2 million deaths, mainly from plasmodium falciparum. Approximately 1,500–2,000 cases of malaria are imported to the UK annually, with up to 20 deaths.

Plasmodium falciparum is responsible for most deaths and severe disease. In contrast to plasmodium vivax and ovale, which only parasitizes very young red cells, and plasmodium malariae, which can only parasitize old red cells, plasmodium falciparum parasitizes red blood cells of all ages leading to high parasitaemia, greater red cell destruction, and anaemia. In turn, macrophages process greater quantities of malaria antigens setting off cytokine cascades and systemic inflammatory response syndrome. Plasmodium falciparum avoids immune clearance, by sequestration, in which it induces changes in parasitized erythrocytes enabling them to adhere to peripheral capillaries, especially in the brain, gut, and placenta. This takes them out of the circulation, avoiding passage through and destruction by the spleen, and facilitates contact with, and thus parasitization of, non-parasitized red cells.

Hypoglycaemia is another marker of severity and an independent risk factor for death in falciparum malaria. Often silent, it occurs especially in children and in pregnant women. It exacerbates coma and lowers the threshold for convulsions, which, in turn, worsen prognosis. Mechanisms for hypoglycaemia are not entirely clear but are thought to include increased glycolysis and decreased gluconeogenesis driven by cytokine pathways, increased glucose metabolism by parasitized red cells (up to 100-fold higher than in non-parasitized cells), and third, treatment with quinine which stimulates pancreatic islet cells to produce insulin.

Hypoglycaemia should be corrected immediately with a rapid infusion of 25 g of glucose. Fifty percent glucose is too irritant to veins, so current guidelines recommend 10% glucose or dilute 50 mL of 50% glucose in 100 mL of any infusion fluid and infuse over three to five minutes. Follow with an intravenous infusion of 200–500 mg/kg per hour using 5% or 10% glucose, and close monitoring of blood glucose, as hypoglycaemia can recur. Antimalarial therapy should be initiated as soon as possible. Patients who have uncomplicated malaria can be treated orally, with either artemether–lumefantrine 4 tablets at 0, 8, 24, 36, 48, and 60 hours (avoid in first trimester of pregnancy). Alternatively quinine 10 mg/kg (max 700 mg) tds for 5–7 days, together with doxycycline, 200 mg od for seven days (if doxycycline is contraindicated, clindamycin can be used as a second agent at 450 mg tds for seven days), or atovaquone–proguanil 4 tablets od for three days is an alternative regimen. If a drug has been used by the patient as prophylaxis, it should not be used to treat.

This patient has several features of severe or complicated malaria (see Table 12.1). She is confused and has a retinal haemorrhage. Although this falls short of the strict definition of cerebral malaria, these signs suggest cerebral involvement. She is also hypoglycaemic and is vomiting.

Immediate correction of hypoglycaemia should be followed by effective parenteral antimalarials, started as soon as possible, with either artesunate or quinine. Artesunate is now the first choice treatment for severe malaria, but may not be immediately available and is currently unlicensed in the UK. In this situation, IV quinine should be used until it is available.

Intravenous quinine should be infused in 250 mL saline over four hours with cardiac monitoring and regular measurement of blood glucose. A second drug should be used, as previously outlined, to complete the treatment of malaria. The dose of quinine is 10 mg/kg quinine (max 700 mg) three times daily, with a loading dose of 20 mg/kg (max 1,400 mg). A loading dose should not be given if the patient has recently had mefloquine. IV therapy is given until well enough to take an oral agent as already indicated.

Quinine has a narrow therapeutic index and can cause arrhythmias. So, to avoid uncertainty about oral dosing, if a patient is vomiting they should receive parenteral quinine so the dose can be assured.

Artesunate is emerging as a favoured agent in severe malaria, with better survival rates and fewer complications. It is given as a bolus of 2.4 mg/kg at 0, 12, 24 hours, and daily until the patient is well enough to switch to an oral agent. It should be considered if quinine is contraindicated.

Severe malaria should be managed in an ITU or HDU setting, with careful monitoring of fluid balance to avoid exacerbating or precipitating pulmonary oedema or ARDS due to increased pulmonary capillary permeability. This complication can occur at any time in the course of the illness and, while it is very important to correct for hypovolaemia, and acidosis, overenthusiastic hydration should be avoided.

Plasmodium vivax, ovale, and malariae are treated with chloroquine. Plasmodium vivax and ovale have dormant liver stages, or hypnozoites, which require eradication with primaquine. Glucose-6-phosphate dehydrogenase deficiency (G6PD deficiency) should be excluded before treating with primaquine to avoid haemolysis in susceptible patients. Malaria is a notifiable disease.

Table 12.1 Markers of severity in falciparum malaria.

Parasitaemia > = 2% or any parasite count in the presence of schizonts
Impaired consciousness or seizures
Hypoglycaemia <2.2 mmol/L
Pulmonary oedema or ARDS
Acidosis (pH <7.3)
Haemoglobin <8 g/dL
Spontaneous bleeding or DIC
Renal impairment (oliguria <0.4 mL/kg or creatinine >265 micromol/L)
Shock (algid Malaria)—may be complicated by gram negative sepsis
Haemoglobinuria (in the absence of G6PD deficiency)

Lalloo D, Shingadia D, Pasvol G et al. (on behalf of the HPA Advisory Committee on Malaria Prevention in UK Travellers). UK Malaria treatment guidelines. Journal of Infection 2007; 54(2): 111–121.

Malaria treatment algorithm. http://www.britishinfection.org

Management of severe malaria: a practical handbook—3rd edn. (WHO)

2. D. Shigella flexneri infection

The clinical picture described is typical for a dysenteric or inflammatory infectious diarrhoeal illness. Shigella infections are most likely to produce this clinical picture, although campylobacter and salmonellae can also present this way. He is young, and the very short incubation period would make clostridium difficile less likely. Katayama fever is described elsewhere.

Gastrointestinal infections are commonly seen in returning travellers. Acute gastroenteritis is notifiable, whether or not an organism is identified. There are two main pathological processes: secretory or non-inflammatory diarrhoea and inflammatory or non-secretory diarrhoea. There is a spectrum and several pathogens can cause one or other or both processes.

Inflammatory diarrhoea is characterized by abdominal pain, fever, and the frequent passage of small-volume stool, often with blood and mucus. It classically affects the distal ileum and colon, and the pathology is mediated by direct invasion of the enterocytes by the pathogen with mucosal inflammation and cell death.

Secretory diarrhoea is characterized by nausea, vomiting, and the passage of large volumes of watery diarrhoea. Pain and fever are not so prominent as in inflammatory diarrhoea. Dehydration is common. Mechanisms include intestinal hurry, osmotic effect of non-absorbable solutes, and toxin.

Shigella infections are exclusive to humans. There are four species: shigella dysenteriae, shigella flexneri, shigella boydi, and shigella sonnei. Shigella dysenteriae is associated with the most severe disease to which it lends its name, and shigella sonnei, which is most commonly seen in the UK, is the mildest. They are highly infectious, with ten organisms sufficient to provide an effective infectious dose, and are spread from person to person or through contaminated food or water. It often leads to outbreaks.

Shigellae cause pathology through direct invasion of the colonic mucosa replicating within colonocytes and macrophages, eliciting an intense local inflammatory response, with cellular destruction. At the severe end of the spectrum this results in necrosis, ulceration, perforation, and strictures may ensue. Bloodstream invasion is rare. Shigella dysenteriae elaborates shiga toxin, which is identical to the toxin elaborated by escherishia coli O15-H7 and can lead to the development of haemolytic uraemic syndrome, usually in the second week of illness. It contributes to the local pathology responsible for the severe manifestations exhibited by shigella dysenteriae.

The incubation period is 1–12 days. A short prodrome, with severe headache as a presenting feature, often leads to a suspicion of meningitis. Symptoms start abruptly with high fever and abdominal cramps. Watery diarrhoea follows, which in the milder forms of disease settles after a few days. In more severe cases, dysenteric symptoms develop with marked abdominal pain, tenesmus, and frequent passage of small-volume bloody stool with mucus and pus. This can lead to rectal prolapse in children.

Complications include electrolyte disturbance, toxic megacolon, bowel perforation, protein-losing enteropathy, convulsions (especially in children), and haemolytic uraemic syndrome. Shigellosis remains a significant cause of death in the tropics.

Diagnosis can be made by stool culture or rectal swab. The organism is fastidious and may die in transit to the laboratory.

Milder disease can be treated supportively with rehydration and correction of electrolytes. Antibiotic therapy shortens the duration of disease. Local susceptibility patterns may vary but useful antibiotics, where sensitivities are known include nalidixic acid, pivmecillinam, ampicillin, septrin, quinolones, and tetracyclines. Antimotility agents should not be used as they predispose to toxic dilatation and bowel perforation. This is a useful general rule for all undifferentiated gastrointestinal infection which presents with fever.

Gagandeep K, Hart C, Shears P. 'Bacterial enteropathogens', Manson's tropical diseases. Edited by Farra J, Hotez P, Junghanns T et al. 23rd edn. Saunders Ltd. 2013.

3. E. Schistosoma mansoni

The patient has a marked eosinophilia, and presents with systemic symptoms, cough, bloody diarrhoea, and splenomegaly eight weeks after exposure to fresh water in Africa. The most likely diagnosis in this scenario is Katayama syndrome, or acute schistosomiasis, caused by infection with a small blood fluke.

Eosinophilia is not a feature of glandular fever, acute dengue, EBV infection, or HIV. The incubation period is too long for leptospirosis and dengue, which typically is 3–14 days.

Katayama syndrome is seen in primary infection with schistosomes. It most often occurs with schistosoma japonicum and schistosoma mansoni infections but can occur with any species. Severity is not necessarily determined by disease burden. It occurs as the flukes mature and begin to lay eggs, exposing the host to egg antigens to which they react. It is characterized by marked eosinophilia, cough, abdominal pain (sometimes associated with bloody diarrhoea), rash, hepatosplenomegaly, and is seen 3–12 weeks after water exposure.

The diagnosis is clinical, although other systemic parasite infections should be excluded, as at this stage of infection ova are not usually seen, and it is too early for a reliable antibody response.

Schistosoma species spend their adult life (of up to 40 years) in mammalian mesenteric venules. The intermediate hosts are species-specific aquatic snails. On maturation, cercaria emerge from the snail, and swim in shallow fresh water ready to penetrate mammalian skin. They then migrate to the mesenteric venules where they mate and stay in a state of permanent copulation. This process takes 6–12 weeks after which they mature and lay eggs which have a single spine. The infection, hitherto silent, may declare itself at this stage as a systemic illness in response to egg antigen as the Katayama syndrome. Typically, eggs find their way through the circulation to the gut or bladder through which they migrate by provoking an inflammatory granulomatous reaction. Once in the lumen, they pass with faeces or urine, hatching when they reach fresh water to complete the life cycle.

The propensity for ova to migrate either to bladder or bowel differs with species, though there is overlap. Schistosoma haematobium eggs favour the bladder, while schistosoma mansoni and japonicum favour the gastrointestinal (GI) tract and liver. Migration to other organs, including lungs, kidneys, uterus, and spinal cord or CNS can cause serious acute local pathology. Over time, chronic fibrotic changes with repeated egg deposition leads to complications such as periportal fibrosis, bladder calcification, and tumours.

Asymptomatic travellers should be screened three months after last water contact, when antibody responses will be positive and ova may be detected on microscopy of stool or terminal urine samples (the last 3–5 mL). At least three samples of each offer the best chance of a positive result. Other clues include haematuria and eosinophilia.

Clinical features of established schistosomiasis can be non-specific and relate to any potential affected organ. Eosinophilia may be present. Haematuria can be a clue to urinary disease. Ova should be sought in stool and terminal urine samples. Eggs may not always be detected despite the presence of infection. Rectal snips or bladder biopsies may demonstrate ova or granulomas surrounding an egg and characteristic granulomata may also be seen in the liver or other affected tissue.

Acute schistosomiasis should be treated with praziquantel 40–60 mg/kg as a single dose and short course of steroids to control the inflammatory reaction. The dose of praziquantel should be repeated after six weeks when flukes are fully mature because immature flukes are relatively resistant to treatment.

Squire B, Stothard R. 'Schistosomiasis', Lecture notes: tropical medicine. Edited by Beeching N, Gill G. 7th edn. Wiley-Blackwell. 2014.

4. C. Loa loa infection

Loiasis is caused by a subcutaneous filarial infection, which is present in West and Central Africa. It is transmitted by the bite of chrysops—a small tabanid fly which bites by daytime. These filarial worms can live up to 18 years, and females give birth to live microfilariae which are most easily detected at around midday to match the feeding habits of the vector.

The adult worm migrates through connective tissues and can sometimes be seen migrating across the conjunctiva. Swellings appear periodically lasting hours to days around an area where the adult is migrating, as a result of immune response to the parasite. These are known as calabar swellings and are characteristic of Loa loa infection, occurring anywhere but most commonly on the hands, wrists, and forearms. Pruritus is another common symptom. Migration of adults through the CNS can lead to serious local complications. When adults die, they sometimes calcify and can be seen on X-ray. Dying adults can elicit an acute inflammatory response and abscess formation. Other complications include nephropathy and complications of hypereosinophilia.

Diagnosis can be confirmed by seeing microfilariae on blood films. Blood should be taken between 10:00 and 15:00 hours to coincide with the periodicity of the parasite. Serology is non-specific with filarial antibodies cross-reacting across the different species.

Treatment is with dieythyl carbamazine (DEC) 10 mg/kg for 2–4 weeks. Before treatment, it is important to determine the filarial load, the possibility of CNS or eye involvement, and whether there is any possibility of concurrent onchocerciasis to avoid acute local reactions on treatment.

DEC is rapidly microfilaricidal, but is not as effective on adult worms. Side effects include allergic reactions, including angioedema, pruritus, rash, systemic symptoms, and encephalopathy, especially with high parasite burdens. Small incremental doses of DEC covered with corticosteroids reduce the incidence and severity of complications. If there has been recent eye migration, treatment should be delayed. Albendazole can also be used to treat Loa loa infection.

Further treatments may be required to kill the adult worms. Alternatively, adults can be surgically removed if seen.

In the case of onchocerciasis co-infection, treatment with DEC can lead to an unintended severe Mazzotti reaction-an intense pruritic rash, sometimes associated with serious systemic reaction through the death of subcutaneous microfilariae of onchocerca volvulus (a controlled Mazzotti reaction with a small dose of DEC has been used as a last resort diagnostic test for onchocerca volvulus but is not recommended). Treatment is with ivermectin, but here it is important to exclude Loa loa infection as inadvertent treatment of Loa loa with ivermectin can cause fatal encephalopathy where the filarial load is high.

Because of the various complications that can occur on management of these filarial infections, it is always important to ensure that patients are managed at a specialist centre.

O'Dempsey T. 'Onchocerciasis, filariasis and loiasis', Lecture notes: tropical medicine. Edited by Beeching N, Gill G. 7th edn. Wiley-Blackwell. 2014.

5. D. Serology

The clinical picture is typical for hepatic amoebiasis.

This is caused by infection with entamoeba histolytica—a human intestinal pathogen spread though the faecal oral route, and endemic in areas of poor sanitation. It usually gives rise to asymptomatic intestinal cyst carriage, but has the ability to cause invasive disease in about 10% of cases. It is morphologically indistinguishable from entamoeba dispar, a non-pathogenic amoeba which also affects man. Molecular techniques can distinguish between the two, unless there is concurrent invasive disease, when the presence of trophozoites with ingested red blood cells on rectal scrapes, or examination of fresh stool confirms entamoeba histolytica.

In invasive disease, amoebic trophozoites initially colonize and invade the colonic mucosa, inducing inflammatory changes. Onset of symptoms is usually insidious, with abdominal discomfort, loose motions, and low-grade temperature. This can progress to severe amoebic dysentery with blood and slime in the stool, and fulminant colitis. It may mimic ulcerative colitis, and as incubation period may be several months to years, it is important to consider the possibility before starting steroids in suspected ulcerative colitis.

Haematogenous spread causes distant infection. Amoebae are capable of invading any tissue, causing necrosis and abscess formation. It most commonly invades the liver via the portal circulation where it usually causes a single abscess, most commonly in the right lobe. It is usually thin-walled with a centre that is composed of necrotic liver tissue which on aspiration has the appearance of thick brown 'anchovy sauce'. Twenty percent of patients give a history of past dysentery. Ten percent have diarrhoea on presentation.

Onset is abrupt with swinging high fevers, rigors, profuse sweats, anorexia, and vomiting, often with no localizing symptoms, unless the abscess is large, when there may be pain in the right upper quadrant. On examination, the liver is enlarged and tender, with tenderness in the right intercostal spaces. A large abscess may rupture into the pleural spaces and the lung, occasionally forming broncho-hepatic fistulae with expectoration of abscess material.

Chest X-ray may reveal an elevated right hemidiaphragm, sometimes with a reactive effusion and atelectasis. Blood count typically demonstrates a neutrophil leucocytosis with anaemia. Inflammatory markers are elevated. Liver function tests may be normal. Alkaline phosphatase may be elevated. Jaundice is uncommon.

Diagnosis is usually possible with the typical ultrasound appearance of a solitary abscess in the right lobe of the liver (5–20% appear on the left). They are usually hypoechoic and round or oval, with thin walls and don't have enhanced echoes. Serology is positive in 95% of cases.

The prognosis has markedly improved since the availability of ultrasound, allowing rapid diagnosis and management. Aspiration may be necessary to exclude bacterial infection. Amoebic 'pus' is thick, sterile, and inoffensive. Smell, or thin pus, indicates secondary or primary bacterial infection. Microscopy reveals acellular necrotic debris. Amoebae are rarely found in the aspirate, but may be found at the edge of the abscess.

Stool microscopy may or may not reveal amoebic cysts.

Treatment for amoebic liver abscess is with metronidazole 800 mg three times daily for ten days or tinidazole 2 g daily for three to five days. This treats the invasive trophozoites. Treatment for intestinal cysts should follow with diloxanide furoate 500 mg three times daily for ten days.

Unless the diagnosis is in doubt, or there is concern of imminent rupture, aspiration should be avoided. Response to metronidazole should help confirm the diagnosis.

Differential diagnosis is of pyogenic infection, hydatid disease, and hepatocellular carcinoma, although they have characteristic appearances that should help distinguish them from amoebic liver abscess.

Complications include contiguous spread or rupture into lung, peritoneum, pericardium, kidney, skin, and biliary tree. Abscesses can sometimes present in the brain and bone.

O'Dempsey T. 'Amoebiasis', Lecture notes: tropical medicine. Edited by Beeching N, Gill G. 7th edn. Wiley-Blackwell. 2014.

6. E. Splenomegaly

The patient has Epstein–Barr virus (EBV) infection—a human herpes virus transmitted via infected saliva through close contact. The incubation period is about 5–6 weeks. Infection is usually asymptomatic in children—severity increases with age. The virus initiates infection in the pharyngeal mucosa and salivary glands infecting B lymphocytes, immortalizing them. Haematogenous dissemination of the B lymphocytes follows. Symptoms start with fever, anorexia, malaise, a fleeting rash, periorbital oedema, and facial puffiness. Pharyngitis develops, with pharyngeal oedema, and petechiae at the junction between the soft and hard palate. The tonsils are swollen with a cheesy exudate. Lymphadenopathy is present in almost 100% of cases, and is generalized, particularly affecting the posterior triangle of the neck. Sometimes, one large node predominates. Splenomegaly is detected in week 2. Several other rashes are associated with glandular fever, including urticaria, maculopapular or purpuric rashes, erythema multiforme, and drug rashes, especially with ampicillin or amoxicillin, usually given for presumptive tonsillitis. This does not imply allergy to these drugs and rashes do not recur after the acute infection.

The illness lasts two to three weeks, with a short convalescence. Only in a very few instances does fatigue persist for longer. Resolution coincides with the development of specific immunity. Cytotoxic T cells destroy the immortalized B cells.

Complications include hepatitis, meningoencephalitis, peripheral neuropathy, autoimmune thrombocytopenia, autoimmune haemolytic anaemia, splenic rupture, haemphagocytic lymphohistiocytosis, and a spectrum of autoimmune phenomena arising from the polyclonal activation of large numbers of B lymphocytes which secrete immunoglobulin.

Cytotoxic T lymphocytes, which appear as atypical lymphocytes on blood film, as an effective immune response develops, destroy the infected B lymphocytes. X-linked lymphoproliferative disease (or Duncan's syndrome) is a rare and fatal complication resulting from a specific defect in T cell immunity with failure to control the infection.

Latent EBV infection within B lymphocytes persists within the host for life. Low-level or intermittent reactivation allows secretion of live virus into saliva, and provides the opportunity to infect others. Chronic low-level reactivation in immunocompromised patients can cause mutations within the genome of the B lymphocytes giving rise to various neoplasms including B cell lymphoma, Hodgkin's and Burkitt's lymphomas, post-transplant lymphoproliferative disease, and nasopharyngeal carcinoma. This is seen typically in association with repeated malaria infections, HIV infection, transplant patients, and in other forms of immunosuppression.

Laboratory diagnosis includes the heterophile antibody test first described by Paul and Bunnell. Heterophile antibodies agglutinate red cells from various animals, and persist after absorption with guinea pig kidney, but not after absorption with beef red cells. They are present in 90% of infected adults, but this is a less sensitive test in children.

Blood film shows atypical lymphocytes, appearing after the first week. These are the reactive T cells. Other conditions which can cause atypical lymphocytes include:

- Cytomegalovirus infection
- HIV infection
- Rubella
- Toxoplasmosis

Specific diagnostic tests include viral capsid IgM antibodies which appear early and disappear in convalescence. Viral capsid antibody (VCA) IgG appears shortly after the IgM and persists. Epstein–Barr nuclear antigen IgG appears after six weeks and also persists.

Virus can be detected by PCR in blood, or when relevant in CSF (see Table 12.2).

Table 12.2 Table showing viral capsid antibody (VCA) IgM/IgG and Epstein–Barr nuclear antigen (EBNA) IgG along with interpretation of results.

VCA IgM	VCA IgG	EBNA IgG	Interpretation
Neg	Neg	Neg	No serological evidence of EBV infection
Pos	Neg	Neg	Early EBV infection, or false +ve IgM– repeat in 2–6 weeks to confirm (or PCR for viral DNA in plasma)
Pos	Pos	Neg	Recent acute EBV infection
Neg	Pos	Neg	Fairly recent EBV infection or past infection – As no EBNA IgG detectable repeat in six weeks to clarify
Neg	Pos	Pos	Past EBV infection (>eight weeks)
Pos	Pos	Pos	EBV at some time. Late primary infection or reactivation of latent infection. IgM may be false +ve. Consider testing CMV and parvovirus IgM, or EBV, CMV or parvovirus PCR to clarify

Adapted from 'Epstein–Barr Virus Serology', *Virology*, UK Standards for Microbiology Investigations, 2014, 26, 4.1. This information is licensed under the terms of the Open Government Licence (http://www.nationalarchives.gov.uk/doc/open-government-licence/version/3).

Epstein M, Rickinson A. 'Epstein-Barr virus', Oxford textbook of medicine. Edited by Warrell D, Cox T, Firth J. 5th edn. Oxford: OUP, 2010.

7. D. Start quadruple antituberculous therapy and notify as tuberculosis

This patient has primary pleural tuberculosis (TB) until proven otherwise. This occurs when a tuberculous focus in the periphery of the lung ruptures into the pleural space, and is most often seen in primary tuberculous infection.

Symptoms of TB typically include fever, night sweats, and weight loss, with additional symptoms according to the organ affected. Pulmonary TB occurs in about 80%, and a cough lasting for longer than three weeks that fails to respond to standard antibiotics with or without haemoptysis should arouse suspicion. Usually, the upper lobes are affected and there may be cavitation on chest X-ray.

Sites of infection in descending order of frequency:
- Pulmonary
- Pleural
- Adenopathy (localized/generalized)
- Genitourinary (17% white UK; 4% in Asian)
- Miliary or disseminated
- Bone and joint (10–15%)
- Abdominal (ileocecal and peritoneal)
- CNS (95% meningeal or tuberculoma)
- Pericardial
- Cutaneous TB or lupus vulgaris
- Cryptic disseminated TB

Any organ can be affected, and symptoms and onset may be indolent or dramatic.

Primary infection can be associated with a variety of hypersensitivity syndromes to TB proteins. Erythema nodosum is the most commonly encountered. More rarely the tuberculides including erythema induratum and phlyctenular conjunctivitis are associated with cryptic disease and resolve on TB therapy. PCR may be positive. They are usually associated with a strong cellular response.

This patient should be commenced on quadruple antituberculous chemotherapy with rifampicin, isoniazid, pyrazinamide, and ethambutol.

There is a statutory duty to notify the patient to the proper officer and there are specific enhanced surveillance TB notification forms which should be used.

Notification should be performed once the decision to treat tuberculosis is made. Culture confirmation is not a prerequisite. Bronchoalveolar lavage is not necessary now as there is a positive culture from pleural fluid, though it would have been an important initial investigation to increase the chance of positive yield, as only 60–80% of patients with tuberculosis have positive cultures.

She has been exposed to an area where there is multidrug resistant TB. Mycobacterial PCR can be used to help confirm mycobateria tuberculosis while awaiting further identification from culture. Gene probes can determine the presence of genes associated with rifampicin resistance, which although not 100% sensitive may give early warning of the possibility of multi-drug resistant (MDR) TB (the definition of MDR TB is resistance to both rifampicin and isoniazid). A Mantoux test or gamma interferon release assay measure the T cell mediated immune response to TB, and indicate exposure, but not necessarily active disease. The Mantoux cross-reacts with BCG, so may be positive in people who have been vaccinated. Interferon–Gamma Release Assays (IGRAs) do not react to BCG and are more specific to TB.

Culture can take up to eight weeks, though liquid broth techniques are typically positive within three weeks.

Standard TB chemotherapy involves quadruple therapy for the first two months. This ensures at least two active drugs within the regimen while sensitivities are awaited, avoiding inadvertent monotherapy (with the risk of further resistance) if there is resistance to one or more agents. After two months, the continuation phase of the regimen can be started, determined by antimicrobial sensitivities. If fully sensitive, mycobacteria tuberculosis is cultured then a further four months of isoniazid and rifampicin is given.

If there is resistance to one or more of the first-line drugs, alternative regimens should be given. MDR TB or extremely multi-drug resistant TB (XDR TB) should be discussed with experts in the management of resistant TB. It usually involves the additional use of an injectable agent for six months such as a quinolone, protionamide, or cycloserine. Duration of therapy can be two years or more, as these agents are not as powerful as first-line treatment, and close monitoring with directly observed therapy should be offered.

All patients with TB should be offered an HIV test. HIV greatly increases the risk of developing active TB compared with the non-HIV infected population. There is also a greater risk of death or complications if HIV remains undetected, which can be reduced by detection and treatment of the HIV.

Squire B. 'Tuberculosis', Lecture notes: tropical medicine. Edited by Beeching N, Gill G. 7th edn. Wiley-Blackwell. 2014.

8. E. Bite from a trombiculid mite

The initial symptoms are non-specific and the differential diagnosis could include dengue fever, malaria, typhoid, rickettsial infection, HIV seroconversion, meningococcal infection, and leptospirosis.

She has a rash, an eschar, and enlarged regional nodes, making rickettsial infection most likely. Scrub typhus, a rickettsial spotted fever occurring in Thailand, is caused by Orientia tsutsugamushi. It is transmitted by the bite of a trombiculid mite. The incubation period is 5–10 days. Illness starts abruptly with fever, headache, myalgia, nausea, vomiting, and cough. Rash appears on day five to seven, on the trunk and limbs. It can be complicated by meningoencephalitis, myocarditis, and shock can ensue with ARDS. Diagnosis can be confirmed by serological detection of the agent by PCR in blood.

Empirical treatment with doxycycline is warranted; 200 mg stat usually suffices, alternatively in severe infection this may be continued for five days.

Gill G. 'Rickettsial infections', Lecture notes: tropical medicine. Edited by Beeching N, Gill G. 7th edn. Wiley-Blackwell. 2014.

9. E. The intermediate host is the pig

She has neurocysticercosis. This is the second-commonest cause of epilepsy worldwide, with TB as the first. It is caused by the tissue stage of Taenia solium or the 'pork tapeworm', and acquired by ingestion of ova in food contaminated by infected human faeces.

Taenia solium is actually a human tapeworm, with the pig as an intermediate host. The tapeworm inhabits the human gut, and is contracted by ingestion of undercooked pork, in which the intermediate stage encysts. On reaching the human gut the cyst develops and matures into an adult tapeworm, and eggs or segments are passed in faeces.

If humans ingest these eggs they can, like the pig, become an intermediate host. Eggs hatch within the gastrointestinal tract and pass into the bloodstream, and encyst in skeletal muscle, bone, eye or brain, persisting for many years. On dying they can elicit an acute inflammatory response, leading to acute symptoms. The most common presentation is with epilepsy. Other complications include hydrocephalus, focal neurological signs, psychiatric disease, encephalopathy, and cognitive impairment.

Diagnosis may be made by identifying characteristic lesions on MRI or CT. Plain radiographs may show rice-grain shaped calcified cysts in skeletal muscle, as in this case. Serology may be of help. Often the diagnosis is clinical.

Anticonvulsants and steroids are important in reducing acute symptoms, before and during antihelminthic therapy with praziquantel 50mg/kg for 15 days, albendazole 15 mg/kg daily for 15 to 30 days (or a 10-day course with both agents). This is avoided if there is active encephalopathy for fear of exacerbating the inflammatory response on killing the cysts. Steroids reduce the inflammatory response in this situation during antihelminthic therapy.

Surgical excision of intraventricular cysts should also be considered.

O'Dempsey T. 'Intestinal cestode infections (tapeworms) including cysticercosis', Lecture notes: tropical medicine. Edited by Beeching N, Gill G. 7th edn. Wiley-Blackwell. 2014.

10. A. Borrelia burgdoferi infection

Borrelia burgdorferi is the organism responsible for Lyme disease, a zoonosis transmitted to man by the bite of an Ixodes tick. Ticks may take two to three days to feed, and transmission occurs after the tick has been feeding for at least 24 hours, so can be prevented by early removal of the tick.

There are three stages of clinical disease: early localized infection, early disseminated disease, and late disease.

Early localized infection refers to erythema migrans, the typical rash that occurs at the site of the bite, and spreads centrifugally, usually with clearing in the middle, and resembling a bull's eye target. This occurs 3–30 days after the original bite and can be asymptomatic, mildly pruritic, or tender. It is sometimes associated with low-grade fever, mild headache, and arthralgia. At this stage, the immune response may not have developed, and serology is often negative. The diagnosis is clinical and treatment is indicated without antibody testing. Eighty percent of patients with Lyme disease will have erythema migrans.

Early disseminated disease follows on from localized infection and presents with various manifestations. At this stage, antibodies to borrelia burgdorferi can be detected.

Cutaneous disease: disseminated erythema migrans (several smaller erythema migrans patches appear), borrelia lymphocytoma—a firm purplish nodule, usually on the earlobe).

Neurological manifestations:

- Meningitis—lymphocytic pleocytosis
- Cranial nerve palsies—usually VIIth—most fully recover
- Peripheral neuritis
- Painful radiculopathy

Muscle weakness

Cardiac manifestations:

- Heart block and arrhythmias

Joint manifestations (more frequently seen in the USA):

- Arthralgia, mono-oligoarthritis, which is migratory and affects large joints, typically the knee

Late Lyme disease can present months to years after the initial infection with peripheral neuropathy which responds poorly to antibiotics. Chronic meningoencephalitis, chronic arthritis, which has an association with HLADR4, and usually responds to antibiotic therapy, and acrodermatitis chronica atrophicans, which may present over several years, especially in older women, where it is often confused with venous changes are also seen.

Post-Lyme syndromes: a variety of non-specific sequelae have been attributed to Lyme disease. On occasions, patients may develop chronic fatigue syndrome following Lyme disease.

Two-stage serological testing is performed for early disseminated or late disease. Screening tests with enzyme immunoassay (IgG/IgM) are highly sensitive, but are prone to false positives.

All positives are sent for second-stage immunoblot assays in response to various borrelia antigens, and a positive result is given according to the pattern of positive bands present.

Cerebrospinal fluid can also be sent for antibody testing. Oligoclonal bands may be present in CSF, but these are usually matched by identical bands in plasma, indicating a systemic inflammatory response and not indicative of intrathecal IgG production.

Culture and PCR are not routinely available for diagnostic purposes.

Treatment

Early Lyme disease can be treated with a two-week course of amoxicillin 500 mg three times daily, or doxycycline 100 mg twice daily, or cefuroxime 500 mg twice daily.

Late Lyme disease can be treated with intravenous ceftriaxone 2 g daily for 28 days. Evidence is emerging that oral doxycycline 100 mg twice daily for 28 days is equally effective. Occasionally, with Lyme arthritis, a second 28-day course is required.

Prolonged antibiotic courses beyond one month have no place in the management of Lyme disease. Residual neurological sequelae and fatigue may persist for several months. Recovery may be slow and is usually complete after a few months, though late neuroborreliosis may not recover completely.

Generally the prognosis is excellent.

Aguero-Rosenfeld M, Wang G, Schwartz I et al. Diagnosis of lyme borreliosis. Clinical Microbiology Reviews 2005; 18(3): 484–509.

11. D. Staphylococcal toxic shock syndrome

Streptococcal and staphylococcal toxic shock syndrome, and Kawasaki disease share similarities. Kawasaki disease (mucocutaneous lymph node syndrome) is typically seen in children—a vasculitis. Features include fever, conjunctivitis, mucositis (red chapped lips and strawberry tongue may be confused with toxic shock or scarlet fever), rash which may be maculopapular, lymphadenopathy, oedematous extremities, lasting approximately two weeks, and peeling of the skin occurring in convalescence. It may be complicated by coronary aneurysms. Treatment is with intravenous immunoglobulin.

Streptococcal toxic shock syndrome is caused by the superantigen toxin of group A streptococcal infection. There are three toxins (streptococcal pyrogenic exotoxins) A, B, and C. A and B are associated with toxic shock syndrome. They share close homology with staphylococcal superantigen toxins, namely toxic shock syndrome toxins 1 (TSST-1) and enterotoxins A–E. Streptococcal toxic shock is associated with a mortality of up to 80%, and is seen in situations where there is invasive streptococcal disease with bacteraemia, like necrotizing fasciitis, wound infections, pneumonia, etc. Diarrhoea does not feature and a rash may or may not feature.

Staphylococcal toxic shock syndrome is mainly driven by the staphylococcal superantigen toxins TSST-1, most often associated with menstrual toxic shock, and in contrast to streptococcal toxic shock, is associated with colonization, or trivial infection, with the syndrome eclipsing the source wound/site which is usually cutaneous, such as an infected chicken pock (originally described by Todd J, Fishaut M, Kapral F, Welch T. 'Toxic-shock syndrome associated with phage-group-1 staphylococci'. Lancet 1978; 2: 1116–1118). The other situation in which staphylococcal toxic shock is seen is in association with tampon use where the vagina is colonized with toxin-producing staphylococci.

Staphylococcal toxic shock syndrome typically presents with abrupt fever. Nausea, vomiting and watery diarrhoea are common features, as are confusion, headache, and sore throat. Myalgia is prominent. There is conjunctival suffusion, and erythema of the mucosae, including a 'strawberry tongue' and vaginal hyperaemia, and a diffuse blanching erythematous rash (like sunburn), hypotension, confusion, but no meningeal signs. Peeling of the extremities occurs in convalescence, after two weeks or so.

Blood tests show thrombocytopenia, abnormal liver function, abnormal renal function, hypocalcaemia, and elevated creatine kinase. Blood cultures are usually sterile, but the pathogen and toxin can be detected from swabs of the suspected lesion, vagina, or tampon. Toxin production is likely to be influenced by different microenvironments. Highly absorbent tampons are particularly associated with staphylococcal TSST-1.

Superantigen toxins can stimulate large numbers of B cells (up to 30%) by their ability to bridge the variable beta region of the T cell receptor. This leads to a cytokine storm which characterizes superantigen-mediated disease.

Treatment is antistaphylococcal antibiotics together with supportive therapy, and removal of tampons (where relevant). Mortality is about 3%.

Silversides J, Lappin E, Ferguson A. Staphylococcal toxic shock syndrome: mechanisms and management. Current Infectious Disease Reports September 2010; 12(5): 392–400.

12. A. Measles

Measles is a highly infectious viral infection caused by a paramyxovirus. It has an incubation period of 10–14 days, and is characterized by a severe catarrhal prodromal stage lasting 3–4 days with the triad of cough, coryza, and conjunctivitis.

The patient feels ill and is miserable with high fever and coryzal symptoms. Koplik spots, seen in 80%, appear just before the rash appears and disappear on the first or second day of the rash. They are pathognomonic, and are seen on the buccal surface at the margin of the molars, and look like granules of salt. Occasionally, they can appear on the tongue, palate, and rectal mucosa. The face has a characteristic puffiness.

A maculopapular rash appears behind the ears on the fourth day, and the rash progresses onto the face and downwards until it reaches the legs after two to three days, stopping just below the knees. As it passes down the chest, lower-respiratory symptoms may become more pronounced with crackles on auscultation.

This relatively slow progression is another hallmark of measles. It fades from the face downwards, and the marked inflammation leads to diapedesis, and staining remains visible for six weeks or so.

Complications include giant-cell pneumonia, which may be severe in malnourished and immunocompromised patients. Post-infectious encephalitis occurs in the first week after the appearance of the rash in 1 in 1,000 cases, causing encephalopathy, seizures, and altered consciousness. It carries a good prognosis. Fifty percent of children with measles will have an abnormal EEG.

Measles carries a high mortality in the tropics (20%), exacerbated by malnutrition and vitamin A deficiency. Severe giant-cell pneumonitis, secondary bacterial pneumonia, PCP infection, reactivation of TB, noma (cancrum oris), and prolonged diarrhoea contribute to mortality. Measles is profoundly immunosuppressive; an effect which stays for several weeks to months. Subacute sclerosing panencephalopathy occurs in 1 in 1,000,000 cases, usually seven years after the onset of measles, where there is persistence of virus, and is fatal.

Administration of vitamin A during the acute illness shortens the duration of the disease and reduces morbidity and mortality, especially in malnourished children, where it should be administered at a dose of 40,000 IU.

Measles is preventable with a live attenuated vaccine which is usually administered in combination with mumps and rubella vaccines.

Parvovirus infection causes slapped cheek syndrome in children. In adults it presents with rashes, fever, transaminitis, and arthralgia. It causes marrow arrest and in patients with haemolytic anaemia can cause anaemia. In pregnancy it is a cause of fetal loss and hydrops fetalis.

Pharyngoconjunctival fever caused by an adenovirus causes a triad of rash, conjunctivitis, pharyngitis, cervical adenopathy, with or without a rash.

Mycoplasma infection can cause a variety of rashes, but none of these, nor the rash of rubella, have the characteristic slow descent down the body that characterizes that of measles.

Whittle H, Aaby P. 'Measles', Oxford textbook of medicine. Edited by Warrell D, Cox T, Firth J. 5th edn. Oxford: OUP, 2010.

13. E. Primary herpes gingivostomatitis

This is primary herpes gingivostomatitis. Herpes simplex infection is a ubiquitous human herpes virus. There are two serotypes of herpes simplex virus (HSV)—type 1 predominates in infections in the oropharynx, and type 2 predominates in genital lesions. There is a 10–15% crossover.

Primary HSV 1 infection is usually acquired in infancy or childhood, and by adulthood 90% of the population has become infected. Infections are often asymptomatic. Symptomatic primary infection is characterized by the triad of fever, cervical lymphadenopathy, and shallow ulcers which appear after a few days on the oropharyngeal mucosa, including tongue, gums, palate, and lips. Swallowing is difficult because of pain and oedema and drooling with virus-laden saliva often leads to secondary spread of the virus and vesicles appear on the chin.

The incubation period is about ten days and transmission is through contact with saliva from symptomatic and asymptomatic carriers.

Recovery occurs after 5–14 days. The virus establishes latency in the dorsal root ganglia by ascent through axons, and can reactivate periodically as a cold sore, typically occurring at the junction between the vermillion border of the lip and the skin.

Other sites of infection include:
- Finger through autoinoculation in primary infection—herpetic whitlow
- Skin through abrasions—often through contact sport—herpes gladiatorum
- Disseminated skin infection in patients with eczema—eczema herpeticum
- Corneal infection—stellate ulcer on conjunctiva, which may lead to blindness
- 'PORN' syndrome (progressive outer retinal necrosis, usually seen in HIV infection)

Sometimes, HSV reactivation can trigger erythema multiforme or Stevens–Johnson syndrome. This may be recurrent and is treated acutely with aciclovir.

HSV 1 can cause encephalitis, which untreated has an 80% mortality within two weeks and a high incidence of neurological sequelae in survivors. Aciclovir has reduced mortality to 10%. The incidence of sequelae remains high at 60%.

HSV 2 most often manifests as genital ulceration. Primary infection may be asymptomatic, but often causes severe systemic symptoms associated with genital ulceration and inguinal adenopathy, and discharge. It sometimes can present with aseptic meningitis. This can be recurrent and is the commonest cause of recurrent aseptic meningitis (Mollaret's meningitis).

Diagnosis is through virus isolation from lesions, saliva, CSF, or brain biopsy. Antibodies may be present. PCR is very sensitive and can be used to exclude the diagnosis of HSV meningitis.

Treatment is with aciclovir 5–15 mg/kg (higher doses for meningitis or encephalitis).

Sissons J. 'Herpes viruses (excluding Epstein–Barr virus)', Oxford textbook of medicine. Edited by Warrell D, Cox T, Firth J. 5th edn. Oxford: OUP, 2010.

14. B. Enterocyte sodium chloride co-transport mechanism is inhibited

This is cholera. It is caused by vibrio cholerae, a curved motile gram-negative rod, which is spread by faecal contamination of drinking water. It is a human gastrointestinal pathogen.

Vibrio cholerae induces secretory diarrhoea caused by the toxin acting on enterocytes. The toxin irreversibly binds adenylate cyclase causing a rise in cAMP. Chlorine channels open in crypt cells, actively transporting chlorine into the gut lumen. Water and sodium ions follow. The sodium and chloride co-transport mechanism in villi is inhibited so sodium chloride reabsorption is reduced.

After an incubation period of a few hours to three days, there is abrupt painless watery diarrhoea, up to 30 litres a day (like 'rice-water'). With the massive loss of water and electrolytes, muscle cramps are common, and arrhythmias can ensue.

There can be evidence of hypovolaemic shock, with tachycardia, absent peripheral pulses, and profound dehydration ('washerwoman hands', sunken eyes, and reduced tissue turgor). Electrolytes show low sodium, chloride, and bicarbonate along with a metabolic acidosis because of loss of bicarbonate in the stool. Full blood count may show haemoconcentration. Stool culture requires specific culture medium—TCBS (thiosulfate citrate bile salts sucrose).

Treatment requires accurate fluid balance. Ninety eight percent respond to oral rehydration solution (ORS) alone. This activates the brush-border glucose–sodium co-transport mechanism, which is unaffected by cholera toxin. With every molecule of glucose transported, 260 molecules of water are coupled, which enhances water absorption by the gut by enabling 260 water molecules to enter the brush-border cell with each glucose sodium transport cycle.

One litre of ORS when reconstituted with potable water contains:

- 20 g glucose
- 3.5 g NaCl
- 2.5 g NaHCO$_3$
- 1.5 g KCl

Amino acids have additive effect on co-transport mechanism (glycine, alanine, and lysine). Thus, *real* rice water has a role to play (not 'rice-water' stool).

Antibiotics reduce stool volume, duration of illness, and infectiousness of the stool. Prognosis is excellent with treatment and support. Oral rehydration solution has reduced mortality of severe cholera from 50% down to 1%, although in Africa mortality is around 4%.

Shears P. 'Cholera', Lecture notes: tropical medicine. Edited by Beeching N, Gill G. 7th edn. Wiley-Blackwell. 2014.

15. D. Doxycyline

The most likely diagnosis described in this scenario is of mycoplasma pneumoniae infection. The incubation period is about three weeks. Symptoms can develop gradually, or more abruptly. It usually begins with coryzal symptoms and a sore throat with a cough that is characteristically persistent, leading to the retrosternal pain and tracheitis that also characterizes this condition. Bullous myringitis is a rare but pathognomonic feature. Cold agglutinins are often present against the antigen on erythrocytes. They are often there at presentation and titres peak about two months after onset, but rarely lead to clinically apparent haemolytic anaemia. Other features which can be associated with this infection include erythema multiforme, and various other rashes, transverse myelitis, and myocarditis.

Chest auscultation may be normal, but the chest X-ray can reveal bilateral fluffy shadowing.

Mycoplasma pneumoniae infection is diagnosed by the presence of antibodies to this infection. It can be cultured, but growth is slow. Treatment is usually started on an empirical basis to cover 'atypical pneumonias'. Mycoplasma pneumoniae lacks a cell wall, so beta lactam antibiotics will have no activity against it. The treatment of choice is either with a macrolide antibiotic (clarithromycin, azithromycin, etc.) or the tetracyclines (tetracycline, doxycycline, etc.) The fluoroquinolones also have activity against mycoplasma pneumoniae.

Scott A. 'Pneumococcal Infections', Oxford textbook of medicine. Edited by Warrell D, Cox T, Firth J. 5th edn. Oxford: OUP, 2010.

16. D. She should receive broad-spectrum antibiotics

This patient has chickenpox. This is a herpes virus infection which is highly infectious and spread mainly by the respiratory route, but also from virus particles from chickenpox vesicles.

The severity of chickenpox increases with age, immune suppression, smoking, and also late pregnancy. This may be partially due to the immunomodulatory effects of pregnancy, and also through splinting of the diaphragm in late pregnancy, which reduces respiratory reserve.

Each spot is derived from a viraemic focus. So the severity of the rash correlates with the degree of viraemia and is a marker of severity. The spots can occur anywhere, but tend to have a centripetal distribution, affecting the trunk and face more severely. Each fever heralds a viraemic wave, which in turn is followed by a new crop of spots. Oropharyngeal spots, when present, indicate likely pulmonary involvement. Spots start off as macules, which quickly vesiculate, and resemble drops of water on the surface of the skin. They are oval, the long axis of which lies along the skin creases. There is a variable erythematous halo around each spot. After a few hours they become cloudy pustules. They crust over after a day or so, starting with a small central crust which spreads outwards to cover the entire spot. After the last spot crusts over the patient is no longer infectious.

Chickenpox pneumonitis is a serious complication, occurring around the second to sixth day, and heralded by tachypnoea (oxygen saturations at this stage will be reduced). Symptoms include dyspnoea, chest tightness, and cough, occasionally with pleuritic pain, with or without sputum. It may be complicated by secondary bacterial infection, and like in influenza, staphylococcus aureus is a potential pathogen alongside streptococcus pneumoniae and haemophilus influenzae. For this reason, broad-spectrum antibiotics which cover these organisms should be included in the management of chickenpox pneumonitis. Specific therapy with aciclovir 10 mg/kg three times a day (tds) for 7–10 days is indicated, and commenced within 24 hours where possible. Aciclovir should not be withheld in pregnancy. The mortality from chickenpox pneumonitis has been significantly reduced with this treatment. Extensive experience in its use in pregnancy suggests that it is safe.

Sissons J. 'Herpes viruses (excluding Epstein–Barr virus)', Oxford textbook of medicine. Edited by Warrell D, Cox T, Firth J. 5th edn. Oxford: OUP, 2010.

17. E. Steroids can be a useful adjunct to treatment

This patient has leprosy, a chronic granulomatous condition of skin and nerves, caused by infection with mycobacterium leprae.

There are few conditions which give rise to enlarged peripheral nerves, and the combination of this together with evidence of nerve damage, and hypopigmented anaesthetic macules makes leprosy the most likely diagnosis in this setting. The presence of mycobacteria in slit-skin smears together with these features is diagnostic, though not all cases have easily visible mycobacteria, especially patients with paucibacillary disease.

Mycobateria leprae grows very slowly. It has a doubling time of 12 days. It has fastidious growth requirements, and has never been cultured *in vitro*. Laboratory culture is possible *in vivo* in the foot-pad of laboratory mice, and can infect nine-banded armadillos in the wild, though humans are the main reservoir of infection.

Leprosy is a disease of humans. It is not very contagious, and is probably spread by nasal secretions of patients who have multibacillary disease. Incidence of leprosy in household contacts of cases of multibacillary disease is up to ten times that of the local population.

The clinical manifestations of leprosy are on a spectrum ranging from multibacillary to pauci-bacillary disease, depending on the cell mediated immune response generated within the patient. A strong cell-mediated response is associated with tuberculoid leprosy, or paucibacillary disease. There is asymmetric involvement of peripheral nerves (only one nerve is usually affected) and a few macules, which are anaesthetic. Biopsy demonstrates epithelioid granulomas with neural involvement, and absent to scanty bacteria seen on Ziehl–Nielsen or Wade–Fite staining.

At the other end of the spectrum, lepromatous or multibacillary disease is associated with a poor cell-mediated response, large numbers of symmetrically distributed macules, symmetric nerve infiltration, and widespread infiltration of the skin. Macules may not be anaesthetic, but the patient is likely to have symmetric predominantly sensory loss on testing. Infiltration of the skin on the face and loss of eyebrows may give the characteristic leonine facies.

Patients with lepromatous disease may also have complications in other organs including the eyes, testes, lymph nodes, kidneys, and bones. Management of leprosy not only involves treating the infection, which is curable with multi-drug therapy, but also management of its complications and sequelae, and support to reduce stigma.

Treatment is according to WHO multi-drug-based therapy, based on whether the patient has multi-bacillary or paucibacillary disease. Treatment for paucibacillary disease consists of dapsone 100 mg daily combined with rifampicin 600 mg monthly for six months. Multibacillary disease is treated for 1–2 years with a combination of daily dapsone 100 mg and clofazimine 50 mg daily, and a 300 mg dose once per month, together with monthly rifampicin 600 mg.

Patients can shift in their immunological status, before during and after treatment. This can give rise to acute symptoms, or lepra reactions. If a patient is 'upgrading' towards the tuberculoid end of the spectrum this is known as a type 1 reaction. This can result in sudden inflammatory infiltration of skin and or nerves, leading to acute damage. Treatment of this reaction involves the use of steroids to reduce inflammation and aim to preserve nerve function, alongside the antimicrobial management of the leprosy. Lepra reactions resulting from a shift towards the lepromatous end of the spectrum are known as type 2 reactions, which include erythema nodosum leprosum. These can also be treated with steroids. Sometimes, additional anti-inflammatory agents are needed, including thalidomide. As in paucibacillary disease, multi-drug treatment for leprosy is continued alongside treatment for the reaction.

Nerve damage may not recover following treatment. It is equally important to manage the sequelae of this disease, with good skin care, footwear, prevention of contractures, and care of trophic ulcers, physiotherapy, and occupational therapy.

Lockwood D, Beeching N. 'Leprosy', Lecture notes: tropical medicine. Edited by Beeching N, Gill G. 7th edn. Wiley-Blackwell. 2014.

18. B. Carry out investigations and directly contact the new mother

This is an ethical dilemma as there is conflict between protecting his confidentiality and protecting others from harm. Failure to contact the new mother and inform her would place her and potentially her newborn child at risk of serious harm; therefore, action is required. There is a policy of antenatal HIV testing in the UK but patients can opt out. On reviewing her tests, even if the new mother had been HIV negative at the 12-week stage, she could have easily contracted HIV later in that pregnancy and therefore still may have exposed her newborn to a high risk of HIV during her sero-conversion stage of maximum infectivity. You need further information from her to decide on the next steps. Are they still in a relationship? Has he informed her of his HIV status? He has demonstrated his wish to disengage from the service by no longer answering calls or taking medical advice. Your duty is to test her and if she is HIV positive enable her child to be tested. If he is in an ongoing relationship and not disclosing his HIV status then he is continuing to place her at risk. If he were to infect her then a criminal offence would have been committed according to UK law. In Scotland, it is also an offence to expose others to the risk of infection but in England, Wales, and Northern Ireland this is not the case. The starting point in these difficult cases is to try to persuade the patient to inform his partner and to protect the patient's confidentiality, but in a case where there is ongoing risk this can be overruled to protect others from serious harm.

Geretti A. HIV testing and monitoring. Medicine July 2009; 37(7): 326–329.

19. D. A negative white cell first pass urine dip test

Reactive arthritis requires the inflammation of fewer than five large joints and occurs in response to cross-reacting antibodies generated in response to an infection in the urethra or gastrointestinal tract.

Reiter's syndrome is a specific type of reactive arthritis in which there coexists the triad of the joint inflammation, eye inflammation (a conjunctivitis or uveitis), and urethritis. A negative first pass urine dip for white cells excludes Reiter's syndrome but would not exclude a reactive arthritis.

The infection triggering the cross-reacting immune response usually precedes the joint involvement by 4–6 weeks. The trigger might also include gastrointestinal or urethral infection.

Penn H, Keat A. Post-infective arthritis. Medicine October 2006; 34(10): 413–416.

20. D. HIV test

This man has an X-ray appearance consistent with a diagnosis of pneumocystis pneumonia (PCP). The organism pneumocystis jirovecii is a fungal organism that opportunistically affects those who are severely immunosuppressed. To determine whether he is susceptible to this infection, an HIV test would be the most immediate and useful test available. The majority of AIDS presentations in the UK present with PCP. The treatment required is high-dose co-trimoxazole for a total of 21 days starting initially at 120 mg/kg for three days, then 90 mg/kg for the next 18 days. In the initial stage there can be an acute deterioration as the organisms rupture. Monitoring of blood gases is required and if the pO_2 <9.3 kPa high-dose immunosuppression with steroids is indicated.

Miller R, Huang L. 'Pneumocystis jirovecii', Oxford textbook of medicine. Edited by Warrell D, Cox T, Firth J. 5th edn. Oxford: OUP, 2010.

INFECTIOUS DISEASES AND HIV | ANSWERS

21. D. A sexual-health screen

The commonest infective cause of pelvic inflammatory disease (PID) is chlamydia. A sexual-health screen includes a chlamydia and a gonorrhoea test, as well as serology for HIV and syphilis. The swab can be a self-taken vaginal swab placed into a special transport medium that enables amplification of genetic material. Chlamydia is an intracellular bacteria that infects approximately 10% of the population in this age group. The national chlamydia-screening programme targets those aged 16 (or under) to 25 years old and has been developed specifically to address rising rates. Statistical modelling requires that one-third of the at risk population are screened annually for there to be any impact on national rates. It can masquerade as appendicitis and can even cause hepatic tenderness when infection becomes peritoneal and affects the hepatic capsule. In this situation, it is referred to as Fitz–Hugh Curtis syndrome and can cause hepato-diaphragmatic adhesions.

UK National Guideline for the Management of Pelvic Inflammatory Disease 2011 (updated June 2011). Clinical Effectiveness Group British Association for Sexual Health and HIV.

22. E. Syphilis serology

Secondary syphilis can present in this way. The patient may feel well and the rash itself is usually asymptomatic but can be accompanied by generalized fatigue and muscular aching. The rash is characteristic in that it can affect the palmar and plantar skin. It would be mandatory to perform acute syphilis serology. A sexual history might guide you as the majority of cases occur in men who have sex with men but the absence of this risk factor should not preclude the test. If there were risk factors it would always be worth considering an HIV test. There has been a dramatic resurgence of syphilis over the past 15 years. There are more cases in some clinics than were seen in the whole UK 20 years ago.

Donovan B, Dayan L. 'Syphilis', Oxford textbook of medicine. Edited by Warrell D, Cox T, Firth J. 5th edn. Oxford: OUP, 2010.

23. D. Primary herpes simplex

The most likely diagnosis is herpes simplex virus (HSV); this should be confirmed using a viral PCR test to enable discrimination between HSV1 and 2. Treatment should not be delayed while awaiting the results. The treatment is the same regardless of type but the prognosis varies as HSV 2 causes approximately twice the number of recurrences as HSV 1 per year. She should receive empiric therapy with high-dose aciclovir at 400 mg three times daily for ten days during the primary episode and if she suffers severe recurrences should be treated with just five days of therapy. For those suffering frequent recurrences episodic therapy may be considered enabling a patient to commence therapy at the earliest sign of an attack. If this fails to help, continuous suppressive therapy can be introduced. Development of full immune response usually takes about 12 weeks and recurrences thereafter are usually mild in comparison with the primary attack. It is an irritating condition with no long-term sequelae and referral to sexual health for advice should be considered when it is uncertain whether episodic or continuous prophylaxis is indicated. In this case, there is no mention of a previous attack, and characteristically the primary episode is severe and associated with systemic symptoms that can include pharyngeal ulceration and meningitis. The viral 'transmitter' is usually unaware of their carrier state and often they are entirely unaware of any prior infection as it can be contracted asymptomatically and recurrences remain silent. HSV may precipitate a mucocutaneous reaction in some via a delayed hypersensitivity reaction, usually occurring 10–14 days following a recurrence of HSV. In up to 70% of those presenting with erythema multiforme without a drug cause, recurrent herpes simplex is the underlying trigger.

Farthing P, Bagan J, Scully C. Mucosal diseases series. Number IV. Erythema multiforme. Oral Diseases. 2005; 11(5): 261–267.

Sissons J. 'Herpes viruses (excluding Epstein–Barr virus)', Oxford textbook of medicine. Edited by Warrell D, Cox T, Firth J. 5th edn. Oxford: OUP, 2010.

24. E. Test for immune deficiency

Health Protection Agency statistics show that 3–5% of those living in the UK originating from sub-Saharan Africa are infected with HIV. Presentation to any healthcare professional should prompt a discussion in which HIV testing is offered. The need for extensive pre-test counselling has been removed by the effective treatments now available. Patients need to consent in the same way they should for all medical investigations. Patients who are diagnosed late expect to have been screened and failure to test results in much worse morbidity and mortality. In Australia, cases have been brought by those avoidably infected against physicians who have failed to test index patients with good indications who have subsequently gone on to infect others. In 2011, the National Institute for Health and Care Excellence (NICE) produced public health guidance on increasing the uptake of HIV testing. The two documents concerning men who have sex with men and black African communities repeat a number of the key recommendations in the British HIV Association (BHIVA) and British Society for Sexual Health and HIV (BASHH) guidelines. In all healthcare settings (including general practice, outpatient, and emergency settings), an HIV test should be routinely offered and recommended to men who have sex with men, and all patients originating from high-prevalence countries, or those who have had sexual contact with those from high-risk countries. In addition, a list of HIV indicator conditions has been developed where HIV testing is recommended. The complete list of HIV indicator conditions is available online but the commonest are listed here:

Respiratory—TB and bacterial pneumonia.

Neurology—cerebral toxoplasmosis, aseptic meningitis/encephalitis, primary cerebral lymphoma, cerebral abscess, cryptococcal meningitis, space occupying lesion of unknown cause, progressive multifocal Guillain–Barré syndrome, transverse myelitis, peripheral neuropathy, and dementia.

Dermatology—Kaposi's sarcoma, severe or recalcitrant seborrhoeic dermatitis, severe or recalcitrant psoriasis, and multi-dermatomal or recurrent herpes zoster.

Gastroenterology—persistent cryptosporidiosis, oral candidiasis, oral hairy leukoplakia, chronic diarrhoea of unknown cause, weight loss of unknown cause, salmonella, shigella, campylobacter, and hepatitis B/C infection.

Oncology—Non-Hodgkin's lymphoma, anal cancer or anal intraepithelial dysplasia, cervical intraepithelial neoplasia grade 2 or above, head and neck cancer, and Hodgkin's lymphoma.

Gynaecology—cervical cancer and vaginal intraepithelial neoplasia.

Ophthalmology—cytomegalovirus retinitis, infective retinal diseases including herpes viruses and toxoplasma and any unexplained retinopathy.

ENT—lymphadenopathy of unknown cause, chronic parotitis, and lymphoepithelial parotid cysts.

Other—mononucleosis-like syndrome (primary HIV infection), pyrexia of unknown origin, and any lymphadenopathy of unknown cause.

http://www.bhiva.org/HIV-testing-guidelines.aspx

25. C. Random allocation

The participants were allocated to treatment groups using random allocation. Following recruitment, each participant had an equal probability of 0.5 of being allocated to the probiotic drink group or placebo group. The allocation sequence was not pre-determined but decided at random by the use of, for example, random number tables. Providing the sample size is large enough, random allocation results in the treatment groups having similar baseline characteristics. Therefore, confounding is minimized; any differences between treatment groups in outcome at the end of the study will be due to differences in treatment and unlikely to be due to differences in baseline characteristics (see Sedgwick, 2015b). Random allocation also meant that the trial could be double-blind through the introduction of a placebo, thereby minimizing ascertainment bias (see Sedgwick, 2015a).

Alternate allocation involves assigning trial participants to treatment groups in an alternating sequence as they are recruited. For example, the first patient to probiotic drink, second patient to placebo, third patient to probiotic drink, fourth patient to placebo, and so on. The allocation sequence would therefore be predetermined. Alternate allocation is prone to selection bias and subsequently allocation bias (see Sedgwick, 2013). Following alternate allocation, there is no guarantee that the treatment groups will be similar in baseline characteristics. Therefore, alternate allocation will no doubt lead to confounding—that is, any differences between the treatment groups in outcomes at the end of the study may not be due to differences in treatment but differences in their baseline characteristics (see Sedgwick, 2015b).

Cluster random allocation requires participants to be recruited through cluster sampling; this would involve obtaining a random sample of clusters from the population, with all members of each selected cluster invited to participate (see Sedgwick, 2014a). Clusters are natural groupings of people, for example schools, hospitals, and general practices. The clusters rather than the participants in the clusters would then be randomized to treatment. All the participants in each cluster would then receive the treatment—probiotic drink or placebo—that their cluster had been allocated (see Sedgwick, 2014b). Trials that use cluster random allocation are called cluster randomized controlled trials, and the study design is often used when it is not possible to make the trial double-blind. In such circumstances, cluster random allocation minimizes practical and contamination problems that may arise if simple random allocation was used (see Sedgwick, 2014b). Although the trial above was a multicentre one, with participants recruited from three hospitals, this was for convenience and to ensure a sufficient number of participants were recruited. It also meant the sample was more representative of the population in respect of their demographic characteristics and prognostic factors. Once patients on a ward were recruited, they were then allocated at random to the probiotic drink or placebo.

Systematic allocation involves allocating participants to treatment using a systematic approach. The simplest type of systematic allocation is alternate allocation described above—that is, allocating every other participant to the probiotic drink group as they are recruited, with all remaining participants allocated to the placebo group. Other systematic allocation approaches might include, for example, allocating every third participant to the placebo group, with all remaining participants allocated to the probiotic drink group. This would result in treatment group sizes in the ratio of 2:1 (probiotic drink:placebo). Systematic allocation is prone to selection bias and allocation bias, plus confounding as described above for alternate allocation (see Sedgwick, 2013; Sedgwick, 2015b).

Random sampling is a method by which participants are recruited to a study, not how they are allocated to treatment following recruitment. Random sampling should not be confused with random allocation—random allocation describes how participants are allocated to treatment once recruited (see Sedgwick, 2011). Random sampling would have involved selecting a sample of a fixed size at random from the population of all hospital patients taking antibiotics; all members of the population would have had the same probability of being selected, independently of all others. The probability that a population member would be chosen would have been known in advance. Random sampling requires a sampling frame—that is, a list of all people belonging to the population.

Sedgwick P. Random sampling versus random allocation. *BMJ* 2011; 343: d7453.

Sedgwick P. Cluster randomised controlled trials. *BMJ* 2012; 345: e4654.

Sedgwick P. Selection bias versus allocation bias. *BMJ* 2013; 346: f3345.

Sedgwick P. Cluster sampling. *BMJ* 2014a; 348: g1215.

Sedgwick P. Treatment allocation in trials: cluster randomisation. *BMJ* 2014b; 348: g2820.

Sedgwick P. Bias in randomised controlled trials: comparison of crossover group and parallel group designs. *BMJ* 2015a; 351: h4283.

Sedgwick P. Randomised controlled trials: understanding confounding. *BMJ* 2015b; 351:h5119.

chapter 13

POISONING AND PHARMACOLOGY

QUESTIONS

1. A 68-year-old woman was admitted via the emergency department with shortness of breath and a productive cough. Her symptoms had started three days previously. She visited her GP, who advised her to take amoxicillin and clarithromycin for a suspected lower respiratory tract infection.

   She had a past medical history of depression for which she had been treated with fluoxetine successfully for many years. She was a non-smoker.

   A right-sided lobar pneumonia was confirmed on a chest X-ray and she was admitted to the acute medical unit for intravenous co-amoxiclav and clarythromicin.

   Overnight, she became confused and agitated. On examination, her mini-mental state examination was 5/10. Her temperature was 38.4°C, her pulse rate was 135 beats per minute and blood pressure was 186/104 mmHg. Her respiratory rate was 28 breaths per minute and oxygen saturation 96% on 5 L per minute of oxygen via a Hudson facemask. Her pupils were dilated and sluggish, her tone was significantly increased globally, as were her reflexes, and she had bilateral sustained ankle clonus.

   Blood results were as follows.

   ```
   Investigations:
     haemoglobin                    123 g/L           (130-180)
     white cell count               18.2 × 10⁹/L      (4.0-11.0)
     platelet count                 340 × 10⁹/L       (150-400)
     serum sodium                   132 mmol/L        (137-144)
     serum potassium                4.5 mmol/L        (3.5-4.9)
     serum urea                     11.0 mmol/L       (2.5-7.0)
     serum creatinine               220 mmol/L        (60-110)
     creatinine kinase              150 IU/L          (124-170)
     international normalized       1.1               (<1.4)
       ratio (INR)
     activated partial              38 s              (30-40)
       thromboplastin time
   ```

What is the next best step in her management?

A. Intravenous diazepam 5 mg
B. Intravenous paracetamol 1 g
C. Intravenous sodium chloride 0.9% 500 mL
D. Olanzapine 10 mg orally
E. Referral to critical care

2. **A 24-year-old woman was admitted to the emergency department with a raised temperature and seizure. On arrival, she received oxygen via facemask and 2 mg of intravenous lorazepam. Her seizure terminated.**

   She had a history of overdose and recently changed from venlafaxine to an alternative antidepressant. Paramedics found empty drug strips around her with approximately 70 tablets missing.

   On examination, she was flushed with a temperature of 38°C. Her pulse was 140 beats per minute with a blood pressure of 72/34 mmHg. Her airway was patent. She had a respiratory rate of 26 breaths per minute and oxygen saturation of 100% on 5 L/min oxygen via a Hudson face mask. Her chest was clear. Her pupils were dilated and sluggish; she was intermittently agitated, appearing to have visual hallucinations. When settled, her Glasgow Coma Score (GCS) was 11 (E2, V4, M5).

   ```
   Investigations:
     12-lead ECG—broad complex tachycardia with a QRS of 280 ms
     and a dominant R wave in aVR

     Arterial blood gas:
     PO₂                     13.4 kPa        (11.3-12.6)
     PCO₂                    2.8 kPa         (4.7-6.0)
     pH                      7.08            (7.35-7.45)
     bicarbonate             17 mmol/L       (21-29)
     base excess             -7 mmol/L       (±2)
     lactate                 3.5 mmol/L      (0.5-1.6)
     carboxyhaemoglobin      0.5%            (<2)
     oxygen saturation       100%            (94-98)
     methaemoglobin          0.2%            (<1)
   ```

   What is the most appropriate next step in her management?

   A. Intravenous adrenaline 10 mcg boluses titrate to effect
   B. Intravenous amoxicillin 1 g
   C. Intravenous phenytoin 20 mg/kg
   D. Intravenous sodium bicarbonate 2 mmol/kg bolus
   E. Referral to critical care for dialysis

3. A 54-year-old woman with a history of collapse attended the emergency department after being found unresponsive; the paramedics thought she may have had a stroke. She had a history of hypertension, depression, chronic kidney disease, chronic back pain, and type II diabetes mellitus.

The paramedics brought a recent prescription for her with them. She was advised to take:

- Metformin 500 mg twice daily
- Gliclazide 40 mg once daily
- Ramipril 10 mg once daily
- Furosemide 40 mg once daily
- Temazepam 10 mg at night
- Citalopram 10 mg once daily
- Morphine sulphate modified release 20 mg twice daily
- Tramadol 50 mg three times daily
- Morphine sulphate oral solution 10 mg as required

On examination, she was tolerating a nasopharyngeal airway. Her pulse was 75 beats per minute with a blood pressure of 110/76 mmHg. Her respiratory rate was 8 breaths per minute with an oxygen saturation of 100% on 15 L per minute of oxygen via a reservoir mask. She had quiet breath sounds at both bases. Her pupils were 3 mm and reactive, tone was reduced with normal reflexes and downgoing plantars, and her GCS was 3/15.

```
Investigations:
  CT scan of head was normal
  PO₂                    15.8 kPa         (11.3-12.6)
  PCO₂                   9.6 kPa          (4.7-6.0)
  pH                     7.16             (7.35-7.45)
  bicarbonate            21 mmol/L        (21-29)
  base excess            -2 mmol/L        (±2)
  lactate                1.8 mmol/L       (0.5-1.6)
  carboxyhaemoglobin     0.5%             (<2)
  oxygen saturation      100%             (94-98)
  methaemoglobin         0.2%             (<1)
```

What is the next best step in management?

A. Flumazenil 500 mcg intravenously
B. Naloxone 100 mcg boluses titrated to conscious level and respiratory rate
C. Naloxone 400 mcg and flumazenil 500 mcg intravenously
D. Naloxone 400 mcg intravenously
E. Naloxone 2 mg infusion over four hours

4. A 16-year-old boy was transferred to the acute medical unit from the emergency department having ingested a large quantity of red berries thought to be yew berries. He claimed to be training as a shaman and believed that the berries were hallucinogenic.

Clinical examination was normal and his observations showed a pulse of 45 beats per minute, blood pressure 105/67 mmHg, respiratory rate of 12 breaths per minute, and oxygen saturation of 98% on air.

```
Investigations:
  ECG—PR interval of 360 ms with slight ST depression
  PO₂                     13.4 kPa             (11.3-12.6)
  PCO₂                    4.9 kPa              (4.7-6.0)
  pH                      7.36                 (7.35-7.45)
  bicarbonate             22 mmol/L            (21-29)
  base excess             +1 mmol/L            (±2)
  potassium               6.7 mmol/L           (3-5-4.9)
  sodium                  139 mmol/L           (137-144)
  lactate                 0.9 mmol/L           (0.5-1.6)
  carboxyhaemoglobin      0.5%                 (<2)
  oxygen saturation       97%                  (94-98)
  methaemoglobin          0.2%                 (<1)
```

What is the best next step in his management?

A. Atropine 600 mcg intravenously
B. Calcium chloride 10%, 10 mL intravenously
C. Digoxin-specific FAB fragments 400 mg intravenous infusion
D. Insulin and dextrose intravenous infusion
E. Sodium bicarbonate 8.4%, 50 mL intravenously

POISONING AND PHARMACOLOGY | QUESTIONS

5. A 34-year-old woman came to the emergency department 24 hours after a salicylate overdose. The estimated quantity ingested was 290 mg/kg. She developed symptoms of tinnitus, tachypnoea, vomiting, and mild confusion. She had no past medical history.

    Urinary alkalinization was commenced due to a metabolic acidosis and she was transferred to the acute medical unit. The next day, she remained unwell with similar symptoms. Her blood tests and arterial blood gas were repeated.

    ```
    Investigations:
        PO₂                 11.8 kPa        (11.3-12.6)
        PCO₂                3.9 kPa         (4.7-6.0)
        pH                  7.55            (7.35-7.45)
        bicarbonate         32 mmol/L       (21-29)
        base excess         +5 mmol/L       (±2)
        potassium           2.8 mmol/L      (3.5-4.9)
        chloride            103 mmol/L      (95-107)
        sodium              132 mmol/L      (137-144)
        lactate             3.0 mmol/L      (0.5-1.6)
        oxygen saturation   100%            (94-98)
        salicylate          3.8 mmol/L      (<2.5)
    ```

    What is the most appropriate next step in her management?
    A. 50 mL sodium bicarbonate 8.4% intravenously
    B. 60 mmol potassium chloride intravenously over three hours
    C. Increase rate of sodium bicarbonate infusion
    D. Transfer to critical care for charcoal haemoperfusion
    E. Transfer to critical care for haemodialysis

6. A 76-year-old man attended the acute medical unit with a non-traumatic swelling to his knee. He felt well, was afebrile, and had a cool, non-erythematous right knee with a restricted but reasonable range of movement, which was only mildly painful. One week ago, he attended the hospital with new onset atrial fibrillation and was discharged to the community team who had been overseeing an induction course of warfarin. He was advised to take 2 mg warfarin once daily. His INR after three days was 2.8 (<1.4) and today it is >10. He took no other medication, drank alcohol rarely, and was a non-smoker. He was very clear that he took 'one small tablet' each night.

    Which of the following is the cause of his excessively raised INR?
    A. ATP-binding cassette transporter protein polymorphism
    B. Cytochrome P450 enzyme polymorphism
    C. Enterohepatic recirculation of warfarin
    D. N-acetyletransferase polymorphism
    E. Vitamin K epoxide reductase polymorphism

7. **A 42-year-old man was admitted via the emergency department. He was found collapsed at the bus station by a member of public. He had empty bottles of whisky in his possession. In the emergency department, he was treated with intravenous fluids and vitamin B12 complex, as he appeared intoxicated. He was subsequently transferred to the acute medical unit. Four hours later, he still appeared to be intoxicated.**

   His pulse was 140 beats per minute and blood pressure was 90/50 mmHg. His respiratory rate was 26 breaths per minute with an oxygen saturation of 97% on room air.

   ```
   Investigations:
      PO₂                     11.8 kPa        (11.3-12.6)
      PCO₂                    2.1 kPa         (4.7-6.0)
      pH                      7.08            (7.35-7.45)
      bicarbonate             10 mmol/L       (21-29)
      base excess             -12 mmol/L      (±2)
      potassium               4.6 mmol/L      (3.5-4.9)
      chloride                95 mmol/L       (95-107)
      sodium                  139 mmol/L      (137-144)
      lactate                 3.2 mmol/L      (0.5-1.6)
      serum urea              5.2 mmol/L      (2.5-7.0)
      random plasma glucose   5.6 mmol/L
   ```

   Which two blood assays would be the most useful?
   A. Ethanol and ethylene glycol
   B. Ethanol and serum osmolality
   C. Ethylene glycol and serum osmolality
   D. Methanol and ethanol
   E. Methanol and serum osmolality

8. A 45 year-old man was referred to the acute medical unit by his GP because of a delayed presentation of therapeutic excess use of paracetamol. He had been trying to relieve dental pain from an abscess. He weighed 80 kg and had taken approximately 16 × 500 mg tablets of paracetamol in a 24-hour period. The last time he ingested paracetamol was 36 hours ago. He felt well and had no abdominal pain and no clinical signs of jaundice. No blood sampling had been done yet. Despite his dental pain, he had been able to eat normally and he had no other medical conditions and was taking no other medication.

On examination, he was apyrexial with a pulse of 86 beats per minute and blood pressure 110/68 mmHg. His respiratory rate was 14 breaths per minute and his oxygen saturation was 98% on room air.

```
Investigations:
  ECG: normal sinus rhythm
```

What are the most appropriate next steps in management?

A. Explain that the risk of hepatotoxicity is low and offer methionine orally
B. Measure serum electrolytes, creatinine, bicarbonate, paracetamol, liver functions tests, and INR. Start n-acetylcysteine immediately
C. Measure serum paracetamol level, liver function tests, and INR and assess the need for treatment with the results
D. Reassure him and discharge with advice to avoid paracetamol for 48 hours
E. Start n-acetylcysteine and measure serum electrolytes, creatinine, bicarbonate, paracetamol, liver functions tests, and INR after the infusion is complete

9. A 21-year-old man was brought into the emergency department having been found collapsed in a nightclub. Witnesses reported that he had ingested a clear colourless liquid repeatedly over the evening. On initial triage, he was drowsy with a GCS of 10 (E2, V3, M5) in the emergency department; he had a 12-lead ECG and a venous blood gas, both of which were normal. Shortly after arrival on the acute medical unit, he became unresponsive and was found to be in respiratory arrest. Naloxone was administered but, on your arrival, he was still unresponsive and the anaesthetist was preparing to intubate the patient.

On examination:

Airway: oropharyngeal airway *in situ*

Breathing: respiratory rate of 6 breaths per minute, requiring some ventilatory support with a self-inflating bag and mask. Chest was clear; pulse oximetry 100% on 15 L/minute of oxygen via a reservoir mask

Circulation: pulse 50 beats per minute, blood pressure 134/78 mmHg; heart sounds normal, 12-lead ECG showed sinus bradycardia

Disability: GCS 3, pupils 2 mm and reactive, blood glucose 6.6 mmol/L

Exposure: no injuries found, temperature 37.3°C.

After intubation, he was transferred to the intensive care unit. He had a CT scan of head, which was normal. Three hours later, he woke abruptly and self-extubated.

Which drug most likely caused his collapse?

A. Benzodiazepine
B. Ethanol
C. Gamma-hydroxybutyrate
D. Ketamine
E. Opiate

10. A 22-year-old, non-smoking man was admitted to the acute medical unit following suspected exposure to carbon monoxide. He remained unwell with tachycardia, vomiting, pounding headache, and flushing.

His arterial blood gas breathing air was as follows.

```
Investigations:
    PO₂                     10.7 kPa            (11.3-12.6)
    PCO₂                    5.8 kPa             (4.7-6.0)
    pH                      7.16                (7.35-7.45)
    Bicarbonate             18 mmol/L           (21-29)
    base excess             -5 mmol/L           (±2)
    lactate                 4.5 mmol/L          (0.5-1.6)
    carboxyhaemoglobin      15%                 (<2)
    methaemoglobin          0.2%                (<1)
```

Which of the following statements is most accurate?

A. Carbon monoxide exhibits type A toxicity in binding to haemoglobin and myoglobin
B. Carbon monoxide exhibits type A toxicity in binding to haemoglobin, myoglobin, and mitochondrial cytochrome oxidase
C. Carbon monoxide exhibits type A and B toxicity in binding to haemoglobin, myoglobin, and mitochondrial cytochrome oxidase
D. Carbon monoxide exhibits type B toxicity in binding to haemoglobin, myoglobin, and mitochondrial cytochrome oxidase
E. Carbon monoxide exhibits type B toxicity in binding to mitochondrial cytochrome oxidase

11. A 42-year-old woman was admitted to the acute medical unit following an intentional overdose of 1,600 mg of verapamil three hours previously.

On examination, her pulse rate was 42 beats per minute with a blood pressure of 80/42 mmHg. Initial treatment with fluids, calcium gluconate, and adrenaline had been commenced by the emergency department without improvement. Atropine had been given with no effect.

Her 12-lead ECG showed sinus rhythm at 42 beats per minute with first-degree heart block.

The next most appropriate step in the management of this patient is:

A. 1.5 mg/kg of 20% Intralipid®
B. 3 mg Atropine
C. Further dose of adrenaline
D. High-dose insulin euglycaemic therapy
E. High-dose insulin therapy and Intralipid®

12. An 18-year-old woman was admitted to the emergency department. She had a history of deliberate self-harm and lived with her grandmother who called an ambulance after finding her to be drowsy and complaining of a headache. She denied ingestion of any substances but had been alone in the house all afternoon. Her grandmother took a sleeping tablet and something for 'leg pain at night'.

    On examination, she had a pulse rate of 120 beats per minute and her GCS was 14 (E3, V5, M6).

    Which of the following is most appropriate?
    A. The patient should be given a test dose of flumazenil to establish the cause of her drowsiness
    B. The patient should receive multiple-dose activated charcoal
    C. The patient should receive single-dose activated charcoal
    D. The patient should receive supportive therapy only
    E. A routine toxicology screen will confirm the nature of possible poisoning

13. **A 55-year-old woman was admitted to the emergency department following an overdose of 20 x 80mg sotalol tablets two hours previously (total 1600 mg). On arrival in the emergency department, she complained of weakness and lethargy.**

    Initial examination showed a pulse rate of 50 beats per minute, blood pressure 95/67 mmHg, respiratory rate 18 breaths per minute, oxygen saturation 98% on room air, and a GCS of 15. She was relatively stable so no specific treatment was started other than intravenous 0.9% sodium chloride. She was placed on a cardiac monitor and referred to the acute medical unit.

    Blood results were as follows.

    ```
    Investigations:
        serum sodium              132 mmol/L        (137-144)
        serum potassium           3.0 mmol/L        (3.5-4.9)
        serum urea                4.2 mmol/L        (2.5-7.0)
        serum creatinine          92 mmol/L         (60-110)
        PO2                       12.1 kPa          (11.3-12.6)
        PCO2                      5.0 kPa           (4.7-6.0)
        pH                        7.37              (7.35-7.45)
        bicarbonate               25 mmol/L         (21-29)
        base excess               -1.0 mmol/L       (±2)
        lactate                   2.0 mmol/L        (0.5-1.6)
        carboxyhaemoglobin        0.5%              (<2)
        oxygen saturation         99%               (94-98)
        methaemoglobin            0.2%              (<1)
    ```

    During transfer to the acute medical unit she complained of palpitations then collapsed with loss of consciousness. She had been taken off the monitor for transfer and, during the episode, had a barely palpable very fast and irregular radial pulse. The episode lasted for a couple of minutes and then slowly resolved. Afterwards, she looked pale but was alert and a repeat ECG showed a sinus bradycardia of 50 beats per minute and a QTc of 600 ms.

    What is the most appropriate next step in her management?
    A. External cardiac pacing
    B. Intravenous glucagon 5 mg
    C. Intravenous high-dose insulin/dextrose therapy
    D. Intravenous magnesium sulphate 2 g.
    E. Intravenous sodium chloride 0.9%

14. **A 36-year-old woman was admitted to the acute medical unit having taken an overdose of carbamazepine. It was estimated she had taken 80 tablets of 200 mg of carbamazepine (total 16000 mg) around two hours before arrival. She had no other medical conditions and was taking no regular medication. The tablets belonged to her husband, who had epilepsy.**

    On examination, she was alert and not distressed or agitated. She had a pulse rate of 88 beats per minute, blood pressure of 110/67 mmHg, and a respiratory rate of 16 breaths per minute. Physical examination was normal. She weighed around 50 kg.

    Her ECG was normal and blood results were pending.

    Which of the following is the most appropriate in her management?

    A. She should be admitted to a high-dependency area
    B. She should be admitted to the short-stay ward
    C. She should be discharged
    D. She should be electively intubated and admitted to intensive care
    E. She should receive multiple-dose activated charcoal

15. **A 26-year-old man was admitted to the acute medical unit via the emergency department having ingested an unknown volume of chemical paraffin. On arrival, he was agitated and difficult to manage, so he received 4 mg of intravenous midazolam. He became drowsy with an intermittent cough. He opened his eyes to voice, had confused speech, and localized pain.**

    Which of the following is true?

    A. Endotracheal intubation should be considered at this point
    B. GCS is a validated assessment tool in intoxication
    C. His airway does not require protection
    D. Insert an oropharyngeal airway because of his reduced GCS
    E. There are no symptoms or signs of aspiration

chapter 13

POISONING AND PHARMACOLOGY

ANSWERS

1. A. Intravenous diazepam 5 mg

The most likely cause of her acute delirium is serotonin syndrome resulting from a drug reaction between fluoxetine and clarithromycin. Macrolides inhibit cytochrome P450 enzymes, including CYP3A4 reducing the metabolism of the sertraline causing increased serotonergic side effects and eventually serotonin syndrome. Other causes include deliberate overdose, dose increase of an SSRI, or introduction of an SSRI and concomitant administration of a second serotonergic drug.

Serotonin syndrome

Serotonin syndrome is a clinical triad of altered mental status, neuromuscular dysfunction, and autonomic dysfunction. However, all three may not be present (Table 13.1).

Table 13.1 Clinical features of serotonin syndrome.

Autonomic	CNS	Neuromuscular
Hypertension	Anxiety	Hyperreflexia
Hyperthermia	Agitation	Tremor
Tachycardia	Delirium	Myclonus
Mydriasis	Seizures	Clonus
Diarrhoea	Coma	Increase tone
Sweating		
Hypotension		

Differential diagnosis includes neuroleptic malignant syndrome, malignant hyperthermia, and sympathomimetic agents.

Treatment is supportive in mild cases. Hypertension, delirium, and tachycardia respond well to benzodiazepines. Specific antidotes include cyproheptadine, olanzapine, and chlorpromazine but these are rarely used in the UK. The patient should have continuous monitoring. More severe cases should be managed in a high-dependency area. Severe hyperthermia (>39.5°C) and/or rigidity requires anaesthesia, intubation, and paralysis. Serotonergic agents and interacting drugs should be stopped. In this case the patient could be changed to azithromycin, as this does not appear to inhibit the Cytochrome P450 (CYP450) enzyme system.

Symptoms usually resolve within 24 hours, except in the case of irreversible MAOI interaction where symptoms can be very prolonged.

Examples of serotonergic drugs
- SSRIs
- Tramadol
- Tricylic antidepressants
- Amphetamine
- SNRIs
- Lithium
- MAOIs

Drug interactions

Drug interactions are an adverse reaction leading to increased adverse effects or decreased therapeutic effect. There are two principle mechanisms for drug interactions: pharmacokinetic and pharmacodynamic.

Pharmacokinetic
- Absorption
  - Drug absorption may be affected by another drug altering gastric pH, e.g. with antacids, forming less absorbable compounds or altering gastric motility.
- Metabolism
  - The majority of drugs undergoing enzyme metabolism do so by the CYP450 enzyme system. Where one drug induces the metabolism of another, therapeutic effect may be reduced or toxic metabolites may be increased. Where enzyme inhibition occurs, enhanced therapeutic effect or, more likely, increased adverse effects may be observed (Table 13.2).

Table 13.2 Common enzyme inhibitors and inducers.

Inducers	Inhibitors
Ethanol	Macrolides (except azythromicin)
Phenytoin	Metronidazole
Carbamazepine	Amiodarone
St Johns Wort	SSRIs

- Transport
  - Many drugs are moved across membranes and thus from compartment to compartment by p-glycoproteins (PgP), a family of ATP-binding cassette proteins. Polymorphism can reduce absorption, increase excretion, and alter the availability of drugs at target receptors.
- Excretion
  - Competition for non-specific active tubular secretion may reduce renal excretion leading to elevated plasma levels. Passive tubular uptake can also be altered by changes in pH. A therapeutic example of this is urinary alkalization in salicylate overdose to increase excretion.

Pharmacodynamic
- This occurs when one drug changes the effect of another by acting at the same receptor or at a separate receptor. Drugs acting at the same receptor may cause an agonist or antagonist effect, which can be clinically beneficial, for example naloxone acting as an opiate antagonist. It may also be harmful such as concomitant administration of two serotonergic or opiate drugs.
- Drugs acting at separate sites may cause an additive, synergistic, or antagonist effect.

Thomas A, Routledge PA. 2003. Drug interactions in clinical practice. Pharmacovigilance Bul 34:1–7.2

The Hunter Serotonin Toxicity Criteria: simple accurate diagnostic decision rules for serotonin toxicity. Dunkley EJC et al. Quarterly Journal of Medicine 2003; 96: 635–642.

British National Formulary Appendix 1.

2. D. Intravenous sodium bicarbonate 2 mmol/kg bolus

This is a very typical clinical picture of a large tricyclic antidepressant overdose. The indications for sodium bicarbonate are QRS duration of >120 ms, ventricular arrhythmia, hypotension, and seizure. Sodium bicarbonate should be given as an initial bolus followed by an infusion. Phenytoin is contraindicated, as it is a sodium channel blocker and thus may cause cardiac arrhythmia and seizure by exacerbating sodium channel blockade.

Tricyclic poisoning

Although seen less often in overdose, all tricyclic antidepressants are very toxic in overdose acting on a wide range of receptors including muscarinic, gaba, alpha, and histamine causing an anticholinergic picture. Importantly, though, they cause sodium channel blockade leading to cardiac symptoms, often termed the quinidine action as seen with class I antiarrhythmics.

Patients should be observed for a minimum of six hours for symptoms and discharged only when symptom-free. Overdose of 10 mg/kg or more can produce life-threatening toxicity and symptoms may take up to 24 hours to appear due to delayed absorption. See Table 13.3.

Table 13.3 Symptoms and signs of tricyclic antidepressant poisoning.

Cardiovascular	Central nervous	Other
Sinus tachycardia	Drowsiness	Dilated pupils
Prolonged QRS	confusion	Nausea
Dominant R wave aVR*	Delirium	Dry mouth
Cardiac dysrhythmia	Seizure	Acidosis
Hypotension	Coma	Rhabdomyolysis
Bradycardia		

*An R wave in aVR of 3 mm or greater is suggestive of significant tricyclic antidepressant poisoning

Treatment is supportive, maintain airway, support ventilation if required, correct hypotension, and manage delirium with benzodiazepines. Sodium bicarbonate is required if indicated, as previously outlined. The therapeutic target is correction of hypotension and the prolonged QRS. Blood pH should be maintained at 7.5 to 7.55; this may require a repeat bolus and follow-up infusion.

Seizures should be treated with benzodiazepines and not phenytoin, as this is also a sodium channel blocker. Torsade de pointes can be treated with magnesium sulphate but other antiarrythmic drugs should be avoided. Patients with who do not respond to emergency and supportive treatment will require critical care.

Anticholinergic toxidrome

See Table 13.4 for anticholinergic toxidrome.

Table 13.4 Anticholinergic toxidrome.

Anticholinergic agents	Symptoms/signs
Antimuscarinics	Delirium*
Antipsychotics (including atypical)	Tremor
Antihistamines	Dry mouth
Tricyclic antidepressants	Dilated pupils
Carbamazepine	Flushed dry skin
Oxybutinin	Urinary retention
Ipratropium bromide	Ileus
Plant material (e.g. deadly nightshade)	Hyperthermia
	Tachycardia

*The delirium is often very typical in nature with and agitated confusion that is fluctuant. The patient is usually restless and a can be aggressive. Visual hallucinations are common with the patient repetitively 'picking' at the air or sheets

Sodium bicarbonate

Sodium bicarbonate has two principle indications in the management of the poisoned patient:

1. Cardiotoxicity in sodium channel blockade, for example, with tricyclic antidepressants and type 1 antiarrhythmics.
2. Enhanced elimination in salicylate poisoning.

It has three main mechanisms:

i. Provides a large sodium load overcoming sodium channel blockade while buffering acidosis with bicarbonate ions.
ii. Elevates blood pH, which prevents shift of ionized drugs to the central nervous system (CNS), e.g. aspirin, and aids sodium channel function.
iii. Urinary alkalization, increasing the amount of ionized salicylate in the renal tubules preventing reuptake of salicylate or 'ion trapping'.

Absorption and distribution

While rate of absorption does not affect the amount of drug absorbed, it does influence the time to peak plasma levels and hence the time to maximal expected symptoms of poisoning. Factors influencing absorption in overdose include drug preparation and gastrointestinal motility (anticholinergic drugs, alcohol, opiates). These factors must be considered when risk-assessing the patient.

Distribution will influence the final plasma concentration. Small molecular weight, non-ionized, lipid-soluble drugs distribute widely and have a large apparent volume of distribution. These drugs also have a long half-life of elimination and, therefore, prolonged toxicity. Dialysis is not an effective method of elimination for these drugs, a good example being triclycic antidepressants.

Body R, Bartram T, Azam F et al. Guidelines in Emergency Medicine Network (GEMNet): guideline for the management of tricyclic antidepressant overdose. Emergency Medicine Journal 2011; 28: 347–368.

UK National Poisons Information Service. Guideline for tricyclic antidepressant poisoning. Commissioned by Public Health England. http://www.toxbase.org

3. B. Naloxone 100 mcg boluses titrated to conscious level and respiratory rate

There are two possibilities here; she may have taken an overdose of some or all of her drugs or her chronic kidney disease has deteriorated resulting in a build up of active opiate and benzodiazepine metabolites. Her symptoms are principally central nervous system and respiratory depression suggesting opiates and or benzodiazepine toxicity. Despite remaining well saturated, she has significant respiratory depression and hypercapnia, which also contributes to reduced consciousness. Symptoms and signs can be clouded by the actions of other drugs; for example, pupil size should be pinpoint but the presence of two serotonergic drugs (tramadol and citalopram) may antagonize the opiate effect.

Naloxone is a very effective opiate receptor antagonist and quickly reverses opiate side effects. Patients who have a history of long-term use are at risk of withdrawal if aggressive reversal is given so doses should be carefully titrated to effect. The half-life of naloxone is 60–90 minutes—shorter than opiates—so an infusion may be required.

Flumazenil is a benzodiazepine antagonist but should not be used in polypharmacy toxicity, chronic benzodiazpine use, underlying seizure disorder, or risk of seizure. The half-life of flumazenil is 40–80 minutes.

Opiate/opioid toxicity

Common in the drug-abusing population but must also be considered in any patient receiving opiates presenting with symptoms consistent with an opioid toxidrome; classically respiratory depression, miosis, and central nervous system (CNS) depression. As previously discussed, naloxone is the antidote but consideration must be given to the half-life of elimination of the opioid in use.

There are some opioids which require special consideration.

Tramadol

Structurally related to venlafaxine, tramadol rarely causes classical opioid toxicity. Its toxic effects are related to its serotonergic actions and hence seizures, tachycardia, and delirium are often seen. This should be treated as per a serotonin-type poisoning. Other opiates with serotonergic effects include fentanyl and pethidine.

Dextropropoxyphene

No longer licensed but still used in a small number of long-term users. Dextroproxyphene is the opioid combined with paracetamol in co-proxamol. It is associated with seizure and cardiac arrhythmia.

Methadone

A very long-acting opioid used in drug-addiction treatment. The toxic effects may last 24 hours and patients are at particular risk of respiratory arrest once they fall asleep, even if they appear to have been well while awake. A long period of observation should be considered. These patients are also at risk of acute withdrawal if high doses of naloxone are given by bolus.

Monitoring in opioid toxicity

Caution should be taken when monitoring patients with opioid toxicity. Pulse oximetry readings are used as a surrogate marker for ventilation, but patients on high-flow oxygen may remain oxygenated with significant respiratory and central nervous system depression. Respiratory monitoring must include respiratory rate; ideally, patients should be monitored off oxygen. Patients who become hypoxic should have immediate review and treatment with oxygen while being reassessed. The treatment for respiratory depression in opioid overdose is naloxone, not oxygen.

Factors in risk assessment

Aside from substance, quantity, and timing, other factors must be considered when risk-assessing a poisoned patient. Most drugs undergo hepatic metabolism to inactive metabolites; factors reducing this capacity, such as chronic liver disease, will delay the clearance of such drugs and increase the period of toxicity. Chronic heart failure may reduce hepatic blood flow, having a similar effect. Inactive metabolites are usually excreted via the kidneys but active metabolites (e.g. opiates and benzodiazepines) and unchanged drugs (e.g. digoxin, lithium) are also excreted. Reduction in glomerular filtration rate will reduce this capacity.

The elderly are generally at higher risk of adverse drug effects because of reduced glomerular filtration and polypharmacy. Hepatic metabolism does decline but the significance of this is variable between individuals probably depending on many other factors such as genetic variation. The very young are at increased risk because of a higher blood–brain barrier permeability, lower glomerular filtration rate, and immature enzyme systems.

Changes in physiology during pregnancy influence metabolism. Pregnant women have a higher cardiac output, and thus hepatic flow, and a higher glomerular filtration rate. This increases the rate of drug clearance and may result in sub-therapeutic levels. Lower plasma protein concentrations result in more unbound and, therefore, active drugs when the drug is usually highly protein bound, e.g. phenytoin.

Boyer EW. Management of opioid analgesic overdose. New England Journal of Medicine 12 July 2012; 367(2): 146–155.

UK National Poisons Information Service. Guideline for opioid poisoning. Commissioned by Public Health England. http://www.toxbase.org

4. C. Digoxin-specific FAB fragments 400 mg intravenous infusion

Yew berries contain a cardiac glycoside, which is similar to digoxin, and is also bound effectively by digoxin-specific FAB fragments. The indications for digoxin specific FAB fragments are:

- serum potassium >6 mmol/L
- life-threatening arrhythmia
- cardiovascular compromise (including cardiac arrest)

Calcium chloride should not be given as it may precipitate arrhythmias and cause further deterioration. Sodium bicarbonate and insulin/dextrose may be given for hyperkalaemia if digoxin-specific FAB fragments are not immediately available. Atropine can be used for a compromised bradycardia.

Cardiac glycosides

There are cardiac glycosides present in several plants in the UK including foxglove, lily of the valley, and yew. In Australasia, the common source is oleander, which is a very popular hedge plant. All of these glycosides can cause a digoxin-like toxicity which can be very successfully treated with digoxin-specific FAB fragments. The digoxin assay can be used to detect plant cardiac glycosides and, although levels are less accurate and do not correlate well with toxicity, they give some indication of the amount ingested.

Cardiac glycosides inhibit Na^+/K^+ pump resulting in an increase in intracellular calcium, decreased sympathetic stimulus, and increased vagal stimulus. This results in increased ventricular automaticity, AV conduction block, and bradycardia.

In digoxin ingestion, peak plasma concentration is at around six hours. Cardiac glycosides have a large volume of distribution, thus haemodialysis is not effective. They are mostly excreted unchanged by the kidneys; renal impairment significantly increases the half-life of elimination. See Table 13.5.

Cardiac glycosides commonly cause metabolic disturbance, with hyperkalaemia and hypercalcaemia being very common in acute poisoning. Hypokalaemia and hypomagnesaemia are often seen in

Table 13.5 Clinical features of cardiac glycoside poisoning.

Gastrointestinal	Cardiovascular	CNS
Nausea	AV blockade	Dizziness
Vomiting	Arrhythmia	Xanthopsia
Abdominal pain	Bradycardia	Reduced visual acuity
	Hypotension	Delirium
	Cardiac arrest	

chronic poisoning. Acute hypokalaemia may also occur as a result of treatment of acute poisoning and must be carefully monitored for.

Unless digoxin-specific FAB fragments are indicated, treatment is supportive with careful attention to correction of metabolic disturbances. Patients should have continuous cardiac monitoring; elimination half-life is 30–40 hours.

Kanji S, Maclean RD. Cardiac glycoside toxicity: more than 200 years and counting. Critical Care Clinics October 2012 Oct; 28(4): 527–535.

UK National Poisons Information Service. Guideline for cardiac glycoside poisoning. Commissioned by Public Health England. http://www.toxbase.org

5. B. 60 mmol potassium chloride intravenously over three hours

Urinary alkalinization is indicated in symptomatic salicylate overdose. Enhancing urinary elimination, works by the effect of ion trapping in the renal tubules and can also be considered for phenobarbitone toxicity. A blood pH of 7.5 to 7.55 is achieved with 1–2 mL/kg boluses of sodium bicarbonate 8.4% followed by an infusion of 25 mmol/hour. Urinary pH should be at least greater than 7.5 with a target of 8.5–8.55. Urinary alkalization is not possible in hypokalaemia as K^+ ions are exchanged for H^+ ions in the kidney to prevent potassium loss; this maintains a more acidic urine. Thus, the correct answer is to correct hypokalaemia and not to give more sodium bicarbonate as this may elevate plasma pH >7.6, which could be fatal. Plasma potassium should be monitored four-hourly. If, despite adequate urinary alkalization, symptoms and levels do not improve or features of severe poisoning are present then haemodialysis should be considered, as most of the salicylate is in the free form in overdose and is readily removed. Elevation of plasma pH also increases the amount of ionized salicylate preventing movement into the CNS compartment and neurotoxicity.

Salicylate poisoning

A relatively rare presentation but often underestimated in its potential for harm (see Table 13.6). The three toxic mechanisms of salicylates are:

1. cyclo-oygenase inhibition
2. central respiratory stimulation and respiratory alkalosis
3. oxidative phosphorylation uncoupling

Table 13.6 Clinical features of salicylate poisoning based on dose ingested and plasma concentration of salicyate.

Dose ingested	Levels	Clinical features
<150 mg/kg (mild)	<2.5 mmol/L (350mg/L)	Nil
150–300 mg/kg (Moderate)	2.5–5.1 mmol/L (350–700 mg/L)	Hyperventilation
		Pyrexia
		Sweating
		Tinnitus
		Vomiting
		Hypoglycaemia
		Respiratory alkalosis
>300 mg/kg (severe)	>5.1 mg/L (700 mg/L)	Altered consciousness
		Metabolic acidosis
		Seizures
		Coma

Patients presenting acutely within an hour should receive 50 g of activated charcoal; in patients with large overdoses and severe features this can be repeated. Aspirin tablets are frequently enteric-coated and can have a significantly delayed absorption profile forming tablet bezoars. Serial salicylate levels, for example at 4, 6, 8, 10, and 12 hours, are sometimes necessary to show a declining trend in levels. Repeat blood gases should also be considered to ensure that metabolic acidosis is not missed and to ensure alkalaemia is maintained. Should pH drop (<7.4) then a sudden increase in CNS salicylate can lead to a rapid deterioration. Ventilated patients are at particular risk.

Pearlman BL, Gambhir R. Salicylate intoxication: a clinical review. Postgraduate Medicine July 2009; 121(4): 162–168.

UK National Poisons Information Service. Guideline for salicylate poisoning. Commissioned by Public Health England. http://www.toxbase.org

6. B. Cytochrome P450 enzyme polymorphism

Warfarin is a substrate of cytochrome P450 2C9 (CYP2C9) of which there are several polymorphisms. Two in particular 2C9*2 and 2C9*3 have 12% and 5% of the normal activity resepctively. Approximately 2–3% of patients carry this polymorphism and these patients display excessive sensitivity to warfarin.

Vitamin K epoxide reductase (VKOR) reduces vitamin K epoxide back to vitamin K hydroxyquinone to allow it to activate coagulation factors II, VII, IX, and X. Warfarin inhibits this enzyme to reduce the amount of active clotting factors available. Polymorphism of the VKOR enzyme produces an enzyme that is less inhibited by warfarin and resistance to anticoagulation.

ATP-binding cassette transporter proteins may have a role in reducing bioavailability of warfarin. N-acetyltransferase and enterohepatic circulation do not influence warfarin metabolism or activity.

The treatment of warfarin overdose depends on whether the patient requires therapeutic warfarin or not. In patients not normally on warfarin and without evidence of any bleeding, 10 mg of vitamin K should be given orally if they have ingested more than 0.25 mg/kg or the INR is greater than 4.0. This can be increased to 20 mg in large overdose. If there is a coagulopathy then INR should be measured six-hourly until it has normalized; repeat doses of vitamin K may be required. In patients without bleeding but who require warfarin for therapeutic reasons, more caution is required as aggressive reversal can lead to problems achieving therapeutic anticoagulation. Advice can be sought from a haematologist but generally if the INR is excessively raised, i.e. >8, a small dose of vitamin K (1–2 mg orally or 0.5–1 mg intravenously) should be given to lower the INR to a more acceptable level. Again, INR should be monitored regularly until at a therapeutic level.

Any patient with active or life-threatening haemorrhage should have urgent correction of the coagulopathy with prothrombin complex concentrate or fresh frozen plasma. Dosing advice will be available from a haematologist.

Vitamin K is a very effective antidote. Although warfarin prevents the activation of vitamin K-dependent clotting factors, the production of those factors is unaffected and the plasma levels are normal. Vitamin K works very quickly to activate these dormant factors, as they will take effect within an hour or two (although peak effect will be later).

Pharmacogenetics

Genetic variation significantly influences an individual's drug metabolism. This may result in faster or slower metabolism of an active drug or potentially faster or slower conversion of a pro-drug to an active substance. A rare but very important example of this would be suxamethonium, a depolarizing paralysing agent that is usually rapidly metabolized to inactive substances by plasma pseudocholinesterase. Autosomal recessive inheritance of an abnormal pseudocholinesterase can result in paralysis for hours or days rather than minutes.

Acetylation of drugs varies greatly on a racial basis. Individuals can be classified as slow or fast acetylators, within European populations 40% are fast acetylators compared with 90% of Japanese. Slow acetylation may result in increased drug side effects such as peripheral neuropathy with isoniazid.

Expression of cytochrome P450 isoenzymes also varies greatly. Individuals can be classified as extensive, ultra-rapid, intermediate, and poor metabolizers. The significant effects of this variation are seen in poor metabolizers (PM) and ultra-rapid metabolizers (UM). With PM, sustained plasma levels are seen leading to an increase in side effects of the drug. The opposite occurs in UM, where drug response is sub-therapeutic at standard doses. Again, when a pro-drug is activated by CYP P450, therapeutic effect may be lost if the individual expresses the PM phenotype. A good example of this is the lack of analgesic effect some patients experience with codeine.

Ultimately, any enzyme, receptor, or transport protein may be affected by genetic variation, all of which will influence the therapeutic effect and side effect profile of a drug.

Pirmohamed M. Cytochrome P450 enzyme polymorphisms and adverse drug reactions. Toxicology 2003; 192: 23–32.

Hall AM. Warfarin: a case history in pharmacogenetics. Heart 2005; 91: 563–564.

Royal Society of Medicine. Personalised Medicines: hopes and realities. September 2005.

7. B. Ethanol and serum osmolality

Initially, this patient is assumed to have presented with alcohol (ethanol) intoxication and has been treated as a regular excessive drinker. However, his subsequent clinical course suggests that there may be other causes for his intoxication. He has a severe acidosis with a considerably widened anion gap, suggesting another exogenous acid. High on the list of suspicion in a patient with intoxication and severe acidosis will be ethylene glycol and methanol ingestion. Most hospitals do not routinely perform assays for ethylene glycol and methanol, samples are sent out to other laboratories, and results may take some time. Calculating the osmolar gap can demonstrate the presence of osmotically active substances but does not distinguish between such substances (e.g. ethanol and methanol). If ethanol levels are included in the calculated osmolality then any further gap indicates the presence of a second substance, assumed in this case to be methanol or ethylene glycol. If calcium oxalate crystals are present in urine, ethylene glycol has been ingested; however, they may be absent.

Methanol and ethylene glycol

Commonly used as antifreeze, ethylene glycol is an uncommon but significant poison. Methanol is present in methylated spirits but also had been increasingly found in illegal, counterfeit alcoholic products. Both cause significant toxicity and mortality if untreated. Once ingested, they are metabolized, as shown in Figure 13.1.

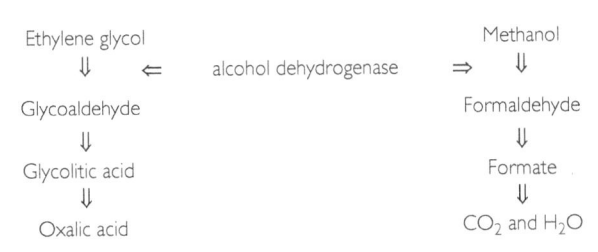

$$
\begin{array}{ccc}
\text{Ethylene glycol} & & \text{Methanol} \\
\Downarrow \quad \Leftarrow \text{alcohol dehydrogenase} \Rightarrow & \Downarrow \\
\text{Glycoaldehyde} & & \text{Formaldehyde} \\
\Downarrow & & \Downarrow \\
\text{Glycolitic acid} & & \text{Formate} \\
\Downarrow & & \Downarrow \\
\text{Oxalic acid} & & CO_2 \text{ and } H_2O
\end{array}
$$

Figure 13.1 Metabolic pathways for ethylene glycol and methanol.

Ethylene glycol and methanol themselves cause a relatively mild CNS effect, presenting with a picture of mild intoxication possibly without the odour of alcohol. However, the metabolites are particularly toxic and result in rapid deterioration. Methanol ingestion results in CNS toxicity, retinal injury, seizures, and coma. Ethylene glycol initially causes renal injury and failure, progressing to multisystem failure and coma. As they are both metabolized by the non-specific enzyme alcohol dehydrogenase (ADH) then inhibition or competition at this enzyme will reduce toxicity by reducing production of metabolites while the methanol or ethylene glycol are cleared unchanged by renal excretion. Thus, treatment for both of these substances is supportive with the use of either fomepizole or ethanol as an antidote. Both act by inhibiting the ADH metabolism of methanol or ethylene glycol. If fomepizole is not available then ethanol can be administered, either intravenously or by nasogastric tube. Guidance regarding dosing and monitoring can be obtained from the UK National Poisons Information Service Toxbase. In severe cases or in those who fail to improve, haemodialysis is effective at removing both substances and their metabolites.

Analytical toxicology

Clinical toxicology often relies on the detection, identification, and quantative measurement of a toxin in a biological system; in this case, the patient. Direct measurement of a specific substance is not always possible routinely and, in such cases, surrogate markers are relied on. In this case, the osmolar gap can be used to confirm the presence of an osmotically active substance but not identify it. Waiting for an external laboratory confirmation of methanol would cause an unacceptable delay in treatment. Another example would be the presence of an anion gap indicating an unmeasured exogenous substance (e.g. salicylate). In some cases, assays will detect a similar substance (e.g. plant cardiac glycosides can be detected and to an extent quantified by the digoxin assay).

Analytical toxicology relies on the correct test on the correct sample at the correct time. Urine is preferred for screening as it is plentiful, easy to collect, and often has a higher concentration of toxin than blood. Timing may be important (e.g. paracetamol levels being done no earlier than four hours to allow for absorption and distribution of the drug). Calcium oxalates take time to form in ethylene glycol poisoning and if looked for too acutely will not be present. Sample must also be collected, stored, processed, and transported correctly.

Commonly used analytical methods include:

- chromatography (gas, thin layer, and liquid)
- enzyme-medicated immunoassay
- radioimmunoassay
- atomic-absorption spectroscopy

Laboratory analyses for poisoned patients: joint position paper.

National Poisons Information Service and Association of Clinical Biochemists. Annals of Clinical Biochemistry 2002; 39: 328–339.

UK National Poisons Information Service. Guideline for methanol and ethylene glycol poisoning. Commissioned by Public Health England. http://www.toxbase.org

8. C. Measure serum paracetamol level, liver function tests, and INR and assess the need for treatment with the results

Single-overdose ingestions are assessed based on a time/plasma level graph which previously used a high-risk and normal-risk curve. This is no longer the case as the National Poisons Information Service (NPIS) paracetamol-overdose guidelines were changed in September 2012. All patients are now assessed on a single-time/dose curve and the NPIS no longer recommends the consideration factors such as starvation and enzyme inducing drugs in treatment decisions.

Uncontrolled dental pain often triggers unintentional excess therapeutic use. Patients who have ingested greater than 150 mg/kg in a 24-hour period should receive a course of n-acetylcysteine. Patients who have ingested 75–150 mg/kg can be assessed clinically. Any patients with symptoms or signs of hepatotoxicity, such as abdominal pain, vomiting, hepatic tenderness, or jaundice should have immediate treatment. In the absence of these features take a venous blood sample for measurement of paracetamol concentration, U&Es, bicarbonate, creatinine, ALT, and INR. If there is detectable paracetamol greater than 24 hours post last ingestion, raised ALT (more than twice normal limits), or increased INR at any time, then treatment should be given. In obese patients, dose and n-acetylcysteine calculations should use a maximum of 110 kg.

Paracetamol overdose

Paracetamol is the commonest agent seen in overdose in the UK accounting for 40–50% of self-poisoning presentations.

At recommended doses, 90% of paracetamol is conjugated with glucuronide and sulphates, 5% is excreted renally, and 5% is metabolized to the highly toxic N-acetyl-p-benzoquinone imine (NAPQI) by cytochrome P450 isoenzymes. This process is increased by cytochrome P450-inducing drugs. Normally, NAPQI conjugates with glutathione but in overdose more NAPQI is produced as the conjugative pathways are saturated. This quickly depletes the liver of glutathione leaving unconjugated NAPQI to cause hepatocellular injury.

N-acetylcysteine

The recommended regime of n-acetylcysteine (Parvolex®) is an extremely effective antidote. It is most effective when given within the first eight hours but continues to be of benefit up to 24 hours post ingestion. N-acetylcysteine acts as a glutathione donor increasing the capacity to conjugate NAPQI and preventing hepatocellular injury. It is also possible that it acts by sulphation of paracetamol.

Reactions to n-acetylcysteine are common, seen in up to 20% of patients receiving it. The typical features are flushing, urticaria, tachycardia, hypotension, and wheeze. The reaction is not an allergic reaction but a dose-dependent direct histaminergic response. If it occurs, the infusion should be stopped and the patient given an antihistamine and a steroid if it is significant. Hypotension can be corrected with fluids and bronchospasm with nebulized salbutamol. Severe reactions are very rare but can require anaphylaxis treatment and critical-care support. The reaction will usually settle within 15–30 minutes at which point the infusion can be recommenced and a slower rate. Evidence does not support slowing down the rate of loading to reduce the incidence of reaction although the recent guideline changes include loading over one hour rather than 15 minutes. Previous reactions are not a contraindication to n-acetylcysteine unless the reaction was severe.

Oral methionine is an alternative antidote in paracetamol overdose; however, it is poorly tolerated and is not effective beyond eight hours. It can be considered in patients who refuse intravenous treatment or admission; however, NPIS now recommends oral use of n-acetylcysteine in those patients.

Liver-unit referral

The Kings College criteria are a prognostic tool for patients with acute liver failure (ALF). The criteria for ALF secondary to paracetamol overdose are: pH <7.30 or

INR >6.5 (PT >100 s) and serum creatinine >300 micromol/L (>3.4 mg/dL) in patients with grade 3 or 4 hepatic encephalopathy.

Bailey et al. Management of anaphylactoid reactions to intravenous n-acetylecysteine. Annals of Emergency Medicine 1998; 31: 710–715.

Kerr et al. The Australasian Clinical Toxicology Investigators Collaboration randomized trial of different loading infusion rates of n-acetylcysteine. Annals of Emergency Medicine 2005; 45: 402–408.

UK National Poisons Information Service. Guideline for paracetamol poisoning. Commissioned by Public Health England. http://www.toxbase.org

9. C. Gamma-hydroxybutyrate

Gamma-hydoxybutyrate (GHB) is a clear and colourless liquid taken as a recreational drug that in overdose typically causes profound coma, airway obstruction, and respiratory arrest. Its mechanism is probably at GABA receptors and its effects are typically short-lived with complete recovery within hours. It is rapidly metabolized to inactive substances. Other features are agitation, nausea, vomiting, bradycardia, and meiosis. A similar drug of abuse is gamma-butyrolactate (GBL), a precursor converted to GHB in the liver. The onset of toxic effect is delayed and inexperienced users may take repeated doses to achieve effect, resulting in subsequent overdose.

In general, most drugs have no specific treatment and after emergency resuscitation the mainstay of toxicological management is good supportive treatment. This is structured using an ABC approach and can be briefly summarized as below:

A   Protect and secure airway
B   Support ventilation and oxygenation
C   Support circulation using volume expansion + /− vasopressors and inotropes. Treat unstable cardiac arrhythmias
D   Manage delirium and seizures. Monitor for and correct hypoglycaemia
E   Manage hypothermia/hyperthermia as required

Drugs of abuse

Opioids

Commonly heroin but may include weaker opiates such as codeine. Caution must be taken over monitoring in long-acting opioids such as methadone. The classic opioid toxidrome is respiratory and central nervous system depression with pinpoint pupils. Effective reversal is achieved with naloxone the half-life of which is usually shorter than the opioid. Ongoing toxicity should be treated with a naloxone infusion. Tramadol, although an opioid, rarely causes classic opioid toxicity but more often serotonergic toxicity.

Cocaine/Amphetamine/MDMA

The toxic mechanism of these drugs is predominantly as a sympathomimetic agent. This produces central nervous system effects such as euphoria but also agitation, delirium, seizures, hallucination, and psychosis. Cardiovascular effects can be profound with tachycardia, hypertension, and arrhythmia. Cocaine causes both arterial vasospasm and increases risk of thrombus resulting in acute coronary syndrome. Patients may become hyperthermic, which again may be severe. Treatment is generally supportive. Central nervous system symptoms may be controlled with benzodiazepines. Severe hypertension may require vasodilators such as glyceryl trinitrate infusion and patients may require cooling for hyperthermia. Occasionally sedation, paralysis, and ventilation are required. Acute coronary syndrome should be investigated and treated as per usual protocols.

Ketamine

Now increasingly used therapeutically, this dissociative anaesthetic drug has become very popular as a cheap drug of abuse. It is usually snorted but also ingested, injected, and occasionally smoked. Its effects include euphoria, agitation, hallucinations, emergence delirium, coma, and seizure. It commonly causes tachycardia, increased blood pressure, tachypnoea, and hypersecretion but can also result in bradycardia and respiratory depression. Treatment is supportive using benzodiazepines to manage delirium. Chronic effects include mental health illness, sleep disturbance, and chronic cystitis.

Stomberg MW, Knudsen K, Stomberg H et al. Symptoms and signs in interpreting Gamma-hydroxybutyrate (GHB) intoxication—an explorative study. Scandinavian Journal of Trauma, Resuscitation and Emergency Medicine 23 April 2014; 22(1): 27.

10. B. Carbon monoxide exhibits type A toxicity in binding to haemoglobin, myoglobin, and mitochondrial cytochrome oxidase

Carbon monoxide (CO) is a clear and odourless gas that rises in the air and accounts for around 40 deaths annually in England and Wales (Table 13.7).

Table 13.7 Clinical features of carbon monoxide inhalation.

Mild	Moderate	Severe
Headache	Weakness	Confusion
Nauasea	Vomiting	Hypotension
Dizziness	Tachypnoea	Arrhythmia
Fatigue	Tachycardia	Cardiogenic shock
	Flushing	Pulmonary oedema
	Drowsiness	Respiratory depression
	Ataxia	Seizure
	Blurred vision	Coma
	Tinnitus	Death
	Mild hypotension	

Aside from supportive therapy, specific treatment is by delivering as high a percentage of inspired oxygen as possible to the patient. The half-life of CO in the body is reduced from four hours in room air to 40 minutes with 100% oxygen. This is difficult to achieve without closed-circuit ventilation; however, inspired fraction of oxygen approaching this can be achieved with a tight-fitting facemask and high-flow oxygen. The half-life can be further reduced with the delivery of hyperbaric oxygen (20 minutes at 3 atmospheres) but the theoretical benefit of this has not been proven. Oxygen therapy should be given until the patient is asymptomatic or carboxyhaemoglobin is below 5%.

CO has several mechanisms of toxicity. CO binds to haemoglobin, reducing oxygen-carrying capacity and release of carried oxygen, a left shift of the oxygen dissociation curve. CO also binds to myoglobin to reduce oxygen-carrying capacity and inhibits cellular respiration by binding to cytochrome oxidase. All of these are examples of type A toxicity, a direct interaction with a target molecule. Type A toxicity is dose related. It can be predicted from a substance's known pharmacology and generally involves agonism or antagonism in a competitive or irreversible manner. Type B toxicity (also termed idiosyncratic or bizarre) is rarer, not predictable, and independent of dose. The mechanisms of type B toxicity are likely to be allergic hypersensitivity or pseudoallergic reactions. Adverse drug reactions can also be categorized in this way. All drugs cause adverse effect when given in excess and these type A effects are often merely an extension of their therapeutic effect and account for 75% of adverse drug reactions.

Risk factors for type A adverse reactions include:

- Extremes of age
- Polypharmacy
- Renal disease
- Liver disease
- Cardiac disease

Type B adverse drug reactions are less common but often more severe.

Mechanisms of type B reactions include:

- Receptor abnormality
- Abnormal drug metabolism
- Immunological
- Drug interactions
- Abnormal enzyme systems

Examples of Type B reactions include:
- Suxamethonium apnoea
- Malignant hypothermia
- Glucose-6-phosphate dehydrogenase deficiency (drug-induced haemolysis)

Garg J, Krishnamoorthy P, Palaniswamy C et al. Cardiovascular abnormalities in carbon monoxide poisoning. American Journal of Therapeutics 10 February 2014.

11. D. High-dose insulin euglycaemic therapy

Verapamil is a phenylalkylamine-derivative selective calcium channel blocker. Phenylalkylamine derivative calcium channel blockers are the most toxic calcium channel blockers. Effects usually occur within two to four hours of ingestion.

Effects of calcium channel blocker toxicity

Cardiac effects:
- myocardial depression
- impaired myocardial conduction
- vasodilation

Metabolic effects:

Under the stress of the drug-induced shock state, cardiac myocytes shift from using free fatty acids, to carbohydrates. Verapamil impairs the uptake of both fatty acids and glucose by cardiac myocytes.

Hypergylcaemia is an important indicator of severity of calcium channel blocker overdose as insulin release is dependent on the influx of calcium into islet beta cells. See Table 13.8.

Table 13.8 Clinical features of calcium channel blocker poisoning.

Mild toxicity	Moderate toxicity	Severe toxicity
Nausea	Vomiting	Bradycardia
Lethargy	Dizziness	Arrhythmia
	Agitation	Conduction defects
	Drowsiness	Severe hypotension
	Hypotension	Hyperglycaemia
		Metabolic acidosis
		Seizures
		Coma
		CVA
		Mesenteric infarction
		Cardiac arrest

Treatment

Initial treatment should be supportive in a monitored environment. Single-dose activated charcoal can be considered in patients presenting within an hour of ingesting a potentially toxic dose. Symptomatic bradycardia should be treated with atropine. Hypotensive patients will require fluid support and should receive high-dose intravenous 10% calcium gluconate/chloride. Where this treatment has failed and hypotension persists then inotropes should be commenced. Following this, high-dose insulin dextrose therapy is recommended in current toxicological guidelines.

POISONING AND PHARMACOLOGY | ANSWERS

High-dose insulin euglycaemic therapy (HIET) is increasingly being used in severe poisoning. There have been numerous case reports documenting the success of HIET. There are numerous possible mechanisms of action:

- Insulin overcomes the metabolic starvation described previously by increasing the myocardial uptake of carbohydrate thereby improving myocardial function without increasing oxygen demand.
- Increases myocardial lactate oxidation, and helps clear the cytosol of glycolytic by-products that impair calcium handling causing diastolic dysfunction.
- Insulin promotes excitation–contraction coupling and contractility because enhanced glycolysis promotes increased sarcoplasmic reticulum-associated calcium ATPase activity and increased cytoplasmic calcium concentrations.
- Increases calcium uptake into the mitochondria.

Insulin has no chronotropic effect and can cause vasodilation; therefore, it may be used in adjunct with catecholamines.

Glucose and potassium should be monitored during HIET and corrected as required.

Intralipid® has been used in parenteral nutrition for years; more recently, Intralipid® has been accepted as an antidote for inadvertent amide local anaesthetic toxicity. Numerous case reports have been published on the use of Intralipid® in the treatment of poisoning of lipophilic medications including verapamil. There are a number of suggested mechanisms for the reversal of calcium channel blocker toxicity with Intralipid®:

- Intralipid® creates a 'lipid sink' (newly created intravascular compartment) for lipid soluble drugs
- Augmentation of cardiac energy supplies
- Direct activation of cardiac voltage gated calcium channels increasing intracellular calcium and restoring myocardial function

As yet, there are very few demonstrated adverse events from high-dose lipid load in human case reports. The research so far, alongside clinical experience, supports the fact that Intralipid® can be a cheap, safe adjuvant therapy for calcium channel blocker overdose.

Engebretsen KM, Kaczmarek KM, Morgan, Holger JS. High-dose insulin therapy in beta-blocker and calcium channel-blocker poisoning. Clinical Toxicology 2011; 49: 277–283.

12. B. The patient should receive multiple-dose activated charcoal

From the background information, there is a strong suspicion of deliberate self-poisoning and there are two likely agents at the patient's disposal; a benzodiazepine and quinine.

Flumazenil should not be used as a diagnostic test in potential mixed overdose. There is a significant risk of seizure in quinine overdose that would be difficult to terminate with benzodiazepines. Toxicology screens are rarely useful in the acute management of poisoning and routine assays would not include quinine. The concern in this case would be that both agents have been taken and establishing the presence of a benzodiazepine would not exclude ingestion of quinine. The indications for decontamination with single-dose activated charcoal (SDAC) are ingestion of a potentially toxic dose, within the last hour of an agent that is adsorbed by activated charcoal and, in the absence of contraindications which are reduced GCS, risk of aspiration, and gastrointestinal perforation. Agents not adsorbed are metals such as iron and lithium as well as alcohol, glycols, esters, strong acids, alkalis, and cyanide.

Multiple-dose activated charcoal is a method of enhanced elimination and can be given in this case. The American Academy of Clinical Toxicology and European Association of Poisons Centres and Clinical Toxicologists recommends the use of multiple-dose activated charcoal (MDAC) if the patient has ingested a life-threatening amount of quinine, phenobarbital, dapsone, or theophylline. Evidence has shown MDAC to be as effective as charcoal haemoperfusion in carbamazepine overdose.

Quinine poisoning is rare but significant. Mild symptoms and signs include headache, drowsiness, and dizziness which progresses to tachycardia, hypotension, tinnitus, and blurred vision in moderate poisoning. The features of severe poisoning are cardiorespiratory collapse, ECG abnormalities, and cardiac arrest. Treatment is predominantly supportive. Decontamination can be achieved with SDAC and MDAC can be effective in enhancing elimination.

American Academy of Clinical Toxicology; European Society of Poisons Centres and Clinical Toxicologists. Position Paper: Single-Dose Activated Charcoal. Clinical Toxicology 2005; 43: 61–87

American Academy of Clinical Toxicology; European Association of Poisons Centres and Clinical Toxicologists. Position Statement and Practice Guidelines on the Use of Multi-Dose Activated Charcoal in the Treatment of Acute Poisoning. Clinical Toxicology 1999; 37(6): 731–751.

13. D. Intravenous magnesium sulphate 2 g

One of the drug-specific adverse effects of poisoning with sotalol is torsade de pointes, the treatment for which is intravenous magnesium sulphate. This is mediated by myocardial potassium channel blocked resulting in a prolonged QT interval. Glucagon is used as a specific antidote in beta-blocker toxicity and high-dose insulin dextrose therapy is described frequently; neither has proven benefit or superiority over standard inotropic or vasopressor support.

Beta-blocker overdose

Beta blockers antagonize noradrenaline beta-adrenergic receptors in the sympathetic nervous system. Of most significance in poisoning $beta_1$ receptors are found in the heart and where adrenergic stimulation result in increased heart rate and contractility. $Beta_2$ receptors are found in vascular and bronchial smooth muscle where stimulation results in vascular and bronchial dilatation. $Beta_2$ receptors are also found in the heart where they exert a positive chronotropic effect. Beta receptors exert effect on the urinary, metabolic, gastrointestinal, skin, and ocular systems. Of particular importance in poisoning is the reduction of glycogenolysis which can result in hypoglycaemia.

Beta blockers can be broadly split into selective and non-selective. This refers to their affinity for a particular beta receptor. Beta blockers that have a predominant effect on $beta_2$ receptors are termed cardioselective; examples include metoprolol and bisoprolol. Propranolol exhibits equal affinity for $beta_1$ and $beta_2$ receptors and is hence non-selective.

Another key distinction between beta blockers is their solubility. Propranolol and metoprolol are lipid soluble and undergo hepatic metabolism which may be significantly extended in hepatic disease or overdose. They are also more likely to cross the blood–brain barrier resulting in central nervous system effects such as drowsiness and dizziness. Water-soluble beta blockers, including atenolol, are renally excreted largely unchanged. Thus, renal impairment will significantly prolong the period of toxicity. See Table 13.9.

Table 13.9 Clinical features of beta-blocker poisoning.

Cardiovascular system	Central nervous system	Other
Bradycardia	Dizziness	Hypoglycaemia
Hypotension	Drowsiness	Bronchospasm
AV block (any)	Lethargy	Non-cardiogenic oedema
Prolonged QRS	Delirium	
Prolonged QT	Seizure	
Ventricular tachycardia	Coma	
(torsade de pointes with sotalol in particular)		

Management

Patients with symptoms or signs of toxicity should be observed for six hours initially but this may need to be extended if there are significant co-morbidities, large overdoses (particularly propranolol), or in sustained-release preparation overdose. Patients with symptoms or signs must be observed on cardiac monitoring until they are fully recovered. Single-dose activated charcoal (SDAC) can be considered within one hour of ingestion. Initially, hypotension should be treated with fluids. If this fails then inotropic and vasopressor support may be required. For severe and resistant hypotension, expert toxicological advice should be sought. Glucagon at an initial bolus of 5 mg followed by an infusion of 2–4 mg/hour can be considered. Other therapy options include high-dose insulin/dextrose therapy and intralipid. Dialysis may be effective in water-soluble beta-blocker toxicity. Symptomatic bradycardia should be initially treated with atropine. Isoprenaline and cardiac pacing can also be considered.

Special considerations

Propranolol has a toxic mechanism similar to tricyclic antidepressant overdose (i.e. sodium channel blockade). For this reason, sodium bicarbonate should be used in QRS prolongation, ventricular arrhythmias, and seizures caused by propranolol toxicity.

Sotalol is a potassium channel blocker (class III antiarrhythmic) resulting in prolonged QT interval and potential torsade de pointes.

Engebretsen KM, Kaczmarek KM, Morgan J, Holger JS. High-dose insulin therapy in beta-blocker and calcium channel-blocker poisoning. Clinical Toxicology 2011; 49: 277–283.

14. A. She should be admitted to a high-dependency area

Carbamazepine overdose is uncommon but has increased in recent years, probably because of its extended use beyond epilepsy for mood disorders. Structurally related to tricyclic antidepressants, its toxic mechanism is sodium channel blockade and anticholinergic effects resulting in neurological and cardiovascular adverse effects.

This case is a very good example where knowledge of a drug's toxicological profile and good risk assessment will allow a clinician to effectively predict the likely outcome of an ingestion. The key elements of the risk assessment are:

1. Substance or substances taken (including type of preparation, e.g. modified release, enteric coated, etc.)
2. Quantity
3. Time of ingestion
4. Clinical features with predicted progress
5. Patient factors (weight, age, co-morbidities, etc.)

This will facilitate early liaison with other clinicians such as intensivists and pre-emptive planning for emergencies such as reduced consciousness, airway problems, and cardiovascular collapse. After the initial assessment by the acute physicians, a summary statement should be documented stating the immediate management plan, likely adverse effects, triggers for clinician review, safe disposal (ward/high-dependency unit, etc.), required period of observation, monitoring requirements, and medical criteria for discharge. Senior or toxicological advice should be documented if required and use of toxicology databases is advised to check current management of specific poisonings. Any other input requirements such as mental health and critical care should be documented and if appropriate a brief mental-capacity assessment should be made.

Carbamazepine is erratically absorbed and the early absence of symptoms and signs should not be interpreted as an insignificant ingestion. There is very good correlation between the dose ingested or serum levels and the clinical course. Ingestion of 50 mg/kg or more and levels of greater than 40 mg/L are highly likely to produce significant neurological toxicity, coma, seizure, and respiratory depression. For this reason, we would expect this patient to become critically unwell and the best option would be admission to a high-dependency area where critical-care management including intubation, ventilation, and cardiovascular support is immediately available. Multiple-dose activated charcoal (MDAC) is indicated in this case (and has been shown to be as effective as haemodialysis) but it is not safe when imminent reduced consciousness is possible because of the risk of aspiration and charcoal pneumonitis. Rapid-sequence induction and intubation should be performed as soon as altered consciousness is evident and at this point MDAC should be commenced. In large overdose, 'cyclical' absorption is possible when anticholinergic effects cause an ileus which slows absorption leading to falling serum levels. The ileus then begins to resolve and gut absorption resumes but because there is still a large drug load in the bowel, levels begin to rise causing subsequent clinical deterioration. Peak levels may be significantly delayed by up to 96 hours. See Table 13.10.

Table 13.10 Clinical features of carbamazepine toxicity.

Anticholinergic	CNS	CVS
Tachycardia	Mydriasis	QRS prolongation
Dry mouth	Nystagmus	Hypotension
Flushing	Ataxia	Ventricular arrhythmia
Urinary retention	Fluctuating delirium	
	Clonus	
	Reduced consciousness	
	Coma	
	Seizure	

Treatment is supportive. Sodium bicarbonate should be given for ventricular dysrhythmias. Dialysis can be considered and has been used but its efficacy in enhancing outcome is unproven.

Anon. Position statement and practice guidelines on the use of multi-dose activated charcoal in the treatment of acute poisoning. Journal of Clinical Toxicology 1999; 37: 731–751.

Graudins A, Peden G, Dowsett RP. Massive overdose with controlled-release carbamazepine resulting in delayed peak serum concentrations and life-threatening toxicity. Emergency Medicine 2002; 14: 89–94.

Soderstrom J, Murray L, Little M, Daly FFS. Toxicology case of the month: carbamazepine. Emergency Medicine Journal 2006; 23: 869–887.

Tapolyai M, Campbell M, Dailey K et al. Hemodialysis is as effective as hemoperfusion for drug removal in carbamazepine poisoning. Nephron 2002; 90: 213–215.

15. A. Endotracheal intubation should be considered at this point

The assessment of the airway in intoxicated patients goes beyond simply scoring a patient's consciousness. GCS is a tool validated for assessment of consciousness in head injury and not intoxication. We commonly quote a cut off with a GCS of 8 as the level at which the airway may become compromised. However, in intoxicated patients there are other factors that must be considered. Airway tone may be reduced because of the substance ingested or drugs given to the patient. Benzodiazepines may reduce tone and airway reflexes in patients whose conscious level may be higher than that usually associated with a loss of airway. In this case, the risk of aspiration is particularly high because of the combination of hydrocarbon encephalopathy, depressed airway reflexes, and the increased risk of silent contamination of the airway with liquid hydrocarbons themselves. The lower the viscosity of liquid ingested, the higher the risk. The patient is coughing, indicating some degree of airway irritation.

An important aspect of the risk assessment is the prediction of potential complications of poisoning and taking preventative steps. In this case, as in others, the consequences of complications may be more significant than the direct toxic effects.

Hydrocarbon pneumonitis presents with cough, bronchospasm, tachypnoea, haemoptysis, and pulmonary oedema, which can lead to respiratory failure requiring full support. Symptoms may take a few hours to appear but are often present very early, accompanied by visible changes on the chest X-ray. They will continue to worsen for up to 72 hours and usually resolve over a period of days.

Hydrocarbons can be divided into three groups:

- Aliphatic—petroleum distillates such as paraffin
- Cyclic aromatic—for example, benzene
- Halogenated cyclical aromatic—for example, carbon tetrachloride

The main routes of toxicity are ingestion and inhalation.

Treatment is simply supportive. See Table 13.11.

Table 13.11 Clinical features of hydrocarbon poisoning.

Gastrointestinal	Respiratory	CNS	Other systemic
Nausea	Choking	Reduced consciousness	Arrhythmia
Vomiting	Cough	Ataxia	Hepatorenal injury
Abdominal pain	Wheeze	Seizure	DIC
GI haemorrhage	Respiratory distress	Coma	
	Haemoptysis		
	Pulmonary oedema		

Shrivastava MS, Palkar AV, Karnik ND. Hydrocarbon pneumonitis masquerading as acute lung injury. British Medical Journal Case Report 15 July 2011.

chapter 14

IMMUNOLOGY AND ALLERGY

QUESTIONS

1. An 18-year-old Iranian man was brought to the emergency department unconscious. He was pyrexial, hypotensive, and had a petechial rash. A computerised tomography (CT) scan of head was normal and he was ventilated on intensive care. He was treated with intravenous ceftriaxone for presumed meningitis and recovered with persistent hearing loss. Blood cultures were positive for Neisseria meningitidis serogroup Y.

    One year later he presented with a rash, headache, and neck stiffness. He was afebrile, conscious, and alert. He was treated with intravenous ceftriaxone for presumed meningitis and blood cultures confirmed Neisseria meningitidis (which was 'not typable' and therefore not serogroup A, B, or C).

    What is the most appropriate investigation to confirm the most likely immunodeficiency?
    A. Classical and alternative pathway complement haemolysis
    B. Complement C1-inhibitor levels
    C. Complement C3 and C4 levels
    D. Immunoglobulin G, A, and M levels
    E. Lymphocyte subset analysis (T, B, and NK cell analysis)

2. A 50-year-old British man presented to the acute medical unit with a cough productive of green sputum and pyrexia. He had a past medical history of right-sided pneumonia 20 years ago and mentioned that he was investigated by the immunology department at the time. On examination, he had bronchial breathing over the right hemi-thorax.

Investigations:

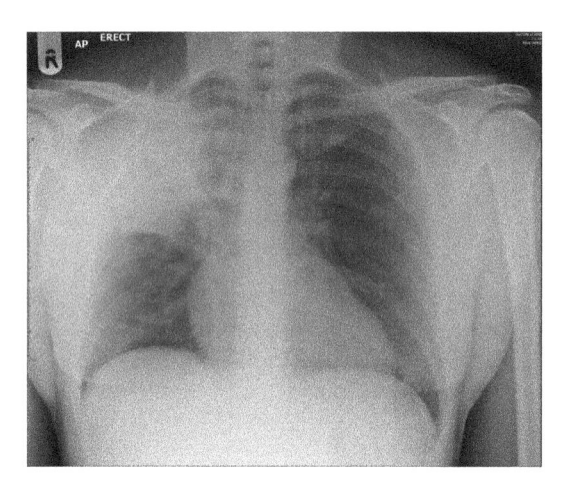

Figure 14.1 Chest X-ray at presentation to the acute medical unit.

```
Previous immunological assessment (20 years ago):
serum IgG                          5.7 g/L              (6.0-13.0)
serum IgA                          <0.07 g/L            (0.8-3.0)
serum electrophoresis normal

His immunological blood tests were repeated on this admission:
serum IgG                          4.85 g/L             (6.0-13.0)
serum IgA                          0.24 g/L             (0.8-3.0)
serum IgM                          0.19 g/L             (0.4-2.5)
serum electrophoresis              no monoclonal protein identified
urine electrophoresis              normal
CD3                                2.4 × 10⁹/L, 89%     (1.1-1.7)
CD4                                1.19 × 10⁹/L, 44%    (0.7-1.1)
CD8                                1 × 10⁹/L, 37%       (0.5-0.9)
CD19                               0.16 × 10⁹/L, 6%     (0.2-0.4)
lymphocyte count                   2.7 × 10⁹/L          (1.5-4.0)
serum C-reactive protein           143 mg/L             (<10)
serum alkaline phosphatase         240 U/L              (40-105)
haemoglobin                        118 g/L              (130-180)
pneumococcal antibodies            9 U/mL               (>20)
```

A CT scan of thorax revealed pleural thickening, bronchiectasis, consolidation of the right lung, and mediastinal lymphadenopathy. Bronchoscopy had easy contact bleeding but no other abnormalities and bronchoalveolar lavage cytology and microbiology was negative.

What is the most likely diagnosis?

A. Bronchiectasis secondary to previous infection
B. Common variable immunodeficiency
C. Hyper IgM syndrome
D. Secondary antibody deficiency
E. Selective IgA deficiency

3. **A 35-year-old British woman presented to the acute medical unit with a three-day history of intense pruritus and rash. The rash consisted of raised pale patches on an erythematous base. She described the patches as 'coming and going' all over her body. She noticed the pruritus on waking, while in bed. She was well without any rash when she went to bed the night before. She did not have any unusual contact during the night and had not changed any of the products used in the house. She did not take any medications regularly.**

   On further questioning, she recalled episodes of a similar rash that was controlled with antihistamines when she was younger.

   She had recently separated from her husband due to domestic abuse and the legal proceedings were due to start next week. Her observations, full blood count, and renal and liver function were all normal.

   What is the most likely diagnosis?

   A. Allergic urticaria
   B. Chronic idiopathic urticaria
   C. Erythema multiforme minor
   D. Idiopathic anaphylaxis
   E. Urticaria pigmentosa

4. A 23-year-old British man attended the emergency department in July with rhinorrhoea, conjunctivitis, and wheeze. The symptoms started in May with rhinorrhoea and conjunctivitis. He had been taking non-sedating antihistamines and intranasal corticosteroids regularly, on the advice of his GP, without significant benefit. His symptoms had occurred on every day over the last two months and had impacted on his sleep and daytime concentration. He had missed ten days of work during the last two months. Today, he developed tightness in his chest and therefore presented to the emergency department. He had no past medical history and had never experienced these symptoms before. His two sisters and his mother had eczema and hay fever.

He was treated with inhaled salbutamol and his wheeze improved. His peak expiratory flow rate returned to the normal predicted for age and height.

```
Investigations:
    total IgE                      120 kU/L      (<120)
    mixed grass-specific IgE        90 kU/L      (0 to 0.4)
    mixed tree-specific IgE         <0.4 kU/L    (0.0.4)
    cat-specific IgE                <0.4 kU/L    (0-0.4)
    dog-specific IgE                <0.4 kU/L    (0-0.4)
    house dust mite-specific IgE    <0.4 kU/L    (0-0.4)
```

What is the most appropriate long-term treatment to consider?
A. Allergen-specific immunotherapy
B. As required bronchodilator
C. Intramuscular corticosteroids before each summer
D. Oral corticosteroids during the pollen season
E. Regular oral antihistamines and intranasal corticosteroids

5. A 25-year-old British man presented to the acute medical unit in September following a collapse while walking with his parents in the countryside. They had been picking blackberries from the hedges. Immediately prior to collapsing he mentioned his hand being pricked by a thorn and he developed shortness of breath and became flushed. Paramedics arrived promptly and administered intramuscular adrenaline. The emergency department administered a further dose of intramuscular adrenaline as he was hypotensive, dyspnoeic, and had significant upper-airway angioedema on arrival. He received high-flow oxygen and intravenous fluids throughout. Antihistamines and corticosteroids were administered later.

What is the most appropriate next step in management?
A. Discharge with oral antihistamines and corticosteroids
B. He is safe to be discharged with general practice follow-up
C. He should be admitted to complete 24 hours' observation
D. He should receive an adrenaline auto-injector and referral to the allergy clinic
E. Mast-cell tryptase blood tests should be sent for analysis

6. An 18-year-old student presented having become acutely unwell at lunch during freshers' week. He had a history of allergy to peanuts, and had adrenaline auto-injectors, which he'd left at home.

   On examination, he was unwell and struggling to breathe. His heart rate was 120 beats per minute, blood pressure 90/55 mmHg, and oxygen saturation 86% breathing room air. He was treated with high-flow oxygen and intravenous crystalloid.

   Which of the following drugs should be administered immediately?
   A. 0.5 mL of 1:1,000 adrenaline intramuscularly
   B. 0.5 mL of 1:1,000 adrenaline intravenously
   C. 10 mg chlorphenamine intravenously
   D. 200 mg hydrocortisone intramuscularly
   E. 200 mg hydrocortisone intravenously

7. An 18-year-old student who suffered a nut-induced episode of anaphylaxis at lunchtime was admitted for overnight observation on the acute medical unit. At 22:00 hours he was mistakenly given intravenous amoxicillin prescribed for the patient in the next bed. There was no previous history of penicillin allergy. At 04:00 hours the following morning he was found in extremis with severe respiratory compromise and hypotension.

   The most likely cause of his deterioration is:
   A. Biphasic allergic response
   B. Inadvertent peanut consumption
   C. Missed peanut aspiration
   D. Previously undiagnosed asthma
   E. Severe type 1 hypersensitivity to amoxicillin

8. A 32-year-old heavily pregnant woman was brought collapsed to the acute medical unit by her husband. She had a history of wasp venom allergy and had been due to start immunotherapy when she discovered she was pregnant.

   On examination, she was unwell with widespread urticaria and angioedema, limited to her face. Her pulse was 135 beats per minute, blood pressure 70/45 mmHg, respiratory rate 28 breaths per minute, and oxygen saturation 89% breathing room air. She received oxygen, intravenous crystalloid fluids, and adrenaline followed by hydrocortisone and chlorphenamine.

   The correct position to nurse the patient in is:
   A. Lay flat on the bed with legs elevated at 45°
   B. Lay on her left-hand side at 15°
   C. Lay on her right-hand side at 15°
   D. Lay on the bed with head down tilt at 25°
   E. Sat up in bed at 60°

9. A 58-year-old man was admitted to the acute medical unit having attended the emergency department the night before with swelling to his face, mouth, tongue, and neck. He had suffered approximately six similar, although milder, episodes over the past 18 months but had not previously sought medical attention. His past medical history revealed hypertension, monoclonal gammopathy of undetermined significance, and mild osteoarthritis. His regular medication was atenolol and paracetamol.

   The day before presentation he had taken his atenolol before lunch. His lunch consisted of beef lasagne and salad (lettuce, tomatoes, and cucumber). Four hours after his lunch he developed swelling of his face. The swelling gradually increased over the following eight hours until he presented to the emergency department. In the emergency department he received adrenaline, chlorphenamine, and hydrocortisone with little improvement so had been admitted for observation. He reported that the swelling to his mouth and tongue had improved while waiting to be seen.

   On examination, he was maintaining his own airway, and although it had been difficult due to his swollen tongue, he had been able to swallow two paracetamol tablets he brought with him. His Early Warning Score was zero.

   The most likely diagnosis is:
   A. Acquired angioedema
   B. Allergy to atenolol
   C. Angiotensin converting enzyme inhibitor related angioedema
   D. Food allergy
   E. Hereditary C1 inhibitor deficiency

10. A 56-year-old man was admitted with sudden onset severe hypotension, widespread urticaria, and angioedema following a wasp sting. Anaphylaxis was suspected and treated appropriately according to the Resuscitation Council guidance. One of the nurses took some extra blood while inserting a spare cannula during resuscitation and asks you if you want any tests done.

    Which blood test should be taken as soon as possible during the management of acute anaphylaxis?
    A. Mast-cell tryptase
    B. Serum histamine
    C. Specific IgE
    D. Specific IgG
    E. Total IgE

chapter 14

IMMUNOLOGY AND ALLERGY

ANSWERS

1. A. Classical and alternative pathway complement haemolysis

This patient has had recurrent meningococcal infections with unusual serogroups of meningococcus. Complement deficiency is the most likely immunodeficiency in cases of recurrent meningococcal infection, although antibody deficiency can occasionally be the cause. Non-immunological causes include anatomical defects (including skull-base abnormalities). Guidelines from the Clinical Working Party of the European Society for Immunodeficiencies in 2006 suggest excluding antibody deficiency and complement deficiency in patients with recurrent meningococcal disease. Complement deficiency in this context requires the testing of the integrity of the entire complement cascade, which is performed on fresh serum by assessing the haemolytic pathways (alternative and classical). Terminal complement (C5, C6, C7, C8, and C9) deficiency, which causes dysfunction of the membrane attack complex, is detected as absent haemolysis on both classical and alternative pathways.

The lifetime risk of meningococcal disease is 1,000 to 10,000 times greater in individuals with terminal complement defects than in the healthy population. Relapse and recurrence of meningococcal disease is 10 and 150 times more likely respectively in terminal complement deficient individuals as compared with healthy controls. Disease tends to occur in older age groups (median age of onset is 3 in healthy controls and 17 in complement deficiency) and is caused by unusual serogroups of meningococcus (W135, X, Y, and non-typable) in complement deficiency.

De Vries E. Clinical Working Party of the European Society for Immunodeficiencies (ESID). Patient-centred screening for primary immunodeficiency: a multi-stage diagnostic protocol designed for non-immunologists. Clinical & Experimental Immunology 2006; 145: 204–214.

Walport MJ. Complement. First of two parts. New England Journal of Medicine 2001; 344: 1058–1066.

2. B. Common variable immunodeficiency

Common variable immunodeficiency (CVID) is the most common clinically significant antibody deficiency disease (1 in 36,000). Patients present with recurrent sinopulmonary infections and often with structural lung and sinus disease. The delay to diagnosis often exceeds two years. The diagnostic criteria for probable CVID include:

1. IgG below reference range (2 SD below mean for age)
2. Marked decrease in IgA and/or IgM
3. Absent/impaired responses to polysaccharide vaccine
4. Onset after 2 years of age
5. Exclusion of defined causes of hypogammaglobulinaemia

Exclusion of secondary and defined causes of hypogammaglobulinaemia is advised by the Clinical Working Party of the European Society for Immunodeficiencies (ESID). The alternative causes include medications (immunosuppression, anticonvulsants, antipsychotics), genetic disorders, infectious diseases (HIV, CMV, rubella, EBV), malignancy (haematological and thymoma), and increased losses (proteinuria, diarrhoea).

This patient has all of the clinical and laboratory features of CVID and the alternative causes have been excluded on clinical features or investigation.

Selective IgA deficiency (IgAD) is the most common antibody deficiency (1 in 600). IgAD is usually asymptomatic but can be associated with infections, autoimmunity, allergy, and transfusion reactions. The other immunoglobulin proteins are normal in IgAD as are responses to vaccination.

Hyper IgM syndrome is a rare antibody deficiency syndrome caused by defective communication between B and T lymphocytes. The most common mutation involves the CD40 ligand molecule and is an X-linked condition. Classically, young boys present with recurrent infections and unusual infections (including pneumocystis). The IgM level is within the normal range or high with low levels of IgG and IgA.

Specific antibody deficiency is similar in presentation to CVID but immunoglobulin levels are normal. The condition is diagnosed by absent response to vaccination with a polysaccharide vaccine (usually the pneumococcal polysaccharide vaccine).

CVID diagnostic criteria. http://esid.org/Working-Parties/Clinical/Resources/Diagnostic-criteria-for-PID2#Q3

Differential diagnosis of hypogammaglobulinaemia. http://esid.org/Working-Parties/Clinical/Resources/Diagnostic-criteria-for-PID2#Q6

Wood P. Primary antibody deficiency syndromes. Annals of Clinical Biochemistry 2009; 46: 99–108.

3. B. Chronic idiopathic urticaria

She describes a classical urticarial rash. Urticaria can arise (with or without angioedema) secondary to allergy, infection, related to medications, or without clear cause (spontaneous or idiopathic). Her features are not consistent with anaphylaxis, which is defined as a severe, life-threatening, generalized, or systemic hypersensitivity reaction. Similarly, type 1 hypersensitivity is not likely as the symptoms started without any related exposure. Type 1 hypersensitivity reactions, including allergic urticaria, usually occur within an hour of exposure to an allergen. In her case, the urticaria could also be precipitated by asymptomatic infection or stress.

Johansson S, Hourihane J, Bousquet J et al. EAACI (the European Academy of Allergology and Clinical Immunology) nomenclature task force. A revised nomenclature for allergy. An EAACI position statement from the EAACI nomenclature task force. Allergy 2001; 56: 813–824.

Powell R, Du Toit L, Siddique N et al. British Society for Allergy and Clinical Immunology (BSACI). BSACI guidelines for the management of chronic urticaria and angio-oedema. Clinical & Experimental Allergy 2007; 37: 631–650.

4. A. Allergen-specific immunotherapy

This patient has allergic rhinitis and has presented with an episode of wheeze. He should be treated with antihistamines and intranasal steroids for his rhinitis. As the pharmacological therapy has failed to control his symptoms and there is clear evidence of grass pollen allergy, he is a good candidate for allergen specific immunotherapy. Inhaled bronchodilators may be necessary currently due to the wheeze. Systemic steroid therapy should be avoided, where possible, in the treatment of allergic rhinitis, particularly intramuscular corticosteroids as the side effects can include avascular necrosis of the femoral neck.

ARIA. http://www.whiar.org/

Walker S, Durham S, Till S et al. British Society for Allergy and Clinical Immunology. Immunotherapy for allergic rhinitis. Clinical & Experimental Allergy 2011; 41: 1177–1200.

5. D. He should receive an adrenaline auto-injector and referral to the allergy clinic

The most appropriate next step is referral to the local allergy clinic for further assessment and advice. He may have insect venom allergy. Mast-cell tryptase blood tests should be taken immediately, 1–2 hours post event and 24 hours post event. Prolonged observation is not required in patients that have recovered completely, but they should be advised of the possibility of a biphasic reaction. Recent NICE guidelines (CG134) recommend an adrenaline auto-injector is given to all patients presenting with suspected anaphylaxis with advice on how and when to use it.

Soar J, Pumphrey R, Cant A, et al. Emergency treatment of anaphylactic reactions – guidelines for healthcare providers. Resuscitation 2008;77:157–69.283.

National Institute for Health and Care Excellence. Clinical Guideline 134. Anaphylaxis: assessment and referral after emergency treatment. December 2011.

6. A. 0.5 mL of 1:1,000 adrenaline intramuscularly

Adrenaline is key to immediate treatment in acute anaphylaxis. The European Resuscitation Council guidance from 2015 emphasizes early treatment with adrenaline and a repeated dose after 5 minutes if no clinical improvement in the patient's condition.

Adrenaline used during anaphylaxis is at a concentration of 1:1,000.

In adults (and in children over the age of 12) the dose is 0.5 mg (a volume of 0.5 mL of the 1:1,000 solution).

Adrenaline for anaphylaxis should be given intramuscularly (IM) by all except for anaesthetists/intensivists experienced in intravenous use. There is a much higher risk of causing harm if intravenous adrenaline is used.

Hydrocortisone 200 mg IM or slow IV and chlorphenamine 10 mg IM or slow IV should be given after the initial resuscitation.

Soar J, Pumphrey R, Cant A, et al. Emergency treatment of anaphylactic reactions – guidelines for healthcare providers. Resuscitation 2008;77:157–69.283.

Truhlár A, Deakin C, Soar J et al. European Resuscitation Council Guidelines for Resuscitation 2015 Section 4. Cardiac arrest in special circumstances ; Resuscitation 95 (2015) 148–201.

National Institute for Health and Care Excellence. Clinical Guideline 134. Anaphylaxis: assessment and referral after emergency treatment. December 2011.

7. A. Biphasic allergic response

The European Resuscitation Council recommends all patients treated for anaphylaxis are observed for at least 6 hours, and in some cases up to 24 hours (e.g. in patients with a severe asthmatic component, previous history of biphasic reactions or patients initially presenting at night). NICE guidance suggests observing adults for 6–12 hours and warning patients about biphasic responses prior to discharge.

The frequency of biphasic reactions is not clear, but may be as high as 20%. They are generally unpredictable, although if there is a history of biphasic reactions, the risk is thought high for future biphasic responses. These can be severe and may result in death.

A review within the resuscitation council guidance found fatal anaphylaxis occurred soon after contact, and never occurred more than six hours after allergen exposure.

Soar J, Pumphrey R, Cant A, et al. Emergency treatment of anaphylactic reactions – guidelines for healthcare providers. Resuscitation 2008;77:157–69.283.

Truhlár A, Deakin C, Soar J et al. European Resuscitation Council Guidelines for Resuscitation 2015 Section 4. Cardiac arrest in special circumstances ; Resuscitation 95 (2015) 148–201 .

National Institute for Health and Care Excellence. Clinical Guideline 134. Anaphylaxis: assessment and referral after emergency treatment. December 2011.

8. B. Lay on her left-hand side at 15°

Pregnant patients beyond 20 weeks' gestation should lie on their left side to prevent caval compression by the pregnant uterus. The European Resuscitation Council guidance recommends a left lateral tilt of 15°.

Truhlár A, Deakin C, Soar J et al. European Resuscitation Council Guidelines for Resuscitation 2015 Section 4. Cardiac arrest in special circumstances ; Resuscitation 95 (2015) 148–201.

9. A. Acquired angioedema

This is angioedema alone, and there are no other features to suggest this is allergy. Additionally, he did not eat food or take atenolol in the period immediately before onset. With episodes starting in his mid-50s, he is unlikely to have hereditary angioedema (hereditary C1 inhibitor deficiency). He is not on an angiotensin converting enzyme inhibitor (ACE-I) for his hypertension. He is in the age range for presentation of acquired angioedema, and has a history of monoclonal gammopathy of undetermined significance (MGUS), one of the major conditions associated with acquired angioedema (AEE).

Allergy—food or drug

IgE-mediated allergy causes immediate allergy. Symptoms include urticaria, angioedema, wheeze secondary to bronchospasm, dizziness secondary to hypotension, and gastrointestinal disturbance. Typically, symptoms appear within minutes of intravenous drug administration and within 30 minutes of food or oral drug ingestion, and may be life-threatening (anaphylaxis).

Cross-linking of the allergen to mast-cell-bound IgE receptors causes mast-cell degranulation, releasing preformed mediators (e.g. histamine, tryptase, and heparin) and newly formed thromboxane, prostaglandin D2, and leukotriene C4. These cause the signs and symptoms of an allergic reaction.

Treatment depends on the severity of the reaction. For anaphylaxis, where potentially life-threatening features are present, adrenaline 0.5 mg intramuscular is essential. Other immediate treatments include oxygen and intravenous fluids followed less urgently by hydrocortisone and chlorphenamine. For milder cutaneous-only reactions, oral antihistamines are usually adequate.

Hereditary angioedema (HAE) (hereditary C1 inhibitor deficiency)

C1 is the initiator of the classical complement pathway, and is made up of C1q, C1r, and C1s. On activation by binding to IgM molecules or to IgG bound to pathogen surface, C1q undergoes a conformational change allowing C1r to activate C1s. C1s then cleaves C2 and C4. Cleavage of C4 means C4 can be used as a screening test for over activation of C1 in this disorder. C1 inhibitor blocks C1 from becoming activated.

C1 inhibitor is also part of the kinin pathway from which bradykinin is produced. C1 inhibitor inhibits plasma kallikrein, which acts on high-molecular weight kininogen produced by the liver to release bradykinin. Bradykinin is a vasoactive peptide that causes vasodilatation and increased vascular permeability via its constitutively expressed B2 receptors. This is the main cause of angioedema in C1 inhibitor deficiency.

HAE is inherited in an autosomal dominant fashion. In females, it may first present around puberty or with commencement of combined oral contraceptives as oestrogen promotes attacks. Episodes may be with overt angioedema, but alternatively patients may present with recurrent episodes of abdominal pain, which may have been extensively investigated by surgical colleagues.

For the treatment of acute attacks of HAE in the UK consider the use of C1 inhibitor concentrate (from donor plasma) or icatibant, a bradykinin B2 receptor antagonist.

Acquired angioedema (AAE) (acquired C1 inhibitor deficiency)

This disorder is identical to HAE except for an older age of onset. It occurs most commonly secondary to MGUS, lymphoproliferative disease, or sometimes in autoimmune diseases such as SLE. A proposed mechanism includes a blocking autoantibody against C1 inhibitor, thereby preventing its action. Higher doses of C1 inhibitor concentrate may be required than for HAE.

ACE-I induced angioedema

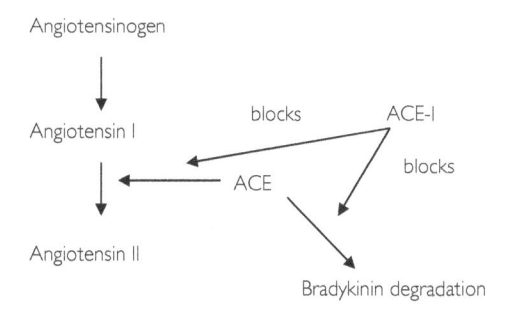

Figure 14.2 Figure showing pathway of ACE-I induced angioedema.

Angiotensin converting enzyme (ACE) acts on the renin–aldosterone system to convert angiotensin I to angiotensin II; however, it also acts to degrade bradykinin (Figure 14.2). Bradykinin is a vasoactive peptide that causes vasodilatation and increased vascular permeability via its constitutively expressed B2 receptors. ACE-I block bradykinin degradation, so increasing levels of bradykinin available.

ACE-I associated angioedema is estimated at occurring in 0.1–0.2% of patients treated with ACE-I, although this is probably an underestimate. The frequency is higher in African Americans. It can appear at any time after starting an ACE-I, and has been reported to occur after patients have tolerated treatment for many years.

There is no universally agreed treatment for ACE-I angioedema and the main aim should be supportive care such as airway protection in laryngeal compromise. Some teams support the use of antihistamines and adrenaline, although these are of unproven benefit. The bradykinin B2 receptor antagonist icatibant, developed for HAE, has recently been reported to be useful and effective in ACE-I induced angioedema, although it is currently not licensed for this use.

ACE-I should be stopped and remain contraindicated for future use. In general, angiotensin II receptor blockers may be used as an alternative, although there have been rare reports of angioedema linked to these too.

Vasekar M, Craig T. ACE inhibitor induced angioedema. Current Allergy and Asthma Reports. Springer, 2011. doi: 10.1007/s11882-011-0238-z

10. A. Mast-cell tryptase

Mast-cell tryptase is pre-formed in the granules of mast cells, and is released into circulation on cross-linking of allergen to mast-cell-bound-specific IgE. It peaks in circulation between 30–120 minutes after onset, and with a half-life of approximately two hours, concentrations return to baseline within about eight hours.

Both the National Institute for Health and Care Excellence and the European Resuscitation Council guidance include measurement of mast-cell tryptase within their recommendations. Both recommend:

1. One sample as soon as possible on presentation (but not delaying resuscitation)
2. A second sample 1–2 hours after onset of symptoms
3. A convalescent sample more than 24 hours after the onset of symptoms

Importantly, the time should be noted on all samples to aid interpretation.

National Institute for Health and Care Excellence. Clinical Guidelines 134, Anaphylaxis: assessment and referral after emergency treatment. December 2011.

Truhlár A, Deakin C, Soar J et al. European Resuscitation Council Guidelines for Resuscitation 2015 Section 4. Cardiac arrest in special circumstances ; Resuscitation 95 (2015) 148–201.

chapter 15

DERMATOLOGY

QUESTIONS

1. A 58-year-old woman was admitted to the acute medical unit with an eight-day history of feeling unwell and a painful spreading rash. It had commenced on her trunk and extended to the limbs. She had missed the last two days of work as a machinist. She had a previous history of slight scalp psoriasis. Two weeks ago, she had commenced medication for joint pains. She had a past medical history of a myocardial infarction and hypertension. Her medication included atenolol, bendroflumethiazide, aspirin, and diclofenac.

   On examination, she had a temperature of 39.2°C, pulse 120 beats per minute, and a blood pressure of 130/92 mmHg. Respiratory, abdominal, and neurological systems were normal. Skin examination revealed sheeted erythema of her back and loins, with areas of superficial skin shedding revealing moist underlying eroded areas on most of her back, the axillae, and beneath the breasts amounting to 20% body surface area. There was patchy redness with purpuric macules on the limbs, palms, and soles. She had painful eyes and small foci of oral mucosal erosion. The genital mucosa was uninvolved, but there was redness of the inguinal and perineal creases with a well-demarcated edge and satellite patches beyond. She had scaling of the scalp.

   ```
   Investigations:
     haemoglobin                      112 g/L            (115-165)
     white cell count                 2.8 × 10⁹/L        (4.0-11.0)
     platelet count                   340 × 10⁹/L        (150-400)
     serum sodium                     137 mmol/L         (137-144)
     serum potassium                  4.5 mmol/L         (3.5-4.9)
     serum urea                       9.5 mmol/L         (2.5-7.0)
     serum creatinine                 174 mmol/L         (60-110)
     serum bicarbonate                18 mmol/L          (22-28)
     serum C-reactive protein         82 mg/L            (>10)
     serum total bilirubin            20 µmol/L          (1-22)
     serum alkaline phosphatase       243 U/L            (45-105)
     serum alanine aminotransferase   158 U/L            (5-35)
     serum albumin                    30 g/L             (37-49)
   ```

What is the most likely explanation for the rash?

A. Erythroderma due to bendroflumethiazide
B. Exacerbation of psoriasis by a febrile illness
C. Infected psoriatic rash with psoriatic arthritis
D. Stevens Johnson syndrome secondary to a herpes infection
E. Stevens Johnson-toxic epidermal necrolysis overlap due to diclofenac

2. A 74-year-old woman presented to the ambulatory care centre with a three-month history of a widespread itchy rash and five-day history of pain and redness of the left leg with blistering. Treatment from her GP had included clobetasone butyrate ointment and emollient. She had a past medical history of a deep vein thrombosis of the left leg five years previously. There was no history of prior skin disease.

On examination, she had a temperature of 38.5°C. Skin examination revealed tense blisters on the trunk and limbs of between 1 and 4 cm on a background of patches of fixed urticated confluent redness. There were widespread scratch marks. The left leg was red and swollen to the knee with blisters and purpura on the dorsum of the foot.

```
Investigations:
    haemoglobin         128 g/L            (115-165)
    platelet count      340 × 10⁹/L        (150-400)
    white cell count    15.2 × 10⁹/L       (4.0-11.0)
    neutrophil count    10.2 × 10⁹/L       (1.5-7.0)
    lymphocyte count    3.2 × 10⁹/L        (1.5-4.0)
    monocyte count      0.6 × 10⁹/L        (<0.8)
    eosinophil count    1.2 × 10⁹/L        (0.04-0.40)
    Skin biopsy of a blister showed the histology of a
      sub-epidermal blister; IgG and complement at the
      dermo-epidermal junction on skin immunofluorescence.
    Doppler ultrasound scan of the left leg was normal.
```

What is the most appropriate initial treatment?

A. Intravenous flucloxacillin and oral prednisolone
B. Intravenous flucloxacillin and topical clobetasol propionate ointment
C. Intravenous vancomycin and oral prednisolone
D. Oral flucloxacillin and clobetasol propionate ointment topically
E. Oral flucloxacillin and oral prednisolone

3. A 43-year-old man was referred to the ambulatory care centre from the genitourinary clinic with a 12-month history of soreness and tightness of the skin of the penis with splitting on intercourse with his male partner. Treatment with a miconazole and hydrocortisone mixed preparation had not improved the condition. His partner had no anogenital skin disease. The patient had no other health problems.

Examination revealed tightness on retraction of the foreskin with 1–2 cm zones of white change on the mucosal aspect of the foreskin most marked around the frenulum. The skin of the frenulum was thickened involving a faint warty plaque extending onto the glans penis. Small foci of purpura were present in the affected area. The rest of the skin and perineum was normal.

```
Investigations:
    haemoglobin          131 g/L              (130-180)
    platelet count       340 × 10⁹/L          (150-400)
    white cell count     9.4 × 10⁹/L          (4.0-11.0)
    HIV viral load       200 copies/mL        (lower detection
                                               limit 40)
    microbiology swab from beneath foreskin: Candida species +
       biopsy of foreskin consistent with lichen sclerosus
```

What is the most appropriate next step in management?

A. Biopsy of glans penis and arrange ultrasound scan of groin
B. Biopsy of glans penis and treatment with oral fluconazole
C. Biopsy of glans penis and treatment with topical clotrimazole
D. Treatment with clobetasol propionate ointment and oral fluconazole
E. Treatment with oral fluconazole and hydrocortisone 1% ointment

4. A 58-year-old man was referred by his GP with a seven-week history of a widespread itchy rash which commenced on the V of his neck towards the end of a ten-day visit to East Africa. He had no history of previous skin disease. GP management had included betamethasone valerate ointment, but the rash had deteriorated such that he could no longer sleep. His medication included candesartan, lisinopril, bendroflumethiazide, aspirin, and a goserelin acetate implant.

On examination, the man was distressed with widespread scaling and redness particularly of the shoulders, upper back, and front of the neck. There were polycyclic scaling lesions. Respiratory, gastrointestinal and neurological examinations were normal.

```
Investigations:
   haemoglobin           136 g/L            (130-180)
   platelet count        320 × 10⁹/L        (150-400)
   white cell count      10.1 × 10⁹/L       (4.0-11.0)
   neutrophil count      7.0 × 10⁹/L        (1.5-7.0)
   lymphocyte count      2.1 × 10⁹/L        (1.5-4.0)
   monocyte count        0.10 × 10⁹/L       (<0.8)
   eosinophil count      0.90 × 10⁹/L       (0.04-0.40)
   serum IgG             7.3 g/L            (6.0-13.0)
   serum IgA             2.4 g/L            (0.8-3.0)
   serum IgM             1.4 g/L            (0.4-2.5)
   serum IgE             340 kU/L           (<120)
   skin biopsy histology: an interface dermatitis with basal
      liquefaction
   stool microscopy examination showed no ova, cysts, or
      parasites
   skin scrapings: negative
```

What additional test would be most likely to clarify whether this was a photosensitive disorder?

A. Anti-Jo1 antibody levels
B. Creatine kinase
C. Photo patch testing
D. Ro and La antibodies
E. Urinary porphyrins

5. A 28-year-old woman presented to the acute medicine clinic with an exacerbation of her long-standing eczema. General examination revealed a flat, pigmented lesion on her lower back, which was irregular in colour and outline with associated inflammation. There was widespread adenopathy. The patient was not aware of the lesion and could not provide any history of change. You decided to increase the potency of her topical steroid and frequency of application of emollient and referred her to dermatology for excision of the pigmented lesion.

```
Investigations:
    haemoglobin                        153 g/L            (115-165)
    platelet count                     224 × 10⁹/L        (150-400)
    white cell count                   13.1 × 10⁹/L       (4.0-11.0)
    neutrophil count                   10.0 × 10⁹/L       (1.5-7.0)
    lymphocyte count                   2.1 × 10⁹/L        (1.5-4.0)
    monocyte count                     0.10 × 10⁹/L       (<0.8)
    eosinophil count                   0.90 × 10⁹/L       (0.04-0.40)
    serum total bilirubin              20 µmol/L          (1-22)
    serum alkaline phosphatase         100 U/L            (45-105)
    serum alanine aminotransferase     28 U/L             (5-35)
    serum albumin                      39 g/L             (37-49)

    chest X-ray: normal

    skin swab: staphylococcus aureus
    skin biopsy histology: superficial spreading melanoma
```

What would be the single most important piece of additional information for prognosis?

A. Diameter of the tumour
B. Lymph node aspirate cytology
C. Ultrasound of abdomen and pelvis
D. Tumour Breslow thickness
E. Tumour ulceration

chapter 15

DERMATOLOGY

ANSWERS

1. E. Stevens Johnson Syndrome-toxic epidermal necrolysis overlap due to diclofenac

There are two possible rashes in this presentation. The patient has a pre-existing rash diagnosed as psoriasis and a further rash which is the presenting complaint. The second rash is painful, widespread, and giving rise to sheets of lost skin revealing an eroded surface beneath. It is associated with sore eyes and mouth and clinically this is characteristic of Stevens John Syndrome-toxic epidermal necrolysis overlap (SJS-TEN). Diclofenac was commenced two weeks prior to presentation, which is within the classic 5–28 days for drug causation with. There is a prodromal febrile illness which is also a common feature. A low white count is sometimes seen. Psoriasis exacerbation by a febrile illness is a recognized clinical pattern, but the description of the rash does not fit, with pain, sloughed skin, and mucosal involvement. The pain and shedding is also against an erythroderma due to bendroflumethiazide, where the time course of events does not suggest this diagnosis. Neither does it fit for this drug as a cause for toxic epidermal necrolysis (TEN). Stevens Johnson Syndrome has clinical overlap with TEN, but is defined as shedding of less than 10% of the skin surface area.

Downey A, Jackson C, Harun N et al. Toxic epidermal necrolysis: review of pathogenesis and management. Journal of the American Academy of Dermatology June 2012; 66(6): 995–1003. doi: 10.1016/j.jaad.2011.09.029

Bastuji-Garin S, Fouchard N, Bertocchi M, Roujeau JC, Revuz J, Wolkenstein P. SCORTEN: a severity-of-illness score for toxic epidermal necrolysis. Journal of Investigative Dermatology. 2000 Aug;115(2): 149–53.

2. B. Intravenous flucloxacillin and topical clobetasol propionate ointment

The clinical description is consistent with the initial phase of pre-bullous pemphigoid, followed by the next phase of blistering combined with the coincidental presentation of bacterial cellulitis of the left leg. Although the blistering of the left leg might have been attributed to the bullous pemphigoid alone, it is not within the distribution of the rest of the bullous change and has other features such as purpura, localized pain, and fever, which is consistent with cellulitis. The likelihood of a deep vein thrombosis is low given the negative ultrasound. Histology of a sub-epidermal blister with positive immunofluorescence for IgG and complement is that of bullous pemphigoid. The eosinophilia is non-specific but also a common finding in bullous pemphigoid. The acute medical disease with priority is the cellulitis and the management of this might be compromised with systemic steroid in an elderly person. This means that initial management might be managed without systemic immune suppression. A large randomized study illustrated that treatment with topical clobetasol propionate was more effective and gave less risk of patient death in the management of bullous pemphigoid when compared with oral prednisolone. There is a range of possible regimens for the treatment of cellulitis, both with different agents and routes of administration. The options here mainly offer flucloxacillin, which in the acute situation, with areas of blistered skin that might also have secondary infection, would be best given intravenously. The use of vancomycin would only be indicated if there were additional complicating factors such as bacterial resistance.

Joly P, Roujeau J, Benichou J et al. A comparison of oral and topical corticosteroids in patients with bullous pemphigoid. New England Journal of Medicine 2002; 346: 321–327.

3. C. Biopsy of glans penis and treatment with topical clotrimazole

This histology of the foreskin and clinical account is consistent with the diagnosis of lichen sclerosus. This is a disease with the potential for evolution to squamous cell carcinoma. The description highlights a thickened area of change on the frenulum and glans penis, which would be the type of change seen when lichen sclerosus is undergoing malignant change. Squamous cell carcinoma at this site is also associated with human papilloma virus (HPV), although HPV is not specifically implicated in lichen sclerosus-related squamous cell carcinoma. HPV is more common in patients with HIV or other forms of immune impairment. The initial priority is to clarify the diagnosis at the most abnormal focus of the disease and to treat the Candida species that has been identified. A light growth of Candida from beneath the foreskin would not warrant systemic treatment unless there was an associated clinical complaint and the clinical description does not match that of mucosal thrush, hence topical therapy is adequate. Both hydrocortisone and clobetasol propionate might be used at some point in the management of lichen sclerosus, but not before malignancy had been fully explored. Equally, there would be no indication for inguinal staging with ultrasound unless there was a confirmed diagnosis of squamous cell carcinoma.

Edmonds E, Hunt S, Hawkins D et al. Clinical parameters in male genital lichen sclerosus: a case series of 329 patients. Journal of the European Academy of Dermatology and Venereology June 2012; 26(6): 730–737. doi: 10.1111/j.1468-3083.2011.04155.x

Neill S, Lewis F, Tatnall F et al. British Association of Dermatologists. British Association of Dermatologists' guidelines for the management of lichen sclerosus 2010. British Journal of Dermatology October 2010; 163(4): 672–682. doi: 10.1111/j.1365-2133.2010.09997.x

4. D. Ro and La antibodies

The patient presented with a history that suggests a rash associated with travel to a hot destination. He has no previous history of rash and has two elements in the description to suggest photosensitivity. First, he is taking a range of medications, some of which are associated directly with photosensitivity (quinine and bendroflumethiazide), or indirectly (bendroflumethiazide) through contributing to other diseases such as sub-acute cutaneous lupus erythematosus. Second, the rash started on the light exposed areas, then spread to the trunk and back. The skin biopsy demonstrated a lichenoid pattern of inflammation which can be seen in lichen planus, lupus, and dermatomyositis. The latter two often have an element of perivascular inflammation, but no mention is made of that. All three are tenable diagnoses, but lichen planus is rarely photosensitive and would not be elucidated by any of the tests offered in the answers. Urinary porphyrins are a useful screening test for porphyria cutanea tarda, but the presentation does not resemble that diagnosis. Photopatch testing is relevant for an allergic contact sensitivity that is elicited by light and there are very few clues consistent with that pattern in this description. Anti Jo1 antibody would be useful for a putative diagnosis of dermatomyositis and, although that is a possible diagnosis here, the neurological examination was normal and the sensitivity for this test is only about 20%. This contrasts with the sensitivity of 50–80% of anti Ro antibody in sub-acute cutaneous lupus erythematosus. This latter diagnosis also fits with the pattern, character, and manner of onset of the rash. He is also taking bendroflumethiazide, which is recognized as a drug that is associated with sub-acute cutaneous lupus erythematosus. Checking the Ro antibody would be the most likely to clarify whether this was a photosensitive disorder by establishing the diagnosis.

Lowe G, Henderson C, Grau R et al. A systematic review of drug-induced subacute cutaneous lupus erythematosus. British Journal of Dermatology March 2011; 164(3): 465–472. doi: 10.1111/j.1365-2133.2010.10110.x

5. D. Tumour Breslow thickness

The most accessible prognosticator is the Breslow thickness. This is a measure of invasion of the melanoma. If the melanoma is limited to within the epidermis without breaching the basement membrane zone, then the tumour is classified as *in situ*, with a Breslow thickness of zero and there is an excellent prognosis. Once invasive, prognosis is gauged at 1 mm steps of invasion up to 4 mm. With no invasion, as long as the histology has been correctly reported, the prognosis is 100% five-year survival. This drops to >90% survival at 1 mm, around 80% survival at 2 mm and 70–80% survival with 3 mm thickness depending on associated ulceration. An ulcerated melanoma with >4 mm thickness results in a five-year survival prognosis for the patient of about 50%. Tumour ulceration is taken as a further element in the prognosis, but is secondary to the thickness of the tumour. Diameter of a pigmented lesion is used in both the ABCDE and Glasgow seven-point scale systems for identifying a pigmented lesion of greater risk of being a melanoma, but it has no bearing on prognostication of a melanoma once it is diagnosed. No form of imaging or node sampling would be appropriate at this point, until the Breslow thickness is established. The presence of widespread adenopathy is likely to represent dermatopathic adenopathy related to the exacerbation of eczema.

Marsden J, Newton-Bishop J, Burrows L et al. British Association of Dermatologists (BAD) Clinical Standards Unit. Revised UK guidelines for the management of cutaneous melanoma 2010. Journal of Plastic, Reconstructive & Aesthetic Surgery September 2010; 63(9): 1401–1419. doi: 10.1016/j.bjps.2010.07.006.

chapter 16

PSYCHIATRY

QUESTIONS

1. A 29-year-old woman on an orthopaedic ward complained of pain following surgery to repair a complex fracture of her right ankle. She was given tramadol and within an hour she became sweaty and agitated. She had a past medical history of bulimia nervosa and was taking fluoxetine 60 mg daily, mirtazepine 30 mg at night, and diazepam 5 mg three times daily as required.

   On examination, her temperature was 38.2°C, her pulse was 102 beats per minute and regular, and her blood pressure was 164/92 mmHg. Neurological examination revealed mydriasis, tremor, hyperreflexia, and increased tone in all limbs but greatest in the lower extremities and clonus induced by rapid dorsiflexion of the left ankle. Additional examination findings included normal skin colour and hyperactive bowel sounds.

   Which medication should not be discontinued?
   A. Diazepam
   B. Metoclopramide
   C. Mirtazepine
   D. Tramadol
   E. Venlafaxine

2. A 69-year-old man presented to the acute medical unit with confusion and drowsiness. He had a history of bipolar disorder and had been mentally stable on treatment with lithium for many years. He also had stage 2 chronic kidney disease and his last glomerular filtration rate two months ago was 62 mL/min/1.73 m². In the past month, he had been suffering with neck pain and had been taking his wife's prescribed arthritis medication, indometacin, frequently. For several weeks, he had been feeling more tired and weak than usual with intermittent nausea. In the last two days, he had become increasingly confused and drowsy.

On examination, he was afebrile, his pulse was 52 beats per minute and regular, and his blood pressure was 126/62 mmHg. He was ataxic, drowsy, and unable to follow commands.

```
Investigations:
    serum creatinine       210 µmol/L     (60-110)
    serum lithium level    4.2 mmol/L     (0.5-1.2)
```

What is the treatment of choice for this patient?

A. Activated charcoal
B. Forced diuresis with loop diuretics
C. Haemodialysis
D. Osmotic diuresis
E. Peritoneal dialysis

3. A 59-year-old woman with chronic obstructive pulmonary disease (COPD) presented to the acute medical unit for the fifth time in two months with a history of sudden onset dyspnoea and palpitations while out shopping. She admitted to having feelings of intense fear that she was dying during these attacks and she was increasingly reluctant to leave her home in case she had another unexpected attack. She did not report an increase in cough, sputum production, or change in sputum colour. On examination, she was afebrile and not cyanosed or dyspnoeic at rest. Her ECG was normal. Her chest X-ray showed no acute changes. She was hoping to once again commence a course of prednisolone and antibiotics to improve her symptoms.

What is the most appropriate next step in management?

A. Arrange an echocardiogram
B. Discharge without further management
C. The reattribution approach
D. Steroid therapy
E. Treatment with 'as required' diazepam

4. **A 21-year-old Somalian man was brought to hospital by his family who were concerned that he had been confused and unwell for the past two days. It emerged that he had been behaving oddly, locking himself in his room, talking and shouting to himself, and today he tried to throw away his brother's mobile phone believing that it was transmitting his thoughts to his persecutors. He had chewed khat intermittently since the age of 16 but his use had increased in the last two weeks.**

   Which of the following is associated with khat psychosis?

   A. A history of war trauma-related symptoms
   B. Confusion and disorientation
   C. Late onset of khat use
   D. Seizures
   E. Use of less than two bundles of khat per day

5. **A 32-year-old man had been admitted to the acute medical unit with a two-week history of hearing voices and a belief that he was being persecuted. He was very suspicious of all staff and was reluctant to talk to anyone and had been very quiet and guarded. Organic causes had been ruled out and he was awaiting assessment by the psychiatric services. He became agitated and angry with a member of the nursing staff.**

   Which is the most appropriate initial management approach for his agitation and anger?

   A. Call security
   B. Confront him with the unacceptability of his behaviour
   C. Insist he take sedative medication
   D. Physical restraint
   E. Redirecting the patient towards a calmer personal space

6. A 70-year-old man was brought to the acute medical unit after being found collapsed at home by his carer who visited daily. He had a past medical history of type 2 diabetes mellitus and hypertension. He was taking aspirin 75 mg once daily, simvastatin 40 mg once daily, amlodipine 10 mg once daily, gliclazide 80 mg twice daily, and metformin 500 mg tds. On admission, he had a Glasgow Coma Score (GCS) of 15. His temperature was 37.0°C, pulse was 98 beats per minute, blood pressure was 145/97 mmHg, and oxygen saturation was 98% on air. Capillary blood glucose concentration was 4.2 mmol/L. Physical examination was normal.

```
Investigations:
  haemoglobin                       146 g/L           (130-180)
  platelet count                    164 × 10/L        (150-400)
  white cell count                  8.3 × 10⁹/L       (4.0-11.0)
  serum sodium                      143 mmol/L        (137-144)
  serum potassium                   4.4 mmol/L        (3.5-4.9)
  serum creatinine                  123 µmol/L        (60-110)
  serum bicarbonate                 27 mmol/L         (20-28)
  serum total bilirubin             8 µmol/L          (1-22)
  serum alanine aminotransferase    56 U/L            (5-35)
  serum alkaline phosphatase        46 U/L            (45-105)
  serum C-reactive protein          5 mg/L            (<10)
  plasma thyroid-stimulating        3.2 mU/L          (0.4-5.0)
    hormone

12-lead ECG: sinus tachycardia
CT scan of head: small vessel disease, an old left parietal
  infarct, but nil acute
chest X-ray: normal
```

Overnight, he became notably anxious. He had not slept at all and was saying that he had done terrible things. He was frightened to leave hospital and had voiced suicidal ideas. Your team could gather only a little more background history and found that he lived alone and had no close family. He was reclusive and stayed indoors a lot. He was currently not under the care of psychiatric services though was seen several years ago for depression. He had been becoming a little more forgetful in the last six months but was still able to live independently with assistance from the carer who provided meals.

Later in the day he became clammy, agitated, and unsteady on his feet. He was fearful and inattentive looking round the cubicle. His responses were inappropriate, and he was now disorientated in time and place.

What is the most likely explanation of this patient's mental state at this point?

A. Acute cerebrovascular event
B. Agoraphobia with panic attacks
C. Delirium tremens
D. Dementia
E. Severe depressive episode

7. A 30-year-old woman was brought to the emergency department after being found by her partner at home surrounded by empty bottles of wine and packets of prescribed and non-prescribed medication, including: aspirin, paracetamol, escitalopram, and omeprazole. She had no significant past medical history except that she had given birth six months ago. The partner informed staff that she had previously been treated at a psychiatric inpatient facility for a severe depressive illness three years ago, but was currently not under mental health services.

    On admission, she appeared to be intoxicated, with a fluctuating GCS of 12–14. Her temperature was 37.5°C, pulse was 90 beats per minute, blood pressure was 110/72 mmHg and her oxygen saturation was 98% breathing air. Capillary blood glucose concentration was 4.2 mmol/L. There were no other abnormalities on physical examination.

    Initial acute medical management of the polypharmacy overdose included intravenous acetylcysteine. The nursing staff reported that she intermittently kept verbalizing that she wanted to be left alone and not to have any treatment but further history from the patient was not possible.

    Medico-legally, how could you proceed if you wanted to implement the acute medical management plan?

    A. The patient has capacity but override her wishes under the Mental Capacity Act 2005
    B. The patient has capacity but override her wishes under the Mental Health Act 1983
    C. The patient lacks capacity and act in her best interests under the Mental Capacity Act 2005
    D. The patient lacks capacity and act in her best interests under the Mental Health Act 1983
    E. Under common law, as you have a duty of care to the patient

8. A 30-year-old woman was admitted to the acute medical unit following a polypharmacy overdose, including paracetamol. She initially agreed to treatment and had so far received 12 hours of intravenous acetylcysteine treatment. The mental health liaison team performed an initial assessment and concluded that she was most likely depressed and would require further assessment and management, so they planned to return when she was medically fit to be discharged. In the meantime, she clearly stated that she did not want anymore treatment with intravenous acetylcysteine, despite highlighting the risks and complications and that she wanted to die. She removed the intravenous cannula and began to leave. She was fully alert, and was orientated to person, place, and time.

    Medico-legally, how could you proceed if you wanted to stop her from leaving hospital?

    A. The patient has capacity but override her wishes under the Mental Capacity Act 2005
    B. The patient has capacity but override her wishes under the Mental Health Act 1983
    C. The patient lacks capacity and act in her best interests under the Mental Capacity Act 2005
    D. The patient lacks capacity and act in her best interests under the Mental Health Act 1983
    E. Under common law, as you have a duty of care to the patient

9. A 65-year-old man presented via his GP to the acute medical unit with shortness of breath and palpitations. He had a significant past psychiatric history of vascular dementia and an organic psychotic disorder. Currently, he was mentally stable and under the care of the community mental health team and was taking amisulpride 150 mg at night. A 12-lead ECG showed atrial fibrillation (AF) with a fast ventricular response, which was not present on an ECG performed two days ago. The QTc was 460 ms.

   With regards to the management of this patient's new onset AF, what is the pharmacological agent of choice?

   A. Amiodarone
   B. Digoxin
   C. Diltiazem
   D. Sotalol
   E. Verapamil

10. A 43-year-old woman attended the emergency department with her brother, following a fit. She had a history of medically unexplained seizures. She was observed frequently going in and out of the waiting room to have a cigarette as she was agitated by having to wait. As she returned to the reception, she collapsed and began convulsing. It was observed that during the seizure she had been incontinent and had hurt her forehead on a chair. She was moved into the resuscitation area and tolerated the insertion of an oropharyngeal airway. The seizure was ongoing at five minutes from onset.

    Which of the following is the most appropriate next step?

    A. CT scan of head
    B. Explain to her brother that the symptoms are self-induced
    C. Intravenous diazepam
    D. Observe but reassure her brother that symptoms will resolve quickly
    E. Reassure the patient that there is definitely not an organic cause

11. The accuracy of a screening test for depression was evaluated in primary care. The screening test involved asking patients two questions about depression and pleasure within the last month. In total, 421 consecutive primary care attendees not taking psychotropic drugs agreed to participate. The two questions could be asked at any time during the consultation. If the patient responded positively to either question, the screening test result was 'positive', and the patient was considered to be at 'high risk' of depression—otherwise, screening was considered 'negative' and the patient was considered to be at 'low risk' of depression. Subsequently, the diagnosis of depression—present or absent was made using a self-completed computerized international diagnostic interview. The sensitivity of screening using the two questions was reported to be 96.6%.*

What is the best interpretation of the sensitivity of the screening test for depression?

A. Of those patients identified at high risk by screening, 96.6% had a diagnosis of depression
B. Of those patients identified at low risk by screening, 96.6% did not have a diagnosis of depression
C. Of those patients with diagnosed depression, 96.6% were identified at high risk by screening
D. Of those patients without a diagnosis of depression, 96.6% were identified at low risk by screening.
E. Screening correctly identified the diagnosis (presence or absence of depression) for 96.6% of all patients.

* Data included in this question is from B Arroll et al., 'Screening for depression in primary care with two verbally asked questions: cross sectional study', BMJ, 2003; 327:1144

chapter 16

PSYCHIATRY

ANSWERS

1. A. Diazepam

The patient is presenting with classical symptoms of serotonin syndrome—a potentially life-threatening syndrome often missed by clinicians. Management should include discontinuing serotonergic drugs, which would include all options apart from diazepam. Indeed, benzodiazepines are recommended for the control of agitation in serotonin syndrome and have been found to improve survival in animal models of serotonin syndrome, perhaps through a blunting of the hyperadrenergic state.

The serotonin syndrome

Serotonergic neurons in the central nervous system (CNS) assist in the regulation of wakefulness, affective behaviour, appetite, thermoregulation, sexual behaviour, nociception, and motor tone. The peripheral serotonergic system helps regulate vascular tone and gastrointestinal motility. The serotonin syndrome is a predictable consequence of excessive serotonergic agonism in the central and peripheral nervous systems. It usually occurs in overdoses of serotonergic drugs or when serotonergic medications are used in combination, although it can occur in patients taking therapeutic doses of serotonergic medications. A large number of medications are associated with the serotonin syndrome, including monoamine oxidase inhibitors, selective serotonin re-uptake inhibitors (SSRIs) and other antidepressants, opiate analgesics, antiemetics, the 'mood stabilizers' valproate and lithium, antihistamines, over-the-counter cough and cold remedy dextromethorphan, and the herbal products tryptophan and St John's Wort. Illicit substances associated with the serotonin syndrome include amphetamines, MDMA ('ecstasy'), and LSD.

Its clinical manifestations range from mild to life-threatening. Mild cases involving only restlessness or tremor and sweating may be easily missed. With increasing severity, there is increasing vital sign and neuromuscular abnormalities. In life-threatening cases, patients may have severe hypertension, tachycardia, agitated delirium, convulsions, muscular rigidity, and core temperatures of more than 41.0°C. No investigations confirm the diagnosis and it must be made on the patient's history and examination. The history should include a full inquiry into all prescribed and over-the-counter medications and illicit substances. The Hunter Serotonin Toxicity Criteria state that in the presence of a serotonergic agent, serotonin syndrome is diagnosed if any of the following are present:

- Tremor and hyperreflexia
- Spontaneous clonus
- Increased muscle tone, temperature >38.0°C, and either ocular clonus or inducible clonus
- Inducible or ocular clonus and either agitation or diaphoresis

The differential diagnosis includes anticholinergic poisoning, malignant hyperthermia, and the neuroleptic malignant syndrome, but clinical differences help to differentiate between each condition, as illustrated in Table 16.1.

Table 16.1 Differentiating serotonin syndrome among common presentations.

Disorder	Causative Agent	Onset/Resolution	Symptoms
Serotonin Syndrome	Postexposure to serotonin agonists	Develops within 24 hours; resolves within 24 hours with treatment	Altered mental status, muscle rigidity (especially in the lower extremities), hyperreflexia, increased bowel sounds, diaphoresis
Neuroleptic Malignant Syndrome	Postexposure to dopamine antagonists	Develops over a period of days to weeks; resolves in approximately 9 days with treatment	Neuromuscular hypoactivity manifesting as rigidity and bradyreflexia
Malignant Hyperthermia	Postexposure to inhalational anesthetics or depolarizing muscle relaxants (succinylcholine)	Develops within minutes or within 24 hours; resolves within 24 to 48 hours with treatment	Rising end tidal carbon dioxide, mottled skin with areas of flushing and cyanosis, rigidity and hyporeflexia
Anticholinergic Toxicity	Postexposure to anticholinergic agents	Develops within 24 hours; resolves within hours to days with treatment	Urinary retention, decreased bowel sounds, hot and dry erythematous skin with normal muscle tone and reflexes

Reproduced from Volpi-Abadie, J et al., 'Serotonin Syndrome', The Ochsner Journal, 13, pp. 533–540. Copyright © 2013 Academic Division of Ochsner Clinic Foundation.

Management includes discontinuation of serotonergic drugs, provision of supportive therapy, control of agitation with benzodiazepines, and consideration of serotonin $_{2A}$ antagonist administration. Cyproheptadine, an antihistamine, is a potent 5-HT$_{2A}$ blocker at higher doses (12–32 mg in a 24-hour period) and case-series evidence supports its use in moderate to severe cases. Bromocriptine and dantrolene use should be avoided. Bromocriptine can precipitate serotonin syndrome and dantrolene is ineffective in animal studies of serotonin syndrome.

Bienvenu OJ, Neufeld KJ, Needham DM. Treatment of four psychiatric emergencies in the intensive care unit. Critical Care Medicine 2012; 40: 2662–2670.

Boyer EW, Shannon M. The serotonin syndrome. N Engl J Med 2005; 352: 1112–1120.

Taylor D, Paton C, Kapur S. The Maudsley prescribing guidelines in psychiatry. 11th edn. Chichester: Wiley-Blackwell, 2012.

2. C. Haemodialysis

Lithium is an element that is dealt with by the body in a similar way to sodium. It is minimally bound to plasma proteins and distributes evenly in the total body water. It is not metabolized and is removed almost exclusively by renal mechanisms.

Lithium is the most effective long-term treatment for bipolar disorder, protecting against both depression and mania. It also reduces suicide risk. It can be used in unipolar depression to augment antidepressant therapy, to treat aggression and self-mutilation, to treat steroid-induced psychosis and mania, and to increase the white blood cell count in patients receiving clozapine. A clinical disadvantage of lithium is its narrow therapeutic range (serum levels between 0.5 and 1.2 mmol/L) with toxic effects seen at levels as low as 1.5 mmol/L. Toxicity has gastrointestinal, neurological, renal, and cardiac effects.

Factors contributing to lithium toxicity in long-term treatment when no acute excess ingestion has occurred include:

- An increase in daily dose
- Long-term high dosage

- Renal impairment
- Any circumstances that predispose to sodium or volume depletion, e.g. dehydration, diarrhoea, vomiting, cardiac failure, surgery
- Drug interactions

Medications that can contribute to lithium toxicity are usually those that alter the handling of sodium by the kidneys. They include angiotensin-converting enzyme inhibitors, diuretics (particularly thiazides), non-steroidal anti-inflammatory drugs (particularly indometacin), and COX-2 inhibitors. The effects on plasma concentrations of lithium are unpredictable but can increase concentrations fourfold. Loop diuretics can increase or decrease serum lithium levels. Propranolol can be used to treat lithium-induced tremor and does not increase serum lithium levels.

The severity of toxicity tends to increase with increasing plasma levels. Mild, moderate, and severe symptoms approximately correlate with lithium levels of >1.5, >2.5, and >3.5 mmol/L respectively. Signs and symptoms of mild toxicity include anorexia, nausea, vomiting, diarrhoea, coarse hand tremor, muscle weakness, and drowsiness. As severity of toxicity increases, neurological effects increase with confusion and ataxia progressing to seizures, coma, and ultimately death. Other effects of severe toxicity include cardiac dysrhythmias and renal failure.

In acute overdose, gastric lavage may be attempted if the patient presents within one hour of ingestion. Lithium does not bind to charcoal and activated charcoal is therefore ineffective. The mainstay of treatment is fluid therapy to normalize the glomerular filtration rate and enhance lithium excretion, and may be sufficient for mild to moderate cases of toxicity. Osmotic or forced alkaline diuresis should be used for more severe symptoms, but never thiazide or loop diuretics. However, in cases of severe toxicity haemodialysis is the treatment of choice and should be considered in all patients with neurological features. There may be a post dialysis rebound increase in levels of lithium and additional haemodialysis may be necessary. Peritoneal dialysis is less effective at eliminating lithium.

Complications of long-term lithium therapy include an increased risk of nephrogenic diabetes insipidus, hypothyroidism (sixfold increased risk), hyperparathyroidism (absolute risk of 10% versus 0.1% in the general population), weight gain, reduction in glomerular filtration rate, possible increased risk of congenital malformations, and aggravation of skin conditions such as psoriasis.

Grandean EM, Aubrey JM. Lithium: updated human knowledge using an evidenced-based approach: part III: clinical safety. CNS drugs 2009; 23: 397–418.

McKnight RF, Adida M, Budge K, Stockton S, Goodwin GM, Geddes JR. Lithium toxicity: a systematic review and meta-analysis. Lancet 2012; 379: 721–728.

Taylor D, Paton C, Kapur S. The Maudesley prescribing guidelines in psychiatry. 11th edn. Chichester: Wiley-Blackwell, 2012.

3. C. The reattribution approach

This patient is describing symptoms suggestive of a panic attack, and a likely history of recurrent un-cued panic attacks points to a diagnosis of panic disorder. Patterns of thinking that can predispose some patients with COPD to develop panic disorder include having catastrophic thoughts about somatic symptoms, a heightened perception of symptoms, and a misinterpretation of physical sensations. Once anxiety symptoms develop, a vicious cycle of anxiety symptoms exacerbating COPD symptoms and vice versa can result: anxiety increases respiratory rate and results in rapid shallow breathing causing symptoms of hyperventilation including light-headedness, numbness, tingling sensations, and breathlessness. In patients with COPD, hyperventilation can also induce bronchoconstriction, probably due to exposure of airways to dry cool air, and can additionally predispose patients to developing dynamic hyperinflation, which further exacerbates dyspnoea. Rates of anxiety disorders in patients with COPD are much higher than in the general population, particularly generalized anxiety disorder and panic disorder. Co-morbid anxiety disorder and COPD lead to significantly reduced quality of life and increased disability, medical treatments, and hospitalization.

The recognition of an anxiety disorder is the first step in devising an appropriate ongoing management plan for this patient that avoids further unnecessary investigations, medical interventions, and future similar presentations. Use of the principles of the reattribution approach then provides a useful framework for the treating doctor to explore with the patient the psychological basis of her recent symptoms and how they link to her physical symptoms. In practice, the reattribution approach involves:

- The patient feeling understood: elicit physical symptoms, mood and anxiety symptoms, beliefs held by the patient about their problem, any social problems, relevant physical examination and investigations
- Broadening the agenda: summarize the physical, psychological, and social findings and negotiate them with the patient
- Making the link: between physical symptoms, psychological symptoms, and any social problems
- Negotiating further treatment: arrange follow-up or treatment of the psychosocial problem or mental disorder

Brenes GA. Anxiety and chronic obstructive pulmonary disease: prevalence, impact and treatment. Psychosomatic Medicine 2003; 65: 963–970.

Bronchoconstriction due to cold weather in COPD. The roles of direct airway effects and cutaneous reflex mechanisms. Chest September 1996; 110(3): 632–636.

Dowrick C, Gask L, Hughes JG et al. General practitioners' views on reattribution for patients with medically unexplained symptoms: a questionnaire and qualitative study. BMC Family Practice 2008; 9: 46.

Livermore N, Sharpe L, McKenzie D. Panic attacks and panic disorder in chronic obstructive pulmonary disease: a cognitive behavioural perspective. Respiratory Medicine 2010; 104: 1246–1253.

4. A. A history of war trauma-related symptoms

The patient is presenting with likely khat psychosis. Khat leaves tend to be chewed by East Africans and contain cathinone, which is structurally related and has similar effects to amphetamine. Early onset of use and heavy consumption are associated with an increased risk of khat psychosis. In Somalia, khat psychosis is also increased in those who have war trauma-related symptoms. It tends to present with a paranoid or schizophreniform psychosis although manic psychoses have also been reported.

Drugs associated with substance-induced psychosis include cannabis and stimulants such as cocaine, amphetamines, and khat. They usually cause a schizophreniform psychosis with typical features that include: paranoid delusions, fear, hostility, persecutory or threatening auditory hallucinations, ideas of reference, and thought alienation. Patients feel under threat and may isolate themselves or become aggressive.

Confusional states are rare and usually psychoses occur in clear consciousness. Confusion and disorientation suggest a state of delirium, perhaps caused by acute drug intoxication or another organic cause of delirium.

There can be difficulties differentiating substance-induced psychosis from a primary psychotic disorder such as schizophrenia, given that symptoms are similar and substance use is extremely common in first episode psychosis (40–70%). However, symptoms of substance-, particularly stimulant-, induced psychosis tend to resolve quickly within days of cessation of the offending substance, while symptoms must persist for at least one month for a diagnosis of schizophrenia. Urinalysis can be useful for identifying offending substances. Other diagnoses in the differential would include delirium and organic psychoses caused by other agents or conditions.

Management of substance-induced psychosis includes stopping the offending substance. If symptoms are severe, early treatment is necessary, or if symptoms do not resolve spontaneously then treatment with an antipsychotic, generally a second-generation antipsychotic, is indicated.

Cox G, Rampes H. Adverse effects of khat: a review. APT 2003; 9: 456–463.

Fraser S, Hides L, Philips L, Proctor D, Lubman DI. Differentiating first episode substance induced and primary psychotic disorders with concurrent substance use in young people. Schizophrenia Research 2012; 136: 110–115.

5. E. Redirecting the patient towards a calmer personal space

Disturbed behaviour can occur in the context of psychiatric illness, physical illness, substance use, and personality disorder. Psychosis increases the risk of violence compared with the general population, and substance use substantially increases the risk. The initial approach to disturbed and agitated behaviour should be psychological and behavioural de-escalation approaches which are techniques to 'defuse' or 'talk down' disruptive behaviours and to prevent violence. Verbal de-escalation includes:

- Avoiding confrontation
- Redirecting the patient towards a calmer personal space
- Observing for signs and symptoms of anger and agitation
- Approaching the patient in a calm, controlled manner
- Giving the patient choices
- Maintaining patient dignity

Observation also helps to prevent violence, watching the patient attentively while avoiding making them feel under surveillance. In this way, early signs of agitation can be identified and defused. It may be necessary to move the patient to a more appropriate environment.

Urgent sedation or 'rapid tranquilization' does not have a strong evidence base, is not without risks, and should be viewed as a treatment of last resort. Oral sedatives should be offered first, usually benzodiazepines to avoid the risks associated with combining antipsychotics if intramuscular (IM) antipsychotic medication is subsequently required. Concomitant use of two or more antipsychotics increases the risk of QTc prolongation common to all antipsychotics, especially where disturbed behaviour predisposes patient to developing cardiac arrhythmias. IM treatment options include lorazepam, midazolam, promethazine, olanzapine, aripiprazole, and haloperidol. Haloperidol should be considered last due to high rates of extra-pyramidal side effects, including acute dystonic reactions in 5% of cases, and its QTc prolongation effects. A pre-treatment ECG is recommended. Studies suggest IM olanzapine is more effective than haloperidol, and that both are more effective than aripiprazole.

National Institute for Health and Care Excellence. Clinical Guideline 10. Violence and aggression: short-term management in mental health, health and community settings. May 2015.

Taylor D, Paton C, Kapur S. The Maudesley prescribing guidelines in psychiatry. 11th edn. Chichester: Wiley-Blackwell, 2012.

6. C. Delirium tremens

Around 40% of older people referred to a mental health liaison service for assessment of depression are actually diagnosed as delirium. Depressive symptoms are as common in the delirious as those diagnosed with actual depression.

People who are physically dependent on alcohol who stop drinking or reduce their alcohol consumption commonly develop an alcohol-withdrawal syndrome. Delirium tremens (DTs) is the most severe manifestation of alcohol withdrawal. Symptoms may appear suddenly but typically develop 2–3 days after cessation of drinking heavily.

No specific findings on physical examination are diagnostic for DTs. However, DTs often presents with a coexisting illness, so careful physical examination should be performed in order to uncover any potentially serious illness that may be present. The patient should be assessed for stigmata of chronic liver disease and a search for signs of trauma should also be included. Clinical findings associated with DTs may include the following: tachycardia, hyperthermia, hypertension, tachypnoea, diaphoresis, tremor, mydriasis, altered mental status, severe psychomotor agitation, fever, positional nystagmus, global confusion, and disorientation.

The most objective and validated tool to assess the severity of alcohol withdrawal is the Clinical Institute Withdrawal Assessment for Alcohol, revised (CIWA-Ar). This tool consists of ten items that can be administered rapidly at the bedside. The tool has high reliability, reproducibility, and validity in detoxification units, psychiatric units, and hospital medical/surgical wards. The CIWA-Ar scale is intended only for patients who have been drinking recently and does rely on patients' ability to respond to questions about their symptoms.

It is important to have a high degree of suspicion of alcohol and other substance misuse issues in patients (of all ages) who present with mental state changes, as this is often unknown or not routinely disclosed. Alcohol and substance misuse by older people is now a growing public health problem. Between 2001 and 2031, there is projected to be a 50% increase in the number of older people in the UK. The percentage of men and women drinking more than the weekly recommended limits has also risen, by 60% in men and 100% in women between 1990 and 2006. Given the likely impact of these two factors on health and social care services, there is a pressing need to recognize and address substance misuse in older people.

In older people, the relationship between cognitive function and alcohol use, and that between functional mental health problems (e.g. anxiety and depression), is complex. The direction of causality is often unclear. Among older people, psychosocial factors (including bereavement, retirement, boredom, loneliness, homelessness, and depression) are all associated with higher rates of alcohol use.

Hales R, Yudofsky S, Talbott J. Textbook of psychiatry (3rd edn). London: The American Psychiatric Press, 1999.

Sullivan JT, Sykora K, Schneiderman J et al. Assessment of alcohol withdrawal: the revised clinical institute withdrawal assessment for alcohol scale (CIWA-Ar). British Journal of Addiction November 1989; 84(11): 1353–1357.

Royal College of Psychiatrists. Who Cares Wins. Improving the Outcome for Older People Admitted to the General Hospital 2005.

Royal College of Psychiatrists. Our Invisible Addicts. Report of the Older People's Substance Misuse Working Group at the Royal College of Psychiatrists 2011.

7. C. The patient lacks capacity and act in her best interests under the Mental Capacity Act 2005

Mental Capacity Act 2005

The Mental Capacity Act states that a person lacks capacity if they are unable to make a specific decision, at a specific time, because of an impairment of, or disturbance, in the functioning of mind or brain.

Assessing capacity

To be able to make a decision, a person should be able to:
- Understand the decision to be made and the information provided about the decision. The consequences of making a decision must be included in the information given.

- Retain the information—a person should be able to retain the information given for long enough to make the decision. If information can only be retained for short periods of time, it should not automatically be assumed that the person lacks capacity. Notebooks, for example, could be used to record information which may help a person to retain it.
- Use that information in making the decision—a person should be able to weigh up the pros and cons of making the decision.
- Communicate their decision—if a person cannot communicate their decision—for example, if they are in a coma—the Act specifies that they should be treated as if they lack capacity. You should make all efforts to help the person communicate their decision before deciding they cannot.

You will need to assess a person's capacity regularly, particularly when a care plan is being developed or reviewed.

Fluctuating capacity

Some patients are intermittently or temporarily unable to make a decision for themselves. It may be possible to wait until the patient has capacity or, where this is not the case, patients must be treated in accordance with their best interests or according to consent given by someone authorized to act on the patient's behalf—someone with parental responsibility in the case of a minor, or a person with a personal welfare lasting power of attorney (LPA).

Advanced decisions

Adults with the capacity to do so can make decisions about how they want to be treated if they later lose their capacity. An advance decision to refuse treatment (ADRT) is legally binding in England and Wales under the terms of the Mental Capacity Act 2005. It must specify the treatments being refused, and in what circumstances, and may be made verbally or in writing. If, however, the refusal relates to life-sustaining treatment, the decision must be in writing, signed, and witnessed. It must also clearly state that the refusal stands even if it will place the individual's life at risk.

Great Britain. Mental Capacity Act 2005. http://www.legislation.gov.uk

8. B. The patient has capacity but override her wishes under the Mental Health Act 1983

Mental Health Act 1983 (key points)

- The Mental Health Act is the law under which someone can be admitted, detained, and treated in hospital against their wishes.
- To be detained or 'sectioned' someone must be suffering from a mental disorder which requires assessment or treatment and this needs to be given in hospital in the interests of their own health or safety or to protect other people.
- There are different sections of the Mental Health Act that have different purposes.
- Anyone detained must be told their rights, including the right to appeal and the right to the assistance of an advocate.
- Someone can be given treatment such as medication, against their will, while under certain sections.

The most likely section used on a general hospital ward is section 5(2), which is a 'holding power'. It is used where the doctor thinks that an assessment under the Mental Health Act ought to be done with a view to detention under section 2 (assessment section for up to 28 days) or section 3 (treatment section for up to six months) of the Mental Health Act.

Section 5(2)

Section 5(2) is a doctor's holding power to authorize detention of an informal patient for up to 72 hours in order for an assessment under the Mental Health Act 1983 to take place.

One can:
- Hold the person in hospital until a Mental Health Act assessment is done

One cannot:
- Give treatment
- Implement another section 5(2) back to back
- Let the section 5(2) lapse
- Use section 5(2) in accident and emergency or outpatients
- Have leave from the section 5(2)
- Transfer a patient to another ward, as they are in a place of safety (unless the patient's life is at risk or there would be irreversible serious harm done)

Department of Health Mental Health Act 1983 information leaflets. https://www.gov.uk/government/publications/code-of-practice-mental-health-act-1983

General Medical Council List of Ethical Guidance. http://www.gmc-uk.org/guidance/ethical_guidance.asp

Medical Protection Society. http://www.medicalprotection.org

9. B. Digoxin

All antipsychotic drugs have the potential to prolong the QTc interval. Serious drug interactions that further prolong the QTc interval (and increase the risk of torsade de pointes) can occur particularly when using cardiac agents in patients taking antipsychotic drugs. Sotalol or amiodarone should never be used in combination with amisulpiride (an antipsychotic); however, alternative beta blockers such as atenolol or bisoprolol are safe and often first-line pharmacological agents in the management of AF. Diltiazem and verapamil when co-prescribed with amisulpiride can increase toxicity by pharmacodynamic synergism and also increase the risk of QTc prolongation. In this situation, therefore, digoxin, which does not interact with psychiatric drugs, would be the safest and preferred rate-controlling medication of choice.

Taylor D, Paton C, Kapur S. The Maudesley prescribing guidelines in psychiatry. 11th edn. Chichester: Wiley-Blackwell, 2012.

10. C. Intravenous diazepam

Dissociative seizures (DSs) or 'pseudoseizures' are psychologically mediated episodes of altered awareness and behaviour that may mimic any type of epilepsy. The prevalence of DSs has been estimated as between 2 and 33 per 100,000. Around three-quarters of patients are female. Seizures typically begin in the late teens or early twenties, but there is a wide range. Seizures have typically been present for three or four years before the correct diagnosis is made. Probably no more than 15 or 20% of patients with DSs also have epileptic seizures.

Clinical assessment

No single clinical feature can be relied upon to distinguish DSs from epileptic seizures with anything approaching 100% accuracy. The most helpful features, as well as some important pitfalls along with symptoms that are commonly mistaken as strong evidence for epilepsy are listed in Table 16.2. Epileptic seizures are brief, highly stereotyped, paroxysmal alterations in neurological function that conform to a number of now well-described syndromes. Broadly speaking, it is any variation from these clinical pictures—an atypical sequence of events—that will raise the suspicion of DSs. A history of pseudoseizures does not exclude 'organic' seizures, and there is an increased risk of pseudoseizures in people with epilepsy. The history of incontinence and accidental injury are not diagnostic of either type of seizure, but would be more unusual in a pseudoseizure. Insertion of an oropharyngeal airway is not impossible in a pseudoseizure, but would be very unusual (NB: it should not be used as a diagnostic 'tool').

Table 16.2 Comparative semiology of dissociative and epileptic seizures.

	Dissociative seizures	Epileptic seizures
Duration over two minutes	Common	Rare
*Stereotyped attacks	Common	Common
Motor Features		
Gradual onset	Common	Rare
Fluctuating course	Common	Very rare
Thrashing, violent movements	Common	Rare
Side-to-side head movement	Common	Rare
Asynchronous movements	Common	Very rare
Eyes closed	Common	Rare
Pelvic thrusting	Occasional	Rare
Opisthotonus, 'arc de cercle'	Occasional	Very rare
Automatisms	Rare	Common
Weeping	Occasional	Very rare
*Incontinence	Occasional	Common
*Injury		
Biting inside of mouth	Occasional	Common
Severe tongue-biting	Very rare	Common
Recall for period of unresponsiveness	Common	Very rare

Note:

*Three features that are commonly misinterpreted as evidence for epilepsy have been included. Otherwise, the table lists clinical features that are useful in distinguishing DS from ES. Figures for frequency of these features are approximate: common >30%; occasional = 10–30%; rare <10%; very rare <5%. ('Reproduced from Postgraduate Medical Journal, 81, Mellers JDC, 'The approach to patients with "non-epileptic seizures"', copyright (2005) with permission from BMJ Publishing Group Ltd.)

Psychiatric co-morbidity

High rates of depression, anxiety, personality disorder, and post-traumatic disorder have been reported in patients with DS, but findings have varied considerably. A history of previous medically unexplained symptoms is very common. An opportunity to observe a seizure may provide invaluable information. Whether the patient is responsive should be established. Movements should be described carefully. If the patient's eyes are shut (an important observation in itself, suggesting DS), the examiner should attempt to open them noting any resistance. A simple test to look for avoidance of a noxious stimulus is to hold the patient's hand over their face and drop it; in DS, the patient may be seen to control their arm movement so their hand falls to one side. If the eyes can be held open easily, evidence of visual fixation may be sought by holding a small mirror in front of the patient and look for evidence of convergent gaze and fixation on the reflection. This procedure will also often stop the seizure.

Mellers J. The diagnosis and management of dissociative seizures 2007. www.e-epilepsy.org.uk

11. C. Of those patients with diagnosed depression, 96.6% were identified at high risk by screening

It would not be practical to offer all patients in primary care diagnostic testing for depression. It would be time-consuming and not cost-effective. Instead, the two questions about depression and pleasure within the last month can be administered easily and quickly. The two questions were a screening test that identified patients at high (positive result) or low (negative result) risk of depression. However, the questions do not provide a diagnosis. Ideally, the two questions should correctly classify all patients with depression as positive and those without as negative. Unfortunately, as a screening test, the two questions may not be 100% accurate and may incorrectly identify some patients with depression as low risk. Equally, some patients without depression may be incorrectly identified as high risk by the screening test. The performance of the screening test for depression is described by a series of indices, including sensitivity, specificity, positive predictive value, and negative predictive value.

The following table shows the results of the screening test and diagnostic test for depression.

Table 16.3 Cross tabulation of the results of the screening test, categorised as "negative" or "positive," against the diagnosis of depression. (BMJ 2003;327:1144).

Result of screening test	Diagnosed with depression		Total
	Yes	No	
Positive (High Risk) (≥1 'yes' responses)	28	129	157
Negative (Low Risk) (no 'yes' responses)	1	263	264
Total	29	392	421

The sensitivity of the screening test is the percentage of patients with diagnosed depression that were identified correctly by the screening test as high-risk (positive). It is calculated as:

$$\frac{28}{28+1} \times 100\% = 96.6\%$$

The specificity of the screening test is the percentage of patients without diagnosed depression that were identified correctly by the screening test as low risk. It is calculated as:

$$\frac{263}{129+263} \times 100\% = 67.1\%$$

The positive predictive value (PPV) of the screening test is the percentage of patients identified as high-risk by screening, subsequently found to have a diagnosis of depression and therefore correctly identified by screening. It is calculated as:

$$\frac{28}{28+129} \times 100\% = 17.8\%$$

The negative predictive value (NPV) of the screening test is the percentage of patients identified as low-risk by screening, subsequently found not to have a diagnosis of depression and therefore correctly identified by screening. It is calculated as:

$$\frac{263}{1+263} \times 100\% = 99.6\%$$

The percentage of patients correctly identified by screening is the number of patients with diagnosed depression correctly identified as high-risk plus the number without diagnosed depression correctly identified as low-risk, as a percentage of the total number of patients investigated. It is calculated as:

$$\frac{28+263}{421}\times100\% = 69.1\%$$

When evaluating the indices of performance for a screening test, all study participants will undergo the screening and diagnostic tests. However, in clinical practice only those patients that receive a 'high-risk' (positive) screening test result will be offered further diagnostic testing. By doing so, the screening test will reduce the number of patients that require diagnostic testing, thereby reducing costs and inconvenience.

The definitions of the four indices of sensitivity, specificity, positive predictive value, and negative predictive value may not be easy to remember. Sensitivity and positive predictive value are often confused, as are specificity and negative predictive value. In the example above, sensitivity and specificity were concerned with diagnosed depression—present or absent. It is suggested that a clinician may be more likely to concentrate on these two indices as they wish to correctly identify, with as high a certainty as possible, the percentage of patients with and without a diagnosis by screening. Equally, it is suggested that a patient may be more interested in the positive predictive value and negative predictive value. Once a patient has undergone screening, they will want to know what percentage of patients receive a correct test result in respects of their actual diagnosis. In order to avoid confusion when defining an index, it is advised to first state the denominator, and then the percentage of the denominator that demonstrates the characteristic of interest. For example, sensitivity is defined as follows: 'Of those patients with a diagnosis of depression, what percentage were identified as high risk and therefore correctly identified by screening'.

The use of 'negative' and 'positive' when reporting the results of a screening test is commonplace. However, this is best avoided and the terms 'low-risk' and 'high-risk' are recommended. Patients may interpret a 'positive' and 'negative' screening test incorrectly. In particular, a positive result might be interpreted to mean something good, i.e. no risk of a having depression, and a negative result as something bad, i.e. a risk of having depression.

Sedgwick P, Joekes K. Evaluating the performance of a screening test for depression in primary care. *BMJ* 2015; 350: h1801.

Sedgwick P. How to read a receiver operating characteristic curve. *BMJ* 2015; 350: h2464.

INDEX

Notes: Page numbers in *q* refer to Question and *a* refer to Answer.

A
ABCD² 172*a*
abdominal distension 27*q*, 43*a*
abdominal pain 32*q*, 34*q*, 36*q*, 37*q*, 39*q*, 49*q*, 50*a*, 52*a*, 53*a*, 55*a*
ABPA (allergic broncho-pulmonary aspergillosis) 87*a*
ACCEPT 20*a*
ACE-I (angiotensin-converting enzyme inhibitor) induced angioedema 393*a*
acetylcholinesterase inhibitors 171*a*
N-acetylcysteine 373*a*
AchR (anti-choline receptor) antibodies 231*a*
ACPA (anti-citrullinated protein antibody) 274*a*
acquired angioedema (AAE) (acquired C1 inhibitor deficiency) 388*q*, 392–393*a*
acute anaphylaxis 387*q*, 391*a*
acute chest syndrome, sickle cell anaemia 302*q*, 307*a*
acute confusional state 11*q*, 23*a*
acute coronary syndrome 5*q*, 19*a*, 168*q*, 181*a*
 management 101*q*, 117–118*a*
acute dialysis 203–204*a*
Acute Dialysis Quality Initiative 200–201*a*
acute gouty olecranon bursitis 251*q*, 273*a*
acute inflammatory demyelinating polyradiculoneuropathy (AIDP) 213*q*, 214*q*, 232*a*, 233*a*
 treatment 218*q*, 237*a*
acute kidney injury 185*q*, 189*q*, 198–199*a*, 200–201*a*
Acute Kidney Injury Network 201*a*
acute liver failure (ALF) 35*q*, 50–51*a*
acute myelogenous leukaemia (AML) 304*q*, 309–310*a*
acute on chronic type 2 respiratory failure 83*a*
acute phenytoin toxicity 218*q*, 237*a*
acute promyelocytic leukaemia (APL) 309–310*a*
acute pseudogout 253*q*, 274*a*
acute pulmonary oedema 110*q*, 124–125*a*
acute renal transplant dysfunction 190*q*, 201*a*
acute respiratory distress syndrome (ARDS) 73*q*, 88*a*
acute severe asthma 65*q*, 82–83*a*, 82*a*
acute severe migraine headache 225*q*, 247*a*
acute stent thrombosis 93*q*, 111–112*a*
acute stroke 307*a*
acute type 2 respiratory failure 69*q*, 86*a*
ADA (adenosine transaminase) 89*a*
Addison's disease management 141*q*, 155*a*

adenocarcinoma
 caecum 291*q*, 298–299*a*
 oesophageal 41*q*, 57–58*a*
adenosine transaminase (ADA) 89*a*
adenovirus infection 342*a*
adjuvant analgesia 292*a*
adrenaline (epinephrine) 22*a*
 acute anaphylaxis 391*a*
 acute severe exacerbation of asthma 82*a*
advanced decisions 416*a*
Advanced Life Support guidelines (2010) 13*q*, 24*a*
AEDs see anti-epileptic drugs (AEDs)
AF see atrial fibrillation (AF)
AIDP see acute inflammatory demyelinating polyradiculoneuropathy (AIDP)
airway management 8*q*, 21*a*
AKIN diagnostic criteria in kidney injury 198–199*a*
alcoholic cardiomyopathy 35*q*, 51*a*
alcoholic hepatitis 36*q*, 52*a*
alcoholic liver disease (ALD) 4*q*, 18–19*a*, 30*q*, 35*q*, 36*q*, 47*a*, 51*a*, 52–53*a*
 CPR guidelines 21*a*
alcoholism/alcohol dependency 36*q*, 40*q*, 52*a*, 56*a*
alcohol withdrawal, tonic–clonic seizures 40*q*, 56–57*a*
ALD see alcoholic liver disease (ALD)
ALF (acute liver failure) 35*q*, 50–51*a*
allergen-specific immunotherapy 386*q*, 390*a*
allergic broncho-pulmonary aspergillosis (ABPA) 87*a*
allergic response
 biphasic allergic response 387*q*, 391*a*
 insect venom 386*q*, 391*a*
allergic rhinitis 386*q*, 390*a*
alternative pathway complement deficiency 383*q*, 389*a*
Alzheimer's disease 157*q*, 170*a*
 formal capacity assessment 158*q*, 171*a*
American Academy of Clinical Toxicology 377–378*a*
American College of Rheumatology (ACR)
 eosinophilic granulomatosis with polyangiitis 271*a*
 Sjögren's syndrome 274*a*
American National Registry of Cardiopulmonary Resuscitation 16*a*, 17*a*
amiodarone 115*a*
 atrial fibrillation 119*a*
amitriptyline, falls 165*q*, 179*a*

AML (acute myelogenous leukaemia) 304q, 309–310a
amlodipine 118a
  hypertensive emergency 117a
amoebiasis, hepatic 316q, 334–335a
amphetamine overdose 374a
amputations, below-knee 187q, 199–200a
amyloidosis 191q, 202a, 254q, 274–275a, 301q, 306a
anaemia, iron deficiency 29q, 45a, 46a
analgesia
  adjuvant 292a
  malignant mesothelioma 283q, 299a
analytical toxicology 372a
anaphylaxis 9q, 22a, 387q, 391a
  acute 387q, 391a
ANCA testing
  non-visible haematuria 199a
  renal medicine 200a
angina 120a
angina, aortic stenosis 120a
angioedema, acquired *see* acquired angioedema (AAE) (acquired C1 inhibitor deficiency)
angiography, coronary 95q, 113a
angiotensin-converting enzyme (ACE-I) induced angioedema 393a
anion gap metabolic acidaemia 196q, 204a
ankylosing spondylitis 262q, 278a
anorexia nervosa 41q, 57a
anterior STEMI 96q, 114a
antibiotics, broad-spectrum 344a
anti-cancer treatment
  nausea and vomiting 288q, 296–297a
  neutropenic sepsis 286q, 295a
anti-choline receptor (AchR) antibodies 231a
anticholinergic toxicity 365–366a, 411a
anti-citrullinated protein antibody (ACPA) 274a
anticoagulants 68q, 85a
anticonvulsants 339a
anti-embolism stockings 308a
anti-epileptic drugs (AEDs) 227a
  during pregnancy 234–235a
anti-glomerular basement membrane disease 192q, 202a
antipsychotic drugs 408q, 417a
anti-synthetase antibodies 276–277a
a-NVH (asymptomatic non-visible haematuria) 184q, 198a
aortic dissection 99q, 116–117a
  Turner syndrome 148–149a
aortic stenosis 105q, 120a
aortic valve replacement 105q, 120a
APL (acute promyelocytic leukaemia) 309–310a
aplastic crises in sickle cell anaemia 307a
ARDS (acute respiratory distress syndrome) 73q, 88a
artesunate 331a
arthritis
  reactive 346a
  septic 257q, 276a
ascending aorta, dissection flap 99q, 116–117a
ascites 35q, 51a
aspiration pneumonia 258q, 276–277a
asthma 65q, 82a

acute severe 65q, 82–83a, 82a
  cough variant asthma 88a
  discharge from hospital 66q, 83a
asymptomatic non-visible haematuria (a-NVH) 184q, 198a
asystolic cardiorespiratory arrest 2q, 16–17a
atrial fibrillation (AF) 94q, 103q, 104q, 112–113a, 118a, 119a
  antipsychotic drugs 408q, 417a
  management 106q, 120a
  medication risks 109q, 124a
  stroke prevention 108q, 123a
avascular necrosis 259q, 277a
azathioprine-induced pancreatitis 260q, 277–278a

B

back pain, lower 165q, 179a
bacterial contamination, transfusion-associated lung injury 311a
Barthel Index 181a
behaviour, disturbed 414a
Behçet's disease 261q, 278a
below-knee amputation 187q, 199–200a
bendroflumethiazide 154a
benign oesophageal stricture 39q, 54a
benign paroxysmal positional vertigo (BPPV) 164q, 177–178a, 221q, 242a
benzodiazepine overdose 353q, 366–368a
beta-adrenoreceptor blockers 115a
  atrial fibrillation 118a
  overdose 378–379a
bilateral papilloedema 117a
bilateral ptosis 213q, 231a
biopsies, renal 200a
biphasic allergic response 387q, 391a
bipolar disorder 404q, 411–412a
bisoprolol 120a
  diarrhoea causes 42a
  peripartum cardiomyopathy 120a
bisphosphonates 178q
Blatchford bleeding score 32q, 49a
  upper gastrointestinal bleeding 48–49a
bloating 32q, 49a
blood pressure, tilt-table tests 180a
bloody diarrhoea 34q, 50a
bone infarction, sickle cell anaemia 307a
bone metastases
  renal cancer 291q, 298a
  spinal cord compression 298a
Borrelia burgdorferi infection (Lyme disease) 321q, 339–340a
botulism 212q, 230a
BPPV (benign paroxysmal positional vertigo) 164q, 177–178a, 221q, 242a
brain death 235–236a
brainstem tests 17–18a
breathlessness 74q, 75q, 89a
Breslow thickness 402a
British Society for Rheumatology (BSR) 272a
British Society of Gastroenterology 45a
broad-spectrum antibiotics, chickenpox 344a
bronchiectasis 70q, 71q, 87a

INDEX

bronchitis
  chronic 64q, 81a
  eosinophilic 88a
burst suppression, EEG 207q, 226a

C

CAD see coronary artery disease (CAD)
caecal adenocarcinoma 291q, 298–299a
calcium channel blocker toxicity 376a
Campylobacter infections 34q, 50a
Candida infections 400–401a
capacity 407q, 415–416a
  detention 407q, 416–417a
capecitabine 298a
capsule endoscopy 45–46a
carbamazepine overdose 362q, 379–380a
carbimazole 146a
carbon monoxide poisoning 359q, 374–376a
cardiac arrest 6q, 7q, 8q, 20a, 21a
cardiac glycosides 368–369a
cardiac syncope 163q, 176–177a
cardiogenic oedema 311a
cardiology 93–110q, 111–125a
  acute coronary syndrome see acute coronary syndrome
  acute stent thrombosis 93q, 111–112a
  anterior STEMI 96q, 114a
  aortic stenosis 105q, 120a
  aortic valve replacement 105q, 120a
  ascending aorta, dissection flap 99q, 116–117a
  atrial fibrillation see atrial fibrillation (AF)
  cardiac arrest 6q, 7q, 8q, 20a, 21a
  cardiac syncope 163q, 176–177a
  carotid sinus hypersensitivity 166q, 180a
  carotid stenosis 159q, 172a
  central chest pain 93q, 111–112a, 111a
  complete heart block 98q, 116a
  coronary angiography see coronary angiography
  coronary artery disease see coronary artery disease (CAD)
  gestational hypertension 104q, 119–120a
  hypertension see hypertension
  infective endocarditis 94q, 98q, 112a, 115–116a
  ischaemic cardiomyopathy 103q, 118–119a
  ischaemic heart disease 30q, 47–48a, 105q, 120a
  peripartum cardiomyopathy 105q, 120a
  prolonged QT syndrome 96q, 113–114a
  second-degree AV block 102q, 118a
  second-degree heart block, Mobitz type 1, 95q, 113a
  ST depression 93q, 111a
  temporary pacing wire 98q, 116a
  unstable angina 94q, 112a
cardiomyopathy
  hypertrophic 306a
  idiopathic dilated 10q, 23a
  ischaemic 103q, 118–119a
  peripartum 105q, 120a
cardiopulmonary resuscitation (CPR) guidelines 21a
cardiorespiratory arrest 1–14q, 15–25a
  American National Registry of Cardiopulmonary Resuscitation 16a, 17a
  asystolic 2q, 16–17a
  peritonitis 2q, 15a
  ST elevation myocardial infarction see ST elevation myocardial infarction (STEMI)
  ventricular fibrillation 2q, 2q, 7q, 10q, 15–16a, 16–17a, 21a, 23a
cardioverter defibrillator, implantable 118–119a
carotid endarterectomy 172a
carotid sinus hypersensitivity 166q, 180a
carotid stenosis 159q, 172a
carpal tunnel syndrome 249q, 270a
catechol-O-methyl transferase (COMT) inhibitors 239a
catheter-associated urinary tract infections 197q, 205a
CBDS (common bile duct stones) 34q, 50a
cefalexin 202a
cellulitis, lower limb 131q, 145a
central chest pain 93q, 111–112a, 111a
central nervous system infection 209q, 228a
central retinal vein occlusion 224q, 246a
central venous pressure (CVP) measurement 19a
cerebral abscess, meningitis vs., 228a
cerebral performance capacity (CPC) 16a
cerebrospinal fluid (CSF) studies
  acute inflammatory demyelinating polyradiculoneuropathy 232a
  infections 243a
cervical cancer 289q, 297a
CHA$_2$DS$_2$VASC 123a
chemical paraffin ingestion 362q, 380–381a
chemotherapy-induced nausea and vomiting (CINV) 288q, 296–297a
chest pain, central 93q, 111–112a, 111a
chest X-ray 59q
  benign oesophageal stricture 54a
  bronchiectasis 70q
  erythema nodosum 275a
  hepatic amoebiasis 335a
  pleural effusion 61q
chickenpox 325q, 344a
  pneumonitis 344a
Chlamydia infections 347a
chlordiazepoxide 44–45a
chloroquine 331a
CHM (Commission on Human Medicines) 43–44a
cholera (Vibrio cholerae infection) 323q, 343a
chronic bronchitis 64q, 81a
chronic idiopathic urticaria 385q, 390a
chronic kidney disease
  acidosis 204a
  treatment 193q, 202a
chronic obstructive pulmonary disease (COPD) 30q, 47–48a, 63q, 64q, 80a, 81a
  exacerbations 66q, 83a
  explanation of 71q, 87a
  panic attacks 404a, 412–413a
chronic type 2 respiratory failure 66q, 83–84a

Churg Strauss syndrome *see* eosinophilic granulomatosis with polyangiitis
CIAKI (contrast-induced acute kidney injury) 187q, 199–200a
CINV (chemotherapy-induced nausea and vomiting) 288q, 296–297a
classical pathway complement deficiency 383q, 389q
claudication 217q, 237a
clinical trials
  cluster random allocation 349a
  probiotic drinks 329q, 348–349a
  random allocation 348–349a
clopidogrel 48a
Clostridium botulinum infection *see* botulism
Clostridium difficile infection 34q, 41q, 50a, 57a
cluster headache 220q, 240a
cluster random allocation, clinical trials 349a
CMV (cytomegalovirus) infections 198a
coamoxiclav 41q, 57a
co-beneldopa 238a
cocaine overdose 374a
co-careldopa (Sinemet®)
  diarrhoea causes 42a
  Parkinson's disease treatment 238a
co-codamol 292a
coeliac disease 39q, 55a
  undiagnosed 146–147a
coffee-ground vomiting 29q, 30q, 31q, 33q, 40q, 45a, 47–48a, 48–49a, 48a, 50a, 55a
colonoscopy
  iron deficiency anaemia 46a
  ulcerative colitis 40q, 56a
Commission on Human Medicines (CHM) 43–44a
common bile duct stones (CBDS) 34q, 50a
common variable immunodeficiency (CVID) 384–385q, 389–390a
community-acquired pneumonia 67q, 69q, 84a, 86a, 137q, 149–150a, 167q, 181a
  hyponatraemia 140q, 154a
complement deficiency, classical and alternative pathway 383q, 389a
complete heart block 98q, 116a
complex regional pain syndrome (CRPS) 250q, 271–272a
computed tomography *see* CT (computed tomography)
computed tomography pulmonary angiogram (CTPA) 309a
COMT (catechol-O-methyl transferase) inhibitors 239a
confusional state, acute 11q, 23a
conjunctivitis 386q
constipation 41q, 58a
  causes 28q, 45a
continuous positive airways pressure (CPAP) 54a
continuous subcutaneous insulin infusion 138q, 151–152a
contrast-induced acute kidney injury (CIAKI) 187q, 199–200a
COPD *see* chronic obstructive pulmonary disease (COPD)
coronary angiography 95q, 113a
  diagnostic 188q, 200a
coronary artery disease (CAD)
  Helicobacter pylori infection association 107q, 121–122a
  investigations 95q, 113a
  risk evaluation 98q, 116a
  TIMI risk score 111a
corticosteroid therapy 225q, 247a
cough variant asthma 88a
CPAP (continuous positive airways pressure) 54a
CPC (cerebral performance capacity) 16a
CPR (cardiopulmonary resuscitation) guidelines 21a
craniotomy, elective 8q, 21–22a
Crohn's disease 39q, 55a, 265q, 280a
CRPS (complex regional pain syndrome) 250q, 271–272a
cryoprecipitate 47a
CSF *see* cerebrospinal fluid (CSF) studies
C-spine X-ray, ankylosing spondylitis 262q
CT (computed tomography)
  bronchiectasis 70q
  colonoscopy, iron deficiency anaemia 46a
  extradural haemorrhage 229a
  generalized seizures 226–227a
  non-contrast helical CT urography 199a
  pulmonary angiography 21a, 309a
  stroke 212a
  subarachnoid haemorrhage 210q, 228a
  subdural haemorrhage 211q
CURB-65 score 84a
Cushing syndrome 136q, 149a
CVID (common variable immunodeficiency) 384–385q, 389–390a
CVP (central venous pressure) measurement 19a
cyproheptadine 411a
cystic fibrosis 75q, 89a
cytomegalovirus (CMV) infections 198a

D

dapsone 345a
DC cardioversion 114a
DC shock 115a
D-dimers 21a
death, diagnosis of 2q, 17–18a
decompressive hemicraniotomy 160q, 173a
deep vein thrombosis (DVT) 164q, 303q, 308a
defibrillator, implantable 118–119a
deliberate self-harm 360q, 377–378a
delirium 157q, 170a
delirium tremens 406q, 414–415a
demeclocycline 293–294a
dementia
  early onset 157q, 170a
  investigations of 158q, 171a
  treatment 158q, 171a
Denosumab 178a
depression, screening trials 409q, 418–420a
de Quervain's (subacute) thyroiditis 127q, 143a
dermatology 395–399q, 400–402a
  eczema 399q, 401a
  HIV infection 348a
  itchy rashes 398q, 401a
  lichen sclerosus 397q, 401a
  phimosis 397q, 400a
  pre-bullous pemphigoid 396q, 400a

Sevens Johnson Syndrome–Toxic epidermal necrolysis overlap 395–396q, 400a
dermatomyositis 401a
dexamethasone
    acute severe migraine headache 247a
    chemotherapy-induced nausea and vomiting 297a
    superior vena cava obstruction 295a
dextropropoxyphene overdose 367a
diabetes mellitus
    diagnosis 145a
    hyperosmolar hyperglycaemic state 134q, 135q, 148a
    hyperosmolar non-ketotic coma 134q, 135q, 148a
    hypoglycaemia see hypoglycaemia
    initial treatment 145a
    lower limb cellulitis 131q, 145a
        see, also insulin
diabetes mellitus type 1, 129q, 145–146a
    continuous subcutaneous insulin infusion 138q, 151–152a
    ketoacidosis 133q, 147–148a
diabetes mellitus type 2, 134q, 148a
diabetic ketoacidosis (DKA) 133q, 134q, 147–148a
diagnostic coronary angiography 188q, 200a
dialysis, acute 203–204a
diarrhoea 34q, 50a
    bloody 34q, 50a
    drug-induced 27q, 42a
    inflammatory 332a
    secretory 332a
diazepam
    seizures 417–418a
    serotonin syndrome 410–411a
digoxin 120a
DIOS (distal intestinal obstruction syndrome) 75q, 89a
diphtheria 230a
diplopia in botulism 212q
dipyridamole 113–114a
dissociative seizures (DSs) (pseudoseizures) 408q, 417–418a
distal intestinal obstruction syndrome (DIOS) 75q, 89a
disturbed behaviour 414a
Dix–Hallpike test 242a
DKA (diabetic ketoacidosis) 133q, 134q, 147–148a
dofazimine 345a
dopamine agonists 239a
doxycycline 344a
Driving and Vehicle Licensing Authority (DVLA)
    driving restrictions 177a
    seizures 208q, 227–228a
driving restrictions 163q, 177a
drug interactions, serotonin syndrome 364–365a
DSs (dissociative seizures) (pseudoseizures) 408q, 417–418a
Duke's criteria 115a
dumping syndrome 150a
DVLA see Driving and Vehicle Licensing Authority (DVLA)
DVT (deep vein thrombosis) 164q, 303q, 308a
dysarthria, botulism 212q
dyspepsia 37q, 53a
dysphagia
    botulism 212q
    polymyositis 276–277a
dyspnoea, progressive 10q, 22–23a

E
early onset dementia 157q, 170a
Early Warning Score (EWS) 47–48a
Ear-Nose-Throat (ENT) medicine, HIV infection 348a
EBV (Epstein–Barr virus) infection 317–318q, 336a
ECG (electrocardiography), Mobitz type 1 second-degree heart block 95q
echocardiography 109q, 124a
    transthoracic 21a
eclampsia 235a
eczema 399q, 401a
EEG see electroencephalography (EEG)
elderly care 157–169q, 170–181a
    acute coronary syndrome see acute coronary syndrome
    Alzheimer's disease see Alzheimer's disease
    benign paroxysmal positional vertigo 164q, 177–178a, 221q, 242a
    cardiac syncope 163q, 176–177a
    delirium 157q, 170a
    dementia see dementia
    driving restrictions 163q, 177a
    falls see falls
    hypothermia see hypothermia
    lower back pain 165q, 179a
    mental capacity definition 158q, 171a
    normal pressure hydrocephalus 160q, 173a
    osteoarthritis 169q, 181–182a
    postural tachycardia syndrome 165q, 179–180a
    power of attorney 159q, 171–172a
elective craniotomy 8q, 21–22a
elective thyroidectomy 128q, 143–144a
electrocardiography (ECG), Mobitz type 1 second-degree heart block 95q
electroencephalography (EEG)
    burst suppression 207q, 226a
    generalized tonic–clonic seizures 234a
encephalitis, immune-mediated 234a
encephalography 215q, 234a
endocarditis
    ANCA titre 199a
    infective 94q, 98q, 112a, 115–116a
endocrinology 127–142q, 143–157a
    Addison's disease management 141q, 155a
    Cushing syndrome 136q, 149a
    fictitious hypoglycaemia 138q, 150–151a
    hypoglycaemia see hypoglycaemia
    hyponatraemia see hyponatraemia
    hypoparathyroidism 143–144a
    hypothyroidism see hypothyroidism
    nephrogenic diabetes insipidus 141q, 155a
    phaeochromocytoma 142q, 149a, 155a
    primary hyperparathyroidism 137q, 149–150a
    primary hypoadrenalism 132q, 147a
    primary hypothyroidism 131q, 146–147a

endocrinology (continued)
    syndrome of inappropriate diuretic hormone 140q, 154a, 283–284q, 292–294a
    Turner syndrome see Turner syndrome
end-of-life care, stroke 212q, 230a
end-organ failure 14q, 24–25a
endoscopic retrograde cholangiopancreatography (ERCP) 34q, 50a
endoscopy
    with banding 19a
    capsule 45–46a
endotracheal intubation 380–381a
end-tidal CO2 21a
entacapone 239–240a
enterovirus infections 222q, 243a
entrapment neuropathies 246a
eosinophilia, schistosomiasis 333a
eosinophilic bronchitis 88a
eosinophilic granulomatosis with polyangiitis 72q, 87–88a, 249q, 270–271a
epigastric pain 29q, 31q, 33q, 38q, 45a, 48–49a, 48a, 50a, 54a
epiglottitis 10q, 22–23a
epilepsy
    seizures 417–418a
    stable generalized 215q, 234–235a
    sudden unexpected death in epilepsy 234–235a
epinephrine see adrenaline (epinephrine)
Epley manoeuvre 242a
Epstein–Barr virus (EBV) infection 317–318q, 336a
Epworth Sleepiness Scale 89a
ERCP (endoscopic retrograde cholangiopancreatography) 34q, 50a
ERGs see European Resuscitation Guidelines (ERGs)
erythema nodosum 256q, 275a
erythromycin 84a
ESC see European Society of Cardiology (ESC) Guidelines
ESCAPE trial 125a
ethylene glycol ingestion 356q, 371–372a
EULAR (European League Against Rheumatism) 274a
European Association of Poisons Centre and Clinical Toxicologists 377–378a
European League Against Rheumatism (EULAR) 274a
European Resuscitation Guidelines (ERGs) 15a
European Society of Cardiology (ESC) Guidelines
    cardiac syncope 176–177a
    carotid sinus hypersensitivity 180a
euvolaemic hyponatraemia 292–293a
external beam radiotherapy 297a
extradural haemorrhage 229a
exudative effusion 62q, 79–80a

F

facial palsy 217q, 236a
faecal calprotectin 37q, 53a
falls 165q, 166q, 179a, 180a
    risk assessment 163q, 177a
FAST (focused assessment with sonography in trauma) ultrasound 33q, 49–50a

femur neck, fractures 164q, 178–179a
fictitious hypoglycaemia 138q, 150–151a
flecainide 112–113a
flexible sigmoidoscopy 34q, 50a
fluctuating capacity 416a
fluid restriction, syndrome of inappropriate diuretic hormone 293a
flumenazil 69q, 86a
fluoropyrimidine-induced vasospasm 291q, 298–299a
foam mattresses 179a
focused assessment with sonography in trauma (FAST) ultrasound 33q, 49–50a
food allergies 392a
forced air warming blankets 22a
formal capacity assessment, Alzheimer's disease 158q, 171a
4 Hs and 4 Ts 15a
Fracture Risk assessment Tool (FRAX) 179q
fresh frozen plasma transfusions 310a
furosemide 120a
Fusobacterium necrophorum infection 71q, 87a

G

G6PD (glucose-6-phosphate dehydrogenase) deficiency 331a
gamma-hydroxybutyrate (GHB) 358q, 373–374a
gastroenterology 27–41q, 42–58a
    abdominal distension 27q, 43a
    abdominal pain 32q, 34q, 36q, 37q, 39q, 49a, 50a, 52a, 53a, 55a
    acute liver failure 35q, 50–51a
    alcoholic hepatitis 36q, 52a
    anorexia nervosa 41q, 57a
    ascites 35q, 51a
    azathioprine-induced pancreatitis 260q, 277–278a
    benign oesophageal stricture 39q, 54a
    bloating 32q, 49a
    bloody diarrhoea 34q, 50a
    Campylobacter infections 34q, 50a
    Clostridium difficile infection 34q, 41q, 50a, 57a
    coeliac disease 39q, 55a
    coffee-ground vomiting 29q, 30q, 31q, 33q, 40q, 45a, 47–48a, 48–49a, 48a, 50a, 55a
    common bile duct stones 34q, 50a
    common bile duct stones (CBDS) 34q, 50a
    constipation see constipation
    Crohn's disease 39q, 55a
    diarrhoea see diarrhoea
    dyspepsia 37q, 53a
    endoscopic retrograde cholangiopancreatography 34q, 50a
    epigastric pain 29q, 31q, 33q, 38q, 45a, 48–49a, 48a, 50a, 54a
    faecal calprotectin 37q, 53a
    flexible sigmoidoscopy 34q, 50a
    haematemesis 28q, 44–45a
    HIV infection 348a
    inflammatory bowel disease 37q, 53a
    irritable bowel syndrome 32q, 49a
    jaundice 35q, 36q, 51–52a
    nasogastric feeding 41q, 57a

oesophagogastroduodenoscopy 29q, 45a
oesophagus see oesophagus
pancreatitis 38q, 54a
paracentesis 27q, 43a
primary biliary cirrhosis 35q, 51–52a
rectal bleeding 39q, 55a
spontaneous bacterial peritonitis 27q, 43a
ulcerative colitis see ulcerative colitis (UC)
upper gastrointestinal bleeding 30q, 31q, 44–45a, 47–48a, 48–49a, 48a
upper quadrant pain 34q, 50a
upper tract bleeding 30q, 31q, 44–45a, 47–48a, 48–49a, 48a
vomiting see vomiting
gastrointestinal tract
   infections 332a
   upper tract bleeding 4q, 18–19a, 30q, 31q, 44–45a, 47–48a, 48–49a, 48a
GCA (giant cell arteritis) 250q, 272a
GCS see Glasgow Coma Scale (GCS)
generalized convulsive status epilepticus 223q, 244a
generalized seizures 7q, 20a
   tonic–clonic seizures 214q, 233–234a
   treatment 208q, 226–227a
germ cell cancer 290q, 298a
gestational hypertension 104q, 119–120a
get-up-and-go test 177a
GHB (gamma-hydroxybutyrate) 358q, 373–374a
giant cell arteritis (GCA) 250q, 272a
Glasgow Coma Scale (GCS)
   generalized seizures 208q, 226–227a
   pituitary hypoplexy 128q
glioblastoma 304q, 309a
Global Registry of Acute Coronary Events (GRACE) 123a
glucose-6-phosphate dehydrogenase deficiency (G6PD deficiency) 331a
gluten-free food 39q, 55a
GOLD guidance 81a
gout 182a
   acute olecranon bursitis 251q, 273a
GPA (granulomatosis with polyangiitis) 187q, 199a
GRACE (Global Registry of Acute Coronary Events) 123a
grand mal seizures 320q
granulomatosis with polyangiitis (GPA) 187q, 199a
Graves disease 75q, 89a
   elective thyroidectomy 128q, 143–144a
   symptoms 153a
   treatment 139q, 152–153a
Guillain–Barré syndrome see acute inflammatory demyelinating polyradiculoneuropathy (AIDP)
gynaecology, HIV infection 348a

H

H2-receptor antagonists 47–48a
HAE (hereditary angioedema) 392–393a
haematemesis 28q, 44–45a, 305q, 310a
haematology 301–305q, 306–311a
   acute myelogenous leukaemia 304q, 309–310a
haemolytic crises, sickle cell anaemia 307a

haemoptysis 68q, 86a
   lung cancer 78q
haemorrhages
   extradural 229a
   intracerebral 219q, 238a
   massive haemorrhage protocols 4q, 18–19a
   rectal bleeding 39q, 55a
   subarachnoid haemorrhage 2q, 17a, 210q, 217q, 228a, 235–236a
   subdural 157q, 170a, 211q, 229a
Hartmann' solution 204a
HAS-BLED score 117–118a
headaches
   acute severe migraine headache 225q, 247a
   cluster 220q, 240a
head thrust test 242a
hearing voices 405q, 414a
Helicobacter pylori infection 45a
   coronary artery disease association 107q, 121–122a
   myocardial infarction 107q, 121–122a
hemicraniotomy, decompressive 160q, 173a
heparin, low-molecular weight see low-molecular weight heparin (LMWH)
hepatic amoebiasis 316q, 334–335a
hereditary angioedema (HAE) 392–393a
hereditary C1 inhibitor deficiency 393a
herpes simplex virus (HSV) infections 323q, 328q, 342–343q, 347a
HHS (hyperosmolar hyperglycaemic state) 134q, 135q, 148a
high-dose insulin euglycaemic therapy (HIET) 377a
HIV infection 328q, 348a
   ethics 326q, 346a
   tests 327q, 346a
HONK (hyperosmolar non-ketotic) coma 134q, 135q, 148a
horizontal nystagmus 222q, 242a
HPV (human papilloma virus) infection 401a
HSV (herpes simplex virus) infections 323q, 328q, 342–343q, 347a
human papilloma virus (HPV) infection 401a
Huntington's disease 221q, 241a
hydrocarbon pneumonitis 381a
hydrocephalus, normal pressure 160q, 173a
hydrocortisone
   Addison's disease management 155a
   ulcerative colitis 54a
hypercalcaemia 147a
   non-small cell lung cancer 287q, 296a
hyperglycaemia 130q, 146a
hyper IgM syndrome 390a
hyperlactemia 2q, 16a
hyperosmolar hyperglycaemic state (HHS) 134q, 135q, 148a
hyperosmolar non-ketotic (HONK) coma 134q, 135q, 148a
hyperparathyroidism, primary 137q, 149–150a
hypertension
   emergency 100q, 117a
   gestational 104q, 119–120a
hyperthermia, malignant 411a
hypertriglyceridaemia 130q, 146a
hypertrophic cardiomyopathy 306a

hypoadrenalism management 155a
hypoadrenalism, primary 132q, 147a
hypocalcaemia, post-operative 143–144a
hypoglycaemia
    fictitious 138q, 150–151a
    malaria 330a
    non-islet cell tumour 151a
hyponatraemia 140q, 153–154a
    community-acquired pneumonia 140q, 154a
    euvolaemic 292–293a
    management 140q, 141q, 154a
hypoparathyroidism 143–144a
hypophosphataemia 45a, 57a
    constipation 45a
hypotension 33q, 49–50a
    orthostatic 180a
hypothermia 160q, 173a
    rewarming 9q, 22a
hypothyroidism 139q, 152–153a
    primary 131q, 146–147a
    symptoms 153a
hypovolaemia 19a
    occult 13q, 23–24a
hypovolaemic shock 44–45a
hypoxia, non-invasive ventilation 84a

I

IABP (intra-aortic balloon pump) 6q, 20a
IBD (inflammatory bowel disease) 37q, 53q
ICH (intracerebral haemorrhage) 219q, 238a
IDA (iron deficiency anaemia) 29q, 45–46a
idiopathic dilated cardiomyopathy 10q, 23a
idiopathic Parkinson's disease 164q, 178a
idiopathic urticaria, chronic 385q, 390a
IGRAs (Interferon–Gamma Release Assay) 338a
immune deficiency testing 348a
immune-mediated encephalitis 234a
immunoglobulin A (IgA), selective deficiency 390a
immunoglobulin, intravenous 237a
immunology 383–388q, 389–393a
    acute anaphylaxis 387q, 391a
    allergen-specific immunotherapy 386q, 390a
    allergic response see allergic response
    allergic rhinitis 386q, 390a
    alternative pathway complement deficiency 383q, 389a
    anaphylaxis see anaphylaxis
    biphasic allergic response 387q, 391a
    chronic idiopathic urticaria 385q, 390a
    common variable immunodeficiency 384–385q, 389–390a
    insect venom allergy 386q, 391–392a
immunotherapy, allergen-specific 386q, 390a
implantable cardioverter defibrillator 118–119a
indices of performance 420a
infectious diseases 313–329q, 330–349a
    adenovirus 342a
    Campylobacter 34q, 50a
    Candida 401a
    catheter-associated urinary tract 197q, 205a
    central nervous system 209q, 228a
    cerebrospinal fluid studies 243a
    Chlamydia 347a
    cholera 323q, 343a
    Clostridium difficile 34q, 41q, 50a, 57a
    cytomegalovirus 198a
    enterovirus 222q, 243a
    Epstein–Barr virus 317–318q, 336a
    Fusobacterium necrophorum infection 71q, 87a
    gastrointestinal tract 332a
    Helicobacter pylori 45a, 107q, 121–122a
    herpes simplex virus 323q, 328q, 342–343q, 347a
    HIV infection see HIV infection
    human papilloma virus 401a
    latent Epstein–Barr virus 336a
    Legionnaire's disease 67q, 84–85a, 86a
    leprosy 326q, 345–346a
    Loa loa 315q, 334q
    Lyme disease 321q, 339–340a
    malaria 313q, 330–331a
    measles 322q, 341–342a
    Mycobacterium marinum 275a
    Mycoplasma 342a
    Mycoplasma pneumoniae 324q, 344a
    Neisseria meningitidis 276a
    neurocysticercosis 320q, 339a
    non-specific interstitial pneumonia 73q, 88a
    norovirus 34q, 50a
    onchocerciasis 334a
    parvovirus 342a
    respiratory infections 348a
    schistosomiasis 315q, 333–334a
    secondary syphilis 327q
    Shigella flexneri 314q, 332–333a
    streptococci 112a
    tuberculosis see tuberculosis (TB)
    urinary tract 194q, 203a
    of urine 41q, 57a
infective endocarditis 94q, 98q, 112a, 115–116a
inflammatory bowel disease (IBD) 37q, 53a
inflammatory diarrhoea 332a
inpatient permanent pacemakers 118a
insect venom allergy 386q, 391–392a
inspiratory stridor 10q, 22–23a
insulin
    continuous subcutaneous infusion 138q, 151–152a
    high-dose euglycaemic therapy 377a
    see, also diabetes mellitus
insulinomas 150a
INTERACT 2 trial 238a
Interferon–Gamma Release Assay (IGRAs) 338a
intra-aortic balloon pump (IABP) 6q, 20a
intracerebral haemorrhage (ICH) 219q, 238a
Intralipid® 377a
intravenous immunoglobulin (IVIG) 237a
intubation 23a
invasive pulmonary artery catheter 124–125a
ipsilateral Horner's syndrome 244a
iron deficiency anaemia (IDA) 29q, 45–46a, 45a, 46a
irritable bowel syndrome 32q, 49a

ischaemic cardiomyopathy 103q, 118–119a
ischaemic heart disease 30q, 47–48a, 105q, 120a
ischaemic stroke 162q, 174–176a, 223q, 244a
itchy rashes 398q, 401a
IVIG (intravenous immunoglobulin) 237a

J
jaundice 35q, 36q, 51–52a

K
Kawasaki disease (mucocutaneous lymph node syndrome) 340a
ketamine overdose 374a
khat psychosis 413–414a
kidney disease
    chronic see chronic kidney disease
    contrast-induced acute kidney injury 187q, 199–200a
Kidney Disease: Improving Global Outcomes group 201a
Klebsiella pneumoniae 86a
knee pain, mechanical 252q, 273a
Koebner's phenomenon 149q, 269–270a

L
LABA (long-acting beta agonists) 80a
labetalol
    gestational hypertension 119a
    hypertensive emergency 117a
lacking capacity 407q, 415–416a
LAMA (long-acting muscarinic antagonist) 80a
Lambert–Eaton myasthenic syndrome (LEMS) 231a
    myasthenia gravis vs. 231a
Lasting Power of Attorney (LPAs) 171–172a
latent infections, Epstein–Barr virus 336a
laxatives 41q, 58a
left partial ptosis 159q, 173a
Legionnaire's disease 67q, 84–85a, 86a
LEMS see Lambert–Eaton myasthenic syndrome (LEMS)
lepromatous (multibacillary) disease 345a
leprosy (Mycobacterium leprae infection) 326q, 345–346a
levodopa 239a
levofloxacin 84–85a
levothyroxine 146a
lichen planus 401a
lichen sclerosus 397q, 401a
Light's criteria 79–80a
liothyroxine 146a
lithium
    bipolar disorder 411–412a
    toxicity 412a
liver transplants 35q, 50–51a
liver-unit referral, paracetamol overdose 373a
LMWH see low-molecular weight heparin (LMWH)
Loa loa infection (loaisis) 315q, 334q
long-acting beta agonists (LABA) 80a
long-acting muscarinic antagonist (LAMA) 80a
long-term oxygen therapy (LTOT) 64q, 81–82a
lorazepam 56–57a
lower back pain 165q, 179a
lower limb
    cellulitis 131q, 145a
    oedema 186q, 199a
low-molecular weight heparin (LMWH) 55a
    pulmonary emboli 85a
    venous thromboembolism 309a
LPAs (Lasting Power of Attorney) 171–172a
LTOT (long-term oxygen therapy) 64q, 81–82a
lumber canal stenosis 257q, 276a
lung cancer 74q, 88–89a
    non-small cell 287q, 296a
lungs, transfusion-associated lung injury 305q, 310–311a
lupus 401a
Lyme disease (Borrelia burgdorferi infection), 321q 339–340a
lymphadenopathy 149q, 269–270a
    Epstein–Barr virus infection 317q

M
macrogol 57–58a
magnetic resonance imaging see MRI (magnetic resonance imaging)
major congenital malformations (MCM) 235a
malaria 313q, 330–331a
malignant hyperthermia 411a
malignant mesothelioma 283q, 299a
malignant middle cerebral artery syndrome 160q, 173a
massive haemorrhage protocols 4q, 18–19a
mast-cell tryptase 388q, 393a
MDMA overdose 374a
MDR TB (multi-drug resistant tuberculosis) 68q, 85a, 338a
measles 322q, 341–342a
mechanical knee pain 252q, 273a
melaena 305q, 310a
meningitis, cerebral abscess vs. 228a
mental capacity definition 158q, 171a
Mental Health Act (1983) 416–417a
Mental Health Capacity Act (2005) 171a, 415–416a
mesothelioma 76q, 90a
    malignant 283q, 299a
metastatic spinal cord compression (MSCC) 285q, 294a
methadone overdose 367a
methanol ingestion 356q, 371–372a
methionine, paracetamol overdose 373a
methotrexate-induced pneumonia 255q, 275a
methylprednisolone 236a
    Behçet's disease 278a
metronidazole 335a
MG (myasthenia gravis) 231a
MGUS (monoclonal gammopathy of undetermined significance) 306a
Miller–Fisher syndrome 232a
MND (motor neurone disease) 223q, 244–245a
MOA-B (monoamine oxidase B) inhibitors 240a
Mobitz type 1, 96q, 114a
moderate asthma 82a
monoamine oxidase B (MOA-B) inhibitors 240a
monoclonal gammopathy of undetermined significance (MGUS) 306a

INDEX

mortality
  community-acquired pneumonia 67q, 84a
  measles 342a
motor neurone disease (MND) 223q, 244–245a
MRI (magnetic resonance imaging)
  claudication 237a
  generalized seizures 226–227a
  lumber canal stenosis 276a
MS (multiple sclerosis) 214q, 233a
MSCC (metastatic spinal cord compression) 285q, 294a
mucocutaneous lymph node syndrome (Kawasaki disease) 340a
multi-drug resistant tuberculosis (MDR TB) 68q, 85a, 338a
multiple-dose activated charcoal (MDAC) 377–378a
multiple myeloma 182a
multiple sclerosis (MS) 214q, 233a
musculoskeletal medicine 248–267q, 269–281a
  acute gouty olecranon bursitis 251q, 273a
  acute pseudogout 253q, 274a
  ankylosing spondylitis 262q, 278a
  carpal tunnel syndrome 249q, 270a
  complex regional pain syndrome 250q, 271–272a
  erythema nodosum 256q, 275a
  giant cell arteritis 250q, 272a
  lumber canal stenosis 257q, 276a
  mechanical knee pain 252q, 273a
  olecranon bursitis 251q, 273a
  osteomalacia 267q, 281a
  Paget's disease 263q, 279a
  palindromic rheumatism 263q, 279a
  post-traumatic rotator cuff tear 266q, 281a
  psoriatic arthritis 252q, 273a
  relapsing polychondritis 266q, 280a
  septic arthritis 257q, 276a
  Sjögren's syndrome 252q, 273–274a
  Still's disease 248q, 269–270a
myasthenia gravis (MG) 231a
Mycobacteria tuberculosis infection see tuberculosis (TB)
Mycobacterium leprae infection (leprosy) 326q, 345–346a
Mycobacterium marinum infection 275a
Mycoplasma infection 342a
Mycoplasma pneumoniae infection 324q, 344a
myocardial infarction
  Helicobacter pylori infection 107q, 121–122a
myocardial perfusion scan 116a

N

naloxone 367a
nasogastric feeding 41q, 57a
National Institute for Health and Care Excellence (NICE) 48–49a
  chronic obstructive pulmonary disease 80a, 81a
  delirium 170a
  diabetes mellitus 145a
  insect venom allergy 391a
  pulmonary emboli 85a
National Osteoporosis Guideline Group (NOGG) guidelines 179q
National Poisons Information Service (NPIS) 372–373a

nausea and vomiting 195q, 197q, 203–204a
  anti-cancer treatment 288q, 296–297a
NEAD (non-epileptic attack disorder) 220q, 240–241a
near-fatal asthma 82a
nebulized recombinant human DNase 87a
negative predictive value (NPV) 419a
Neisseria meningitidis infection 276a
nephrogenic diabetes insipidus 145q, 155a
nephrotic syndrome 186q, 199a, 306a
nerve conduction studies
  carpal tunnel syndrome 270a
  stroke diagnosis 245q
neurocysticercosis (Taenia solium infection) 320q, 339a
neuroleptic malignant syndrome 411a
neurology 207–225q, 226–247a
  acute inflammatory demyelinating polyradiculoneuropathy see acute inflammatory demyelinating polyradiculoneuropathy (AIDP)
  acute severe migraine headache 225q, 247a
  benign paroxysmal positional vertigo 164q, 177–178a, 221q, 242a
  central nervous system infection 209q, 228a
  cluster headache 220q, 240a
  encephalography 215q, 234a
  enterovirus infections 222q, 243a
  facial palsy 217q, 236a
  generalized convulsive status epilepticus 223q, 244a
  generalized seizures see generalized seizures
  headaches see headaches
  HIV infection 348a
  Huntington's disease 221q, 241a
  intracerebral haemorrhage 219q, 238a
  ischaemic stroke 162q, 174–176a, 223q, 244a
  motor neurone disease 223q, 244–245a
  multiple sclerosis 214q, 233a
  non-epileptic attack disorder 220q, 240–241a
  Parkinson's disease see Parkinson's disease
  partial seizures 207q, 226a
  subarachnoid haemorrhage 2q, 17a, 210q, 217q, 228a, 235–236a
  subdural haemorrhage 211q
  transient vertigo 221q, 242a
  ulnar nerve palsy 224q, 245q
  vestibular neuronitis 222q, 243a
  Wernicke–Korsakoff syndrome 221q, 242a
neuropathies, entrapment 246a
neutropenic fever 302q, 307–308a
neutropenic sepsis 286q, 295a
NICE see National Institute for Health and Care Excellence (NICE)
NIV (non-invasive ventilation) 66q
NNT (numbers needed to treat) 77q, 91–92a
NOACs (novel oral anticoagulation agents) 309a
NOGG (National Osteoporosis Guideline Group) guidelines 179q
non-contrast helical CT urography 199a
non-epileptic attack disorder (NEAD) 220q, 240–241a
non-inflammatory bowel disease, inflammatory bowel disease vs. 37q, 53a

non-invasive ventilation (NIV) 66q
non-islet cell tumour hypoglycaemia 151a
non-small cell lung cancer (NSCLC) 287q, 296a
non-specific interstitial pneumonia 73q, 88a
non-ST elevation
   acute coronary syndrome 117–118a
   myocardial infarction 108q, 123a
non-visible haematuria (NVH) 187q, 199a
   asymptomatic 184q, 198a
normal pressure hydrocephalus 160q, 173a
norovirus infection 34q, 50a
notification, primary pleural tuberculosis 338a
novel oral anticoagulation agents (NOACs) 309a
NPIS (National Poisons Information Service) 372–373a
NPV (negative predictive value) 419a
NSCLC (non-small cell lung cancer) 287q, 296a
nuclear Mi-2 protein 277a
numbers needed to treat (NNT) 77q, 91–92a
NVH see non-visible haematuria (NVH)
nystagmus, horizontal 222q, 243a

O

obstructive sleep apnoea/hypopnoea syndrome
   (OSAHS) 76q, 89–90a
occult hypovolaemia 13q, 23–24a
oedema
   acute pulmonary 110q, 124a
   cardiogenic 311a
   lower limb 186q, 199a
   pitting 191q
oesophagoduodenoscopy 29q, 45a
oesophagus
   adenocarcinoma 41q, 57–58a
   benign stricture 39q, 54a
   stents in situ 40q, 55a
oesophagectomy 58a
OH (orthostatic hypotension) 180a
olecranon bursitis 251q, 273a
omeprazole 42a
onchocerciasis 334a
oncology 283–291q, 292–299a
   acute myelogenous leukaemia 304q, 309–310a
   adenocarcinoma see adenocarcinoma
   bone metastases see bone metastases
   cervical cancer 289q, 297a
   chemotherapy-induced nausea and vomiting 288q, 296–297a
   germ cell cancer 290q, 298a
   glioblastoma 304q, 309a
   HIV infection 348a
   lung cancer see lung cancer
   malignant mesothelioma 283q, 299a
   melaena 305q, 310a
   metastatic spinal cord compression 285q, 294a
   pharmacology 359q, 374–376a
   testicular cancer see testicular cancer
   treatment see anti-cancer treatment
ophthalmology
   bilateral ptosis 213q, 231a
   central retinal vein occlusion 224q, 246a
   conjunctivitis 386q
   diplopia in botulism 212q
   HIV infection 348a
   horizontal nystagmus 222q, 243a
   optic neuritis 217q, 236a
   ptosis see ptosis
   visual loss 224q, 246a
optic neuritis 217q, 236a
oral rehydration solution (ORS) 343a
ORS (oral rehydration solution) 343a
orthostatic hypotension (OH) 180a
OSAHS (obstructive sleep apnoea/hypopnoea
   syndrome) 76q, 89–90a
osteoarthritis 169q, 181–182a
osteomalacia 267q, 281a
osteosarcoma 279a

P

pacemaker, permanent 120a
pacemakers, inpatient permanent 118a
Paget's disease 263q, 279a
pain
   epigastric 29q, 31q, 33q, 38q, 45a, 48–49a, 48a, 50a, 54a
   sickle cell anaemia 307a
palindromic rheumatism 263q, 279a
palliative radiotherapy, cervical cancer 289q, 297a
pancreatitis 38q, 54a
   azathioprine-induced 260q, 277–278a
panhydropituitarism 45a
panhypopituitarism 45a
panic attacks 404q, 412–413a
papilloedema, bilateral 117a
paracentesis 27q, 43a
paracetamol
   diarrhoea causes 42a
   overdose 28q, 35q, 43–44a, 50–51a, 357q, 372–373a
parathyroid hormone (PTH) 144a
   assay 200a
Parkinson's disease
   idiopathic 164q, 178a
   treatment 219q, 220q, 239a
partial anterior circulation stroke 224q, 245–246a
partial seizures 207q, 226a
parvovirus infection 342a
   arthritis 264q, 279–280a
PBC (primary biliary cirrhosis) 35q, 51–52a
PCA (posterior inferior cerebellar artery), ischaemic
   stroke 244a
PCP (pneumocystis pneumonia) 327q, 346a
PCR (polymerase chain reaction), Epstein–Barr virus
   infection 317–318q
PE see pulmonary embolism (PE)
pelvic inflammatory disease (PID) 327q, 347a
percutaneous cervical cordotomy 91a
performance, indices of 420a
peripartum cardiomyopathy 105q, 120a
peripartum myopathy 120a
peritonitis 2q, 15a

permanent pacemaker 120*a*
phaeochromocytoma 142*q*, 149*a*, 155*a*
pharyngoconjunctival fever 342*a*
phenytoin 23*a*
    acute toxicity 218*q*, 237*a*
phimosis 397*q*, 401*a*
phospholipase A2-receptor autoantibodies (PLA2R) 199*a*
photopatch testing 401*a*
phtotsensitive disorders 401*a*
PID (pelvic inflammatory disease) 327*q*, 347*a*
pitting oedema 191*q*
pituitary gland 144*a*
    hypoplexy 128*q*, 144*a*
plasma cell myeloma 306*a*
Plasmodium falciparum *see* malaria
platelet transfusion, alcoholic liver disease 30*q*, 47*a*
pleural effusion 61*q*, 79*a*
pleural fluid amylase, exudative effusion 80*a*
pleurisy, tuberculous *see* tuberculous pleurisy
pleuritic chest pain 59*q*, 78*a*
pneumococcal polysaccharide vaccination 86*a*
pneumocystis pneumonia (PCP) 327*q*, 346*a*
pneumonia
    aspiration 258*q*, 276–277*a*
    community-acquired *see* community-acquired pneumonia
    methotrexate-induced 255*q*, 275*a*
    non-specific interstitial 73*q*, 88*a*
    secondary spontaneous pneumothorax 78–79*a*
pneumonitis
    chickenpox 344*a*
    hydrocarbon 381*a*
pneumothorax 60*q*, 79*a*
poisoning 351–362*q*, 363–381*a*
    benzodiazepine overdose 353*q*, 366–368*a*
    carbamazepine overdose 362*q*, 379–380*a*
    chemical paraffin ingestion 362*q*, 380–381*a*
    ethylene glycol ingestion 356*q*, 371–372*a*
    methanol ingestion 356*q*, 371–372*a*
    opioid overdose 353*q*, 366–368*a*, 374*a*
    paracetamol overdose 28*q*, 35*q*, 43–44*a*, 50–51*a*, 357*q*, 372–373*a*
    paraffin ingestion 362*q*, 380–381*a*
    salicylate overdose 355*q*, 369–370*a*
    sotalol overdose 361*q*, 378–379*a*
    tricyclic antidepressant overdose 352*q*, 365–366*a*
    verapamil overdose 359*q*, 376–377*a*
    warfarin overdose 355*q*, 370–371*a*
    yew berry poisoning 354*q*, 368–369*a*
polychondritis, relapsing 266*q*, 280*a*
polydipsia 142*q*
polymerase chain reaction (PCR), Epstein–Barr virus infection 317–318*q*
polymyositis, dysphagia 276–277*a*
polyuria 142*q*
Pontiac fever 85*a*
positive predictive value (PPV) 419*a*
posterior inferior cerebellar artery (PCA), ischaemic stroke 244*a*
post-operative hypocalcaemia 143–144*a*

post-traumatic rotator cuff tear 266*q*, 281*a*
postural tachycardia syndrome (PoTS) 165*q*, 179–180*a*
pouch of Douglas 33*q*, 49–50*a*
power of attorney 159*q*, 171–172*a*
PPIs (proton pump inhibitors) 47–48*a*, 53*a*
PPV (positive predictive value) 419*a*
prasugrel 112*a*
praziquantel
    neurocysticercosis 339*a*
    schistosomiasis 333*a*
pre-bullous pemphigoid 396*q*, 400*a*
prednisolone 81*a*
pre-eclampsia 235*a*
pregnancy
    acute severe asthma 65*q*, 82–83*a*
    stable generalized epilepsy 215*q*, 234–235*a*
    tonic–clonic seizures 217*q*, 234–235*a*
    wasp venom allergy 387*q*, 392*a*
primary biliary cirrhosis (PBC) 35*q*, 51–52*a*
primary herpes gingivostomatitis 323*q*, 342–343*a*
primary hyperparathyroidism 137*q*, 149–150*a*
primary hypoadrenalism 132*q*, 147*a*
primary hypothyroidism 131*q*, 146–147*a*
primary pleural tuberculosis 318*q*, 337–338*a*
primary spontaneous pneumothorax (PSP) 78*a*, 79*a*
probiotic drinks, clinical trials 329*q*, 348–349*a*
progressive dyspnoea 10*q*, 22–23*a*
prolonged QT syndrome 96*q*, 113–114*a*
propranolol overdose 379*a*
propylthiouracil 152–153*a*
prostate-specific antigen (PSA) 203*a*
prothrombin complex concentrate (PTC) 47*a*, 310*a*
    intracerebral haemorrhage 238*a*
proton pump inhibitors (PPIs) 47–48*a*, 53*a*
PSA (prostate-specific antigen) 203*a*
PsA (psoriatic arthritis) 252*q*, 273*a*
pseudogout 182*a*
    acute 253*q*, 274*a*
pseudoseizures (dissociative seizures) 408*q*, 417–418*a*
psoriatic arthritis (PsA) 252*q*, 273*a*
PSP (primary spontaneous pneumothorax) 78*a*, 79*a*
psychiatry 403–409*q*, 410–419*a*
    antipsychotic drugs 408*q*, 417*a*
    bipolar disorder 404*q*, 411–412*a*
    capacity *see* capacity
    co-morbid conditions 418*a*
    delirium tremens 406*q*, 414–415*a*
    depression 409*q*, 418–420*a*
    dissociative seizures 408*q*, 417–418*a*
    hearing voices 405*q*, 414*a*
    lacking capacity 407*q*, 415–416*a*
    panic attacks 404*q*, 412–413*a*
    seizures *see* seizures
    war trauma-related symptoms 405*q*, 413–414*a*
psychosis 414*a*
PTC *see* prothrombin complex concentrate (PTC)
PTH *see* parathyroid hormone (PTH)

ptosis
  bilateral 213q, 231a
  left partial 159q, 173a
pulmonary artery catheter 124–125a
pulmonary embolism (PE) 67q, 85a, 303q, 309a
  anticoagulants 68q, 85a
pulmonary function testing 75q, 89a
pulmonary oedema, acute 124–125a
pyoderma gangrenosum 280a

Q
quinine 331a

R
radial nerve palsies 245–246a
radiotherapy, cervical cancer 289q, 297a
random allocation, clinical trials 348–349a
random sampling, clinical trials 349a
rasagiline 219q, 239a
rashes, itchy rashes 398q, 401a
reactive arthritis 346a
rectal bleeding 39q, 55a
re-feeding syndrome 57a
Reiter's syndrome 326q, 346a
relapsing polychondritis 266q, 280a
renal calculi 186q, 199a
renal medicine 183–194q, 198–205a
  acute kidney injury 185q, 189q, 198–199a, 200–201a
  acute renal transplant dysfunction 190q, 201a
  acute reversible vs. established chronic disease 188q, 200a
  anion gap metabolic acidaemia 196q, 204a
  anti-glomerular basement membrane disease 192q, 202a
  asymptomatic non-visible haematuria 184q, 198a
  biopsy 200a
  calculi 186q, 199a
  cancer, bone metastases 291q, 298a
  catheter-associated urinary tract infections 197q, 205a
  contrast-induced acute kidney injury 187q, 199–200a
  nephrotic syndrome 186q, 199a, 306a
  non-visible haematuria see non-visible haematuria (NVH)
  renal artery stenting 188q, 200a
  transplants see renal transplants
  urinary sepsis 185q, 198–199a
  urinary tract infections 194q, 203a
renal transplants
  acute dysfunction 190q, 201a
  infections 183q, 198a
respiratory failure
  acute on chronic type 2, 83a
  acute type 2, 69q, 86a
  aspiration pneumonia 258q, 276–277a
  chronic type 2, 66q, 83–84a
respiratory system 59–77q, 78–92a
  acute respiratory distress syndrome (ARDS) 73q, 88a
  acute type 2 respiratory failure 69q, 86a
  asthma see asthma
  bronchiectasis 70q, 71q, 86a, 87a
  bronchitis see bronchitis

chest X-ray see chest X-ray
chronic obstructive pulmonary disease see chronic obstructive pulmonary disease (COPD)
chronic type 2 respiratory failure 66q, 83–84a
community-acquired pneumonia see community-acquired pneumonia
cystic fibrosis 75q, 89a
exudative effusion 62q, 79–80a
Fusobacterium necrophorum infection 71q, 87a
Graves disease see Graves disease
haemoptysis see haemoptysis
HIV infection 348a
Legionnaire's disease 67q, 84–85a, 86a
long-term oxygen therapy 64q, 81–82a
lung cancer see lung cancer
mesothelioma see mesothelioma
multi-drug resistant tuberculosis (MDR TB) 68q, 85a, 338a
non-invasive ventilation 66q
non-specific interstitial pneumonia 73q, 88a
obstructive sleep apnoea/hypopnoea syndrome 76q, 89–90a
pleural effusion 61q, 79a
pleuritic chest pain 59q, 78a
pneumothorax 60q, 79a
pulmonary embolism see pulmonary embolism (PE)
pulmonary function testing 75q, 89a
transfusion-associated lung injury 305q, 310–311a
tuberculosis see tuberculosis (TB)
RF (rheumatoid factor) 274a
rheumatism, palindromic 263q, 279a
rheumatoid effusions 89a
rheumatoid factor (RF) 274a
rhinorrhoea 386q
rhythm control 97q, 115a
rifampicin 345a
RIFLE criteria, acute kidney injury 189q, 200–201a
rivastigmine 171a
Romberg's test 242a

S
SABA (short-acting beta agonists) 80a
SAH (subarachnoid haemorrhage) 2q, 17a, 210q, 217q, 228a, 235–236a
salicylate overdose 355q, 369–370a
salivary gland biopsy, Sjögren's syndrome 273–274a
SANAD trial 227a
SBP (spontaneous bacterial peritonitis) 27q, 43a
SCC see squamous cell carcinoma (SCC)
schistosomiasis (Schistosoma mansoni infection) 315q, 333–334a
screening test sensitivity 419a
SCUBA diving 79a
SDAC (single-dose activated charcoal) 377a
secondary spontaneous pneumothorax (SSP) 78–79a
secondary syphilis 327q
second-degree AV block 102q, 118a
second-degree heart block, Mobitz type 1, 95q, 113a
secretory diarrhoea 332a

seizures 408q, 417–418a
  after stroke 226–227a
  dissociative seizures (pseudoseizures) 408q, 417–418a
  driving restrictions 208q, 227–228a
  epilepsy 417–418a
  generalized see generalized seizures
  grand mal 320q
  partial 207q, 226a
  tonic–clonic seizures see tonic–clonic seizures
selective IgA deficiency 390a
self-harm, deliberate 360q, 377–378a
sepsis 14q, 24–25a
  diagnosis 13q, 23–24a
  severe 3q, 18a
Sepsis Trust 25a
septic arthritis 257q, 276a
serotonin syndrome 351–352q, 363–365a, 403q, 410–411a
serum transferrin receptor (sTfR) 46a
Sevens Johnson Syndrome–Toxic epidermal necrolysis overlap (SJS-TEN) 395–396q, 400a
severe sepsis 3q, 18a
severity markers, malaria 331a
sexual health screens 347a
Shigella flexneri infection 314q, 332–333a
short-acting beta agonists (SABA) 80a
SIADH (syndrome of inappropriate diuretic hormone) 140q, 154a, 283–284q, 292–294a
sickle cell anaemia 302q, 307a
sigmoidoscopy, flexible 34q, 50a
signal recognition peptide (SRP) 277a
simvastatin 42a
Sinemet® see co-careldopa (Sinemet®)
single-dose activated charcoal (SDAC) 377a
sinus tachycardia 8q, 21–22a
SIRS see systemic inflammatory response syndrome (SIRS)
Sjögren's syndrome 252q, 273–274a
SJS-TEN (Sevens Johnson Syndrome–Toxic epidermal necrolysis overlap) 395–396q, 400a
SLE (systemic lupus erythematosus) 195q, 203a
sore throat 10q, 22–23a
sotalol overdose 361q, 378–379a
SpA (spondyloarthritides) 278a
spinal cord compression, bone metastases 298a
spirometry 173a
splenomegaly, Epstein–Barr virus infection 336a
spondyloarthritides (SpA) 278a
spontaneous bacterial peritonitis (SBP) 27q, 43a
squamous cell carcinoma (SCC) 401a
  Candida infections 400–401a
  human papilloma virus 400–401a
SRP (signal recognition peptide) 277a
SSP (secondary spontaneous pneumothorax) 78–79a
stable generalized epilepsy 215q, 234–235a
Staphylococcal toxic shock syndrome 322q, 340–341a
status epilepticus 12q, 23a, 234–235a
ST depression 93q, 111a
ST elevation myocardial infarction (STEMI) 2q, 13q, 15–16a, 24a
  anterior 96q, 114a

stent thrombosis, acute 93q, 111–112a
steroids
  alcoholic hepatitis therapy 52a
  alcoholic liver disease therapy 52–53a
Still's disease 248q, 269–270a
sTfR (serum transferrin receptor) 46a
streptococci infections 112a
stroke
  acute 307a
  diagnosis 224q, 245q
  driving restrictions 163q, 177a
  end-of-life care 212q, 230a
  ischaemic stroke 162q, 174–176a, 223q, 244a
  partial anterior circulation stroke 224q, 245–246a
  prevention in atrial fibrillation 108q, 123a
  seizures 226–227a
  subdural haemorrhage 157q, 170a, 211q, 229a
  thrombolysis 174–176a
strontium 179q
subacute (de Quervain's) thyroiditis 127q, 143a
subarachnoid haemorrhage (SAH) 2q, 17a, 210q, 217q, 228a, 235–236a
subdural haemorrhage 157q, 170a, 211q, 229a
subluxation 182a
sudden unexpected death in epilepsy (SUDEP) 234–235a
sulphonylurea 150a
superior vena cava obstructions (SVCO) 290q, 294–295a
suprapubic catheters, management 205a
Surviving Sepsis Campaign Guidelines (2012) 13q, 23–24a, 24–25a
SVCO (superior vena cava obstruction) 290q, 294–295a
syncope
  aortic stenosis 120a
  episodes 165q, 179–180a
syndrome of inappropriate diuretic hormone (SIADH) 140q, 154a, 283–284q, 292–294a
syphilis
  dementia investigations 171a
  secondary 327q
systematic allocation, clinical trials 349a
systemic inflammatory response syndrome (SIRS) 15a, 23a
  diagnosis of 18a
systemic lupus erythematosus (SLE) 195q, 203a

T

tachyarhythmias 24a
TB see tuberculosis (TB)
temporary pacing wire 98q, 116a
Tensilon test 231a
testicular cancer 298a
  metastases 290q
thiamine 40q, 56a
thrombolysis, stroke 174–176a
thromboprophylaxis 39q, 55a
thymoma 213q, 231a
thyroidectomy, elective 128q, 143–144a
tilt-table tests 166q, 180a
  benign paroxysmal positional vertigo 242a
  blood pressure 180a

TIMI risk scores 93q, 111a
tinidazole 335a
TIPSS (transjugular intrahepatic portosystemic shunt) 43a
tirofiban 112a
tonic–clonic seizures 40q, 56–57a, 207q, 214q, 226a, 233–234a
　pregnancy 217q, 234–235a
　syndrome of inappropriate diuretic hormone 283–284q
torsade de pointes 378a
toxicology, analytical 372a
TRALI (transfusion-associated lung injury) 305q, 310–311a
tramadol overdose 367a
transfer ribonucleic acid (tRNA) synthetases 277a
transfusion-associated lung injury (TRALI) 305q, 310–311a
transient vertigo 221q, 242a
transition point 37q
transjugular intrahepatic portosystemic shunt (TIPSS) 43a
transthoracic echocardiography 21a
tricyclic antidepressants (TCAs)
　falls 179a
　overdose 352q, 365–366a
trombiculid mite bites 319q, 338–339a
tuberculosis (TB) 76q, 90a
　multi-drug resistant 68q, 85–86a, 338a
　primary pleural 318q, 337–338a
　spread of 85–86a
tuberculous pleurisy 74a
　adenosine transaminase 89a
Turner syndrome 135q, 148–149a
　aortic dissection 148–149a
two-level DVT Wells score 308a

U

Uhthoff's phenomenon 214q, 233a
ulcerative colitis (UC) 38q, 53–54a
　colonoscopy 40q, 56a
ulcers, venous leg 2q
ulnar nerve palsy 224q, 245q
ultrasound (US)
　hepatic amoebiasis 335a
　renal medicine 200a
undiagnosed coeliac disease 146–147a
unstable angina (UA) 94q, 112a
upper gastrointestinal bleeding 4q, 18–19a, 30q, 31q, 44–45a, 47–48a, 48–49a, 48a
upper quadrant pain 34q, 50a
uraemia 45a
urinary alkalinization, salicylate overdose 369a
urinary sepsis 185q, 198–199a
urinary tract infections (UTIs) 194q, 203a
urine infections 41q, 57a
urticaria, chronic idiopathic 385q, 390a

V

varenicline, clinical trials 77q, 91a
vaso-occlusive crises in sickle cell anaemia 307a
vasospasm, fluoropyrimidine-induced 291q, 298–299a
venous leg ulcers 2q
venous thromboembolism (VTE)
　glioblastoma 304q, 309a
　therapy 303q, 308a
ventricular fibrillation 2q, 2q, 7q, 10q, 15–16a, 16–17a, 21a, 23a
verapamil overdose 359q, 376–377a
vertigo, transient 221q, 242a
vestibular neuronitis 222q, 243a
Vibrio cholerae infection (cholera) 323q, 343a
visual loss 224q, 246a
vitamin A 342a
vitamin C deficiency 161q, 174a
vitamin D deficiency 161q, 174a
　osteomalacia 267q, 281a
vitamin K 47a
　intracerebral haemorrhage 238a
　warfarin overdose 370a
vitamin K epoxide reductase (VKOR) 370a
VKOR (vitamin K epoxide reductase) 370a
vomiting 37q, 53a
　coffee-ground 29q, 30q, 31q, 33q, 40q, 45a, 47–48a, 48–49a, 48a, 50a, 55a
　see, also nausea and vomiting
VTE see venous thromboembolism (VTE)

W

warfarin overdose 355q, 370–371a
war trauma-related symptoms 405q, 413–414a
wasp venom allergy 388q, 393a
　pregnancy 387q, 392a
waveform capnography 21a
Wegener's granulomatosis. see granulomatosis with polyangiitis (GPA)
Wernicke–Korsakoff syndrome 221q, 242a
Wernicke's encephalography 40q, 56a
wheeze 386q
World Health Organization (WHO)
　diabetes mellitus 145a
　drug trials 345a
　fracture risk 179q
　pain 292a

X

X-ray
　chest see chest X-ray
　C-spine 262q
　germ cell cancer 290q

Y

yew berry poisoning 354q, 368–369a

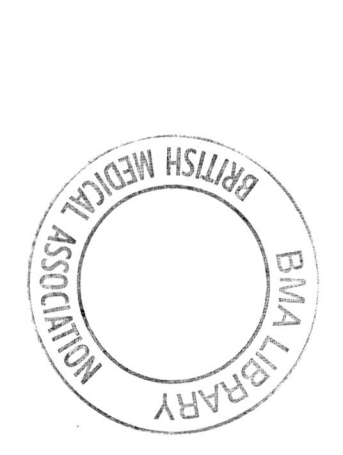